The complete encyclopedia of EXERCISES

The complete

EXER

THE DIAGRAM GROUP

encyclopedia of
CISES

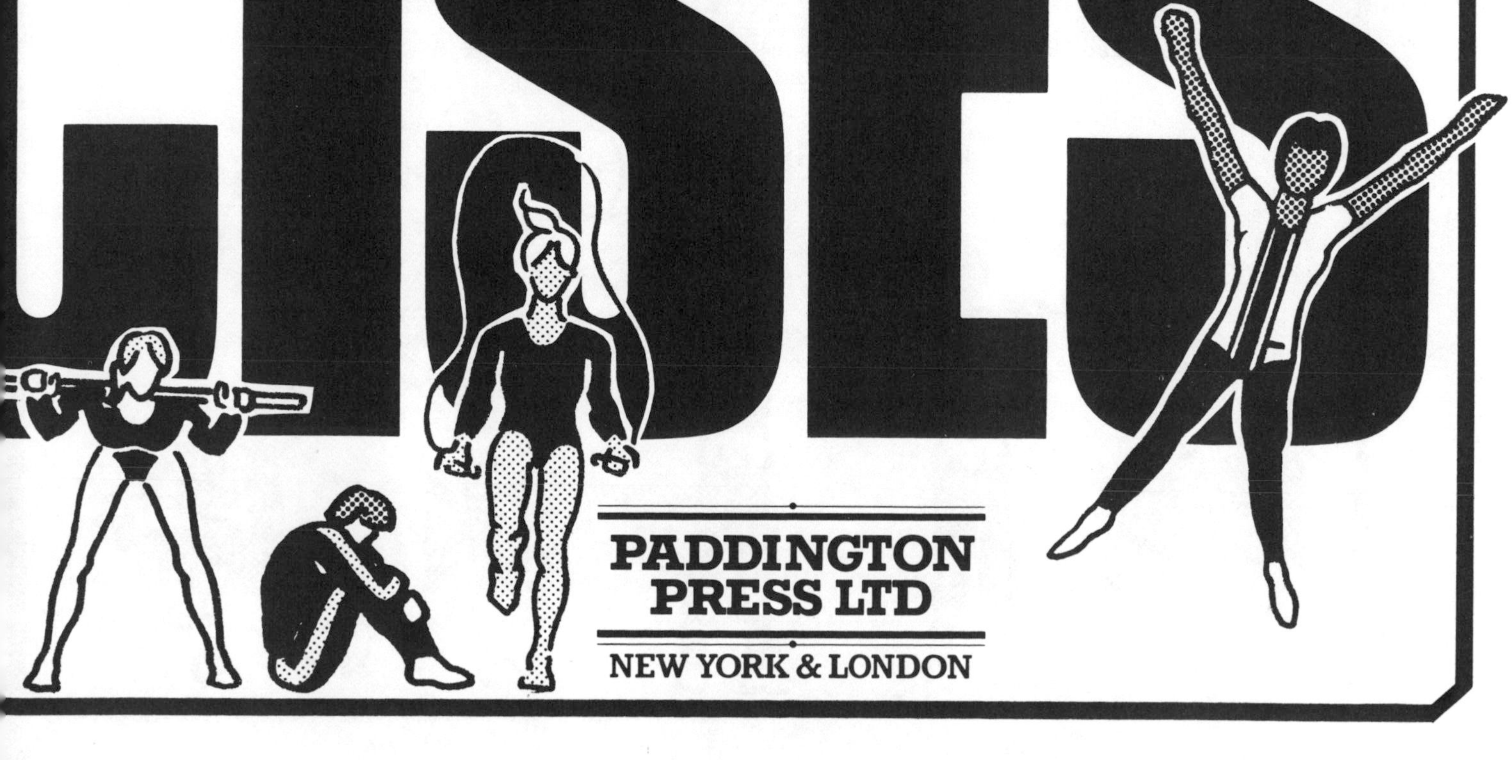

PADDINGTON PRESS LTD

NEW YORK & LONDON

ISBN 0 7092 0157 5
ISBN 0 7092 0156 7 (pbk)
U.S. and Canada only
    ISBN 0 448 22212 4
    ISBN 0 448 22211 6 (pbk)

Filmset in England by Tradespools
Ltd., Frome, Somerset.
Printed and bound in the United States

In the United States
PADDINGTON PRESS
Distributed by
GROSSET & DUNLAP

In the United Kingdom
PADDINGTON PRESS

In Canada
Distributed by
RANDOM HOUSE OF
CANADA LTD.

In Southern Africa
Distributed by
ERNEST STANTON (PUBLISHERS)
(PTY.) LTD.

In Australia and New Zealand
Distributed by
A. H. & A. W. REED

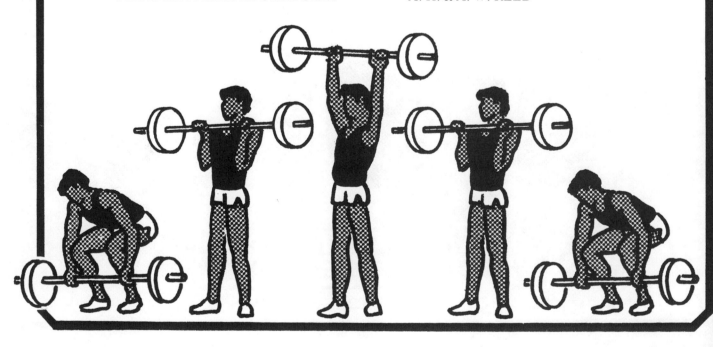

The Diagram Group

Managing editor	Ruth Midgley
Editor	Hope Cohen
Contributors	Gail Besley, Jeff Cann, Marion Casey, Ann Kramer, David Lambert, Bernard Moore
Research	Pamela George, Clair Lonay, Margo Lynn, Linda Proud, Enid Moore, Marita Westberg
Index	Mary Ling
Art director	Diana C. Taylor
Artists	Alan Cheung, Steven Clark, Robin Crane, Pauline Davidson, Brian Hewson, Richard Hummerstone, Susan Kinsey, János Márffy, Graham Rosewarne
Art assistants	Alan Harris, Sarah Joyce, Vanessa Lane, Ray Stevens
Consultants	Sharron Beamer, Dan Donovan, Molly Jennings (obstetric physiotherapist), Dr Gwyneth Lewis MBBS, Al Murray MSRG, Shirley Norman, Susan Rollason

The authors and publishers would like to express their thanks to the following:
Department of Education, People's Republic of China
Health Education Council, United Kingdom
International Wu Shu Association
Mary Ward Centre for Adult Studies, London
President's Council on Physical Fitness and Sports,
United States of America

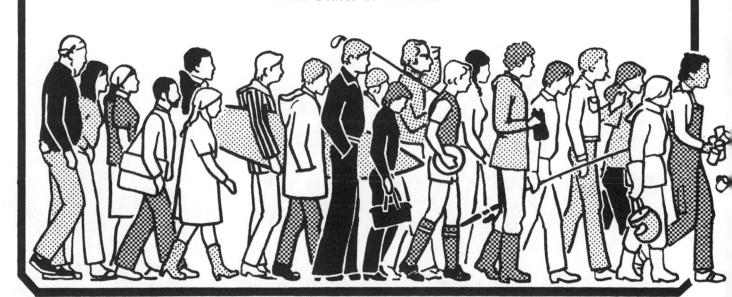

Contents

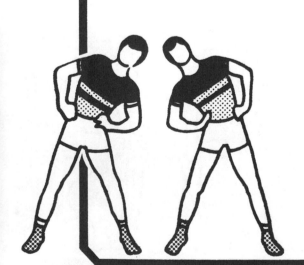

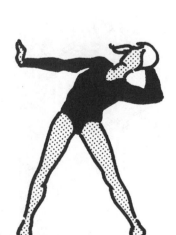

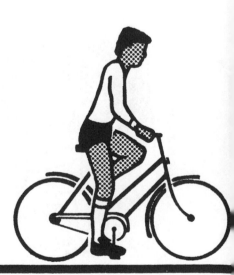

4 5 6

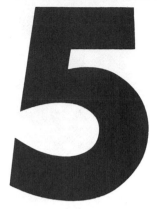
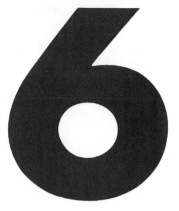

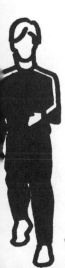
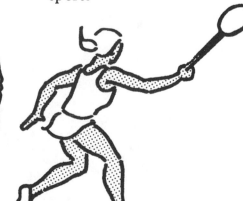

7

Specialty exercises

8

Exercise programs

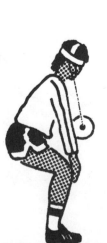
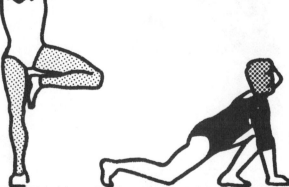
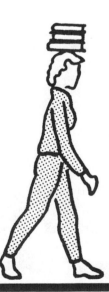

Foreword

As part of a general growing concern for our physical well-being, increasing numbers of people are accepting responsibility for their own fitness. This greater awareness has been strongly evidenced by the recent epidemic of health and exercise books, and the hundreds of different exercise methods publicized everywhere.

Now for the first time over 350 important exercises of every type are described and illustrated within one volume. An explanation of how the body works is combined with step-by-step exercise instructions to enable everyone—of any age or level of fitness—to create and vary their own exercise program to meet individual and changing needs.

The Complete Encyclopedia of Exercises offers tests that allow you to assess and rate your own fitness, explains the reasons for the different forms of exercise, and details the benefits derived from each of them. The exercises range from those for general health, reducing and pregnancy through bodybuilding and sports to yoga and jogging, as well as techniques for mental relaxation to relieve tension and stress. Also included are the official national programs from The President's Council on Physical Fitness and Sports, from the Health Education Council of Great Britain and, with unique cooperation, from the People's Republic of China.

Boldly and attractively presented, the book is divided into self-contained chapters designed to meet everyone's special needs. Each section begins with an introduction explaining the aims, effects and benefits of each form of exercise. Clear figure drawings and concise captions make it easy for the reader to do the various activities while looking at the book.

Each group of exercises has been approved by experts. Activities for children have been used in schools; those for elderly people and pregnant women in clinics; and all specialist exercises have been supervised by appropriate consultants.

The editors, researchers and artists of *The Complete Encyclopedia of Exercises* hope that this book will help you to enjoy both discovering and maintaining the health and vitality that are your natural birthright.

Chapter 1

CHOOSING TO EXERCISE

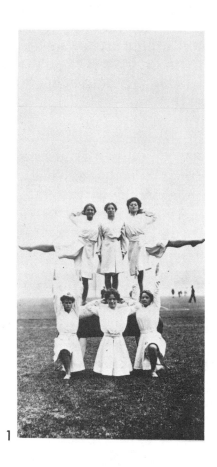

1

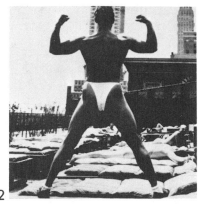

2

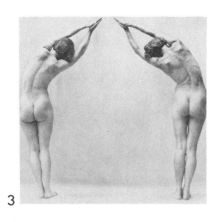

3

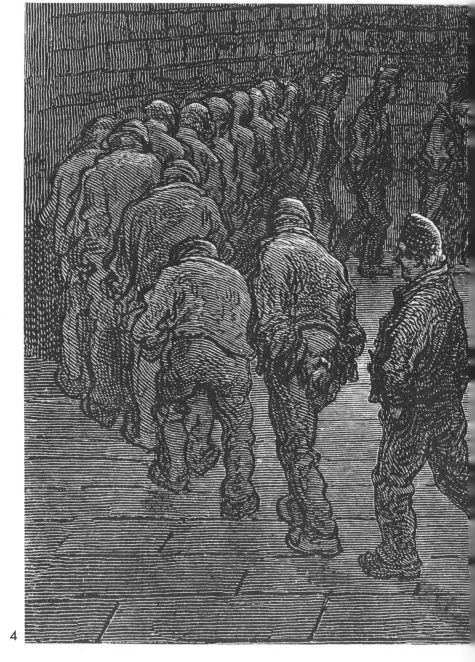

4

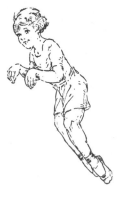 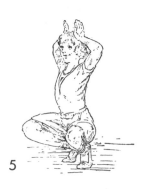 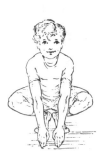

5

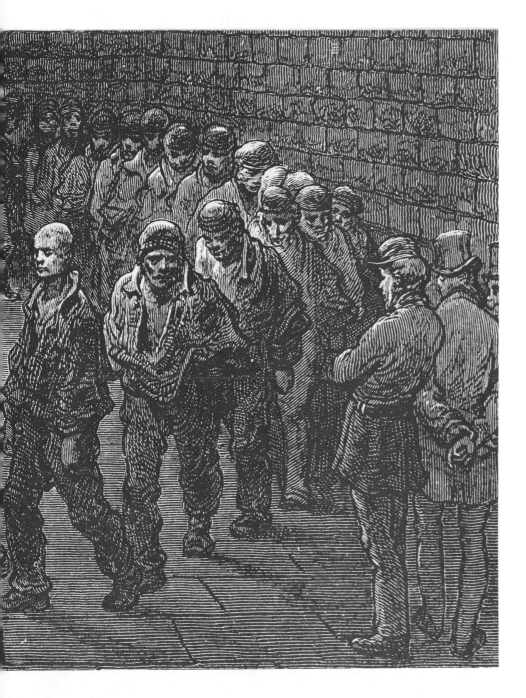

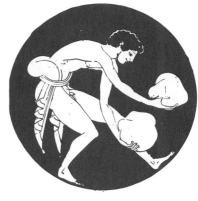

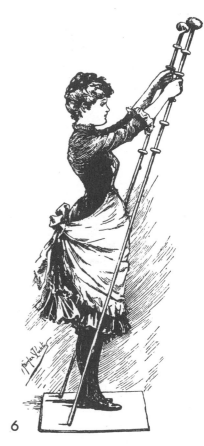

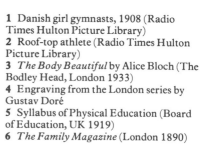

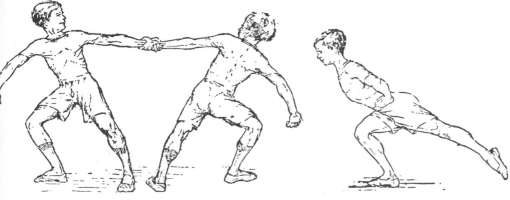

6

1 Danish girl gymnasts, 1908 (Radio Times Hulton Picture Library)
2 Roof-top athlete (Radio Times Hulton Picture Library)
3 *The Body Beautiful* by Alice Bloch (The Bodley Head, London 1933)
4 Engraving from the London series by Gustav Doré
5 Syllabus of Physical Education (Board of Education, UK 1919)
6 *The Family Magazine* (London 1890)

WHY EXERCISE?

Exercise is a basic bodily need. The human body is built for use, and without it will deteriorate. By denying yourself exercise you are functioning below your possible best, and so are denying yourself the chance of getting the most out of life. An unfit body is only about 27% efficient in its exploitation of the energy available for use, but this low rate of efficiency can be raised to over 56% with regular exercise. Such increased efficiency will be appreciated in every area of life. Your work and your leisure will become less tiring and more enjoyable as your capacity for activity

Benefits of regular exercise
Nervous system:
coordination and responses improve;
stress decreases.
Heart:
blood volume per beat increases;
coronary circulation increases;
pulse rate decreases;
pulse recovery rate decreases.
Lungs:
capacity increases;
circulation increases;
efficiency increases.
Muscles:
circulation increases;
size, strength and endurance increase;
oxygen debt capacity increases.
Bones and ligaments:
strength increases;
joint tissues strengthen.
Metabolism:
body fats decrease;
blood sugars decrease.

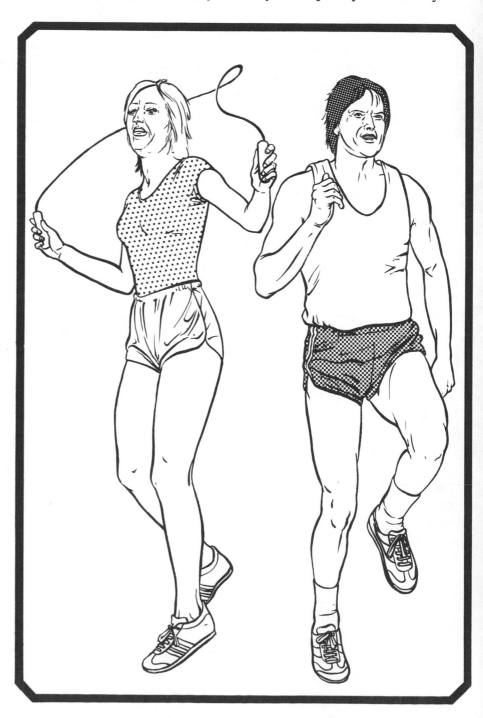

increases. Improved organic efficiency also means that you will be less likely to succumb to illness and organic deterioration; healthy, active life will therefore be extended, and the signs of aging delayed.

Physiologically all your body systems will benefit from regular exercise. Depending upon the degree of exertion and the exercise performed, muscles may increase in size, strength, hardness, endurance and flexibility, with improved reflexes and coordination.

Regular exercise greatly reduces the risk of heart disease. Exercise increases the strength, endurance and efficiency of the heart. A fit heart pumps 25% more blood per minute when at rest and 51.3% more blood per minute during vigorous exercise than an unfit heart. A fit person's heart beats 60–70 times per minute (86,400–100,800 beats per day); an unfit person's heart beats 80–100 times per minute (115,200–144,000 beats per day). The heart of a fit person is obviously more efficient than that of an unfit person and is therefore less subject to fatigue and strain. With exercise the cardio-vascular system (see page 40) improves its carrying ability. More capillaries (small blood vessels) are formed in active tissues to improve the supply of food and oxygen, and exercise burns up excess fats in the system and checks the deposit of fats in the arteries, so reducing the risk of thrombosis.

Exercise also increases the ability of the respiratory system. The lungs' vital capacity (the amount of air taken in at one time) and ventilation (the amount of air taken in over a period of time) are both increased, as is the efficiency of the exchange of gases that takes place in the lungs (see page 42). The nervous system also benefits, becoming more coordinated and responsive. For some people alertness and absence of tension are related to fitness, especially if it is achieved by rhythmic exercise or games that involve enjoyable competition.

In addition to benefiting specific body systems, fitness also brings the following advantages. A fit person may take less time to recover from illness; can withstand fatigue longer; uses less energy for any given job; has a lower metabolic rate and is more likely to sleep well, look well and feel healthy and positive than an unfit person. Exercise, therefore, increases your physical abilities and possibilities. Its positive effects can also help you to fight negative habits such as smoking and excessive eating and drinking, as well as showing you how much better you are without them.

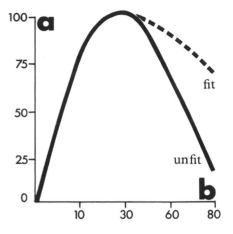

Decline of abilities
Functional abilities decline more slowly with age in a fit person than in an unfit person:
a is the % of function remaining;
b is age in years.

DEMANDS OF LIFE

In performing the tasks of everyday life we use energy which we obtain from food with the help of oxygen (see pp. 44–47). How well we perform those tasks, how much energy they take out of us, and how much pleasure we derive from them depends upon how efficiently our bodies can release, transport and use that energy.

Exercise increases the efficiency of our bodies and therefore allows us extra energy for our leisure time. It also increases our work capacity, which means that we can work harder for longer, or work with less effort and less fatigue. For instance, a person who is used to running a few miles every day will have little trouble running for a bus or coping with the physical demands of an office job, whereas someone whose only activity is to sit at a desk all day will find even that tiring!

Everyone needs a certain amount of exercise to keep his body working properly, but beyond that a person's fitness requirements depend on the demands of his job and the type of life that he leads — or would like to lead!

Energy requirements

Different jobs require different amounts of energy. Therefore minimal fitness requirements vary with your life-style. If you are too tired by the end of the working day to enjoy your leisure in the evenings or at weekends, the chances are that you need to increase your fitness level.

The diagram below shows the energy requirements for a variety of common activities. They are rated on a scale from 1 to 10 (very light to very heavy) to show the level of exertion needed. This will help you see how fit you need to be, and what jobs to do to aid that fitness.

A Digging: 10
B Hoeing: 4–8
C Weeding: 3–6
D Cutting grass with a hand mower: 4–6
E Cutting grass with a power mower: 4–5

F Sawing wood (by hand): 5–10
G Carpentering: 2–7
H Painting: 3–6
I Cleaning the house: 2–4

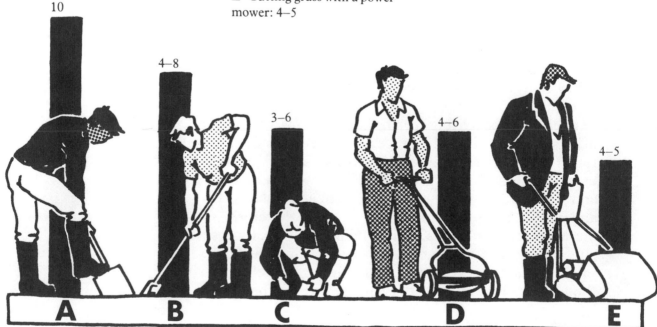

10   4–8   3–6   4–6   4–5

A   B   C   D   E

1

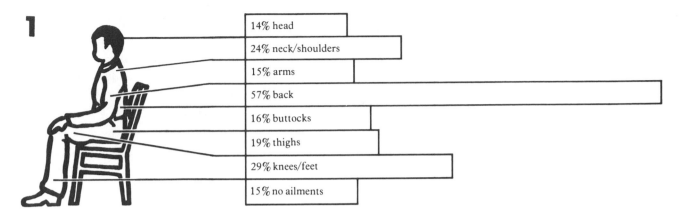

14% head	
24% neck/shoulders	
15% arms	
57% back	
16% buttocks	
19% thighs	
29% knees/feet	
15% no ailments	

2

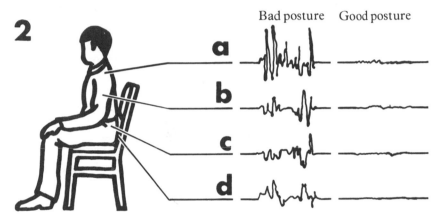

Bad posture   Good posture

a
b
c
d

1 Exercise and ailments
Sedentary (inactive) workers are more likely to suffer from ailments than active workers. The diagram shows the results of a survey of ailments among sedentary workers.

2 Posture and effort
The diagram compares the effort needed to sit with bad posture compared with good posture, measured by the electrical activity of the back muscles:
a Left trapezius
b Left lateral dorsi
c Left sacro spinalis
d Right sacro spinalis

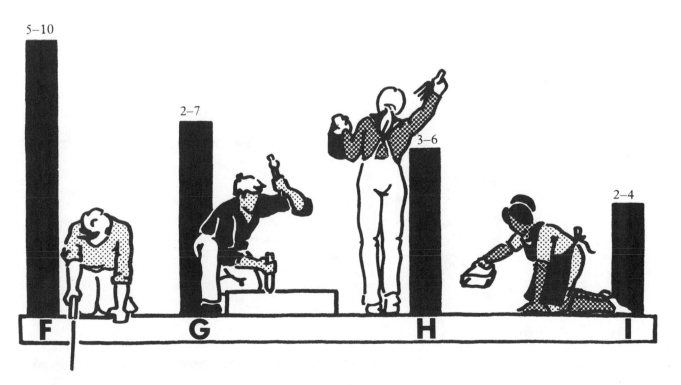

5–10

2–7

3–6

2–4

F   G   H   I

©DIAGRAM

MAKING YOUR CHOICE

The chart below will help you to decide on the ingredients of your exercise program. But first you must decide how fit you want to be. If your aim is only to improve your overall physical capacity within the daily round, you need not train as hard as someone who wants to join in a team sport. Different sports also have different fitness requirements. Softball, for instance, requires a lower level of fitness than football. Incentive is also important. Some people will find it best to find their exercise in a group activity or team sport, while others will prefer to exercise alone. Your environment (town or country, flat or hilly, cold or hot) and the

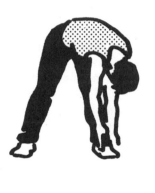

Mobility exercises

These ensure that all the major joints and muscles are moved through their complete range of movements. They are especially good for office workers, dancers, people whose sport has a tightening effect on their muscles (for example, runners and weight lifters), and for anyone who suffers from general "aches and pains."

Exercises that promote mobility and flexibility include yoga (pp. 256–269) and any exercises involving bending, stretching and rotating movements.
Exercises of this type help to loosen stiff joints and muscles and promote smoothness and ease of movement. They can therefore be useful for rehabilitating damaged or aching joints and muscles.

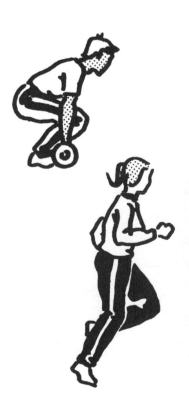

Strength exercises

These are good for everyone. They give the body muscles shape and tone and aid self-confidence. They prepare the body to cope with situations calling for extra effort — carrying a heavy bag, changing a wheel — and help the muscles to protect the joints and internal organs. Such exercises are particularly good for people doing heavy manual work.

Strengthening exercises build up the weight and strength of the muscles by means of repeated actions. The most common and obvious way to increase muscle strength is by the use of weights (pp. 234–245).

Heart and lung exercises

These improve the performance and endurance of the cardio-vascular (circulatory) and respiratory systems. Such "CR" exercises form the basis of good health and all-round fitness (pp 76–77). They will benefit anyone seeking to improve general fitness, irrespective of life-style or sporting activities.

Heart and lung exercises increase the oxygen requirements of the body. They necessitate continued vigorous movement over an extended period of time (10–15 minutes or more).

availability of space or facilities may also influence your choice of activities.

Whatever level of fitness you wish to attain and however you choose to maintain it, you should try for a balanced program of mobility, strengthening, and heart and lung exercises for all-round fitness. Choose the activities most suited to your needs, and remember that the major requirement is that your program helps you to enjoy keeping fit. If you have any health doubts, first check with your doctor.

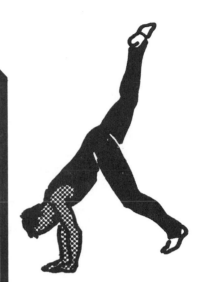

Sports that need and promote mobility include:
Swimming (pp. 206, 214, 216)
Golf (pp. 214, 218)
Gymnastics (pp.212–213, 215, 219)
Squash (pp. 215, 222)
Athletics (pp. 210–211, 214)

Calisthenics are exercises involving rhythmic, repetitious movements. They require little or no equipment, and are often performed to music. They help produce flexibility and strength in programs that are not too strenuous and can be carried out anywhere (pp. 272–281).

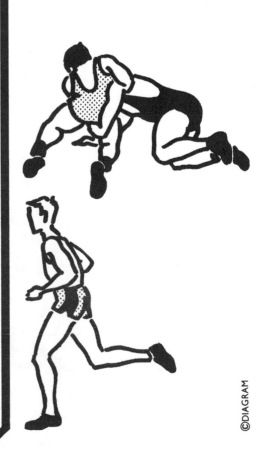

Sports that increase strength are any that involve repeated strain (pushing, pulling or lifting) over a period of time. Most of these sports, such as skiing (pp. 207, 217) or the shot put (p. 211), develop strength in only one set of muscles. Swimming (pp. 206, 214, 216) and wrestling (p. 220) have a greater all-round effect.

Strength/endurance exercises combine strength with endurance and are good for muscle tone and shape. Examples of these are push-ups, squat jumps and sit-ups (pp. 286–288).
Isometric exercises use effort without movement. They apply the force of one set of muscles against another set of muscles or against an immovable object such as a wall (pp.226–233).

Sports exercising the heart and lungs fall into two categories.
a) Group or team sports that involve running, for example racquet sports (pp. 206, 222) and football, etc. (pp. 206, 223).
b) Solo activities such as running and jogging (pp. 206, 320–329), skipping (pp. 190–195), cycling (p. 208), cross-country skiing (pp. 207, 214, 217), and swimming (pp. 206, 214, 216).

©DIAGRAM

EXERCISE ACTIVITIES

When choosing an exercise activity to suit your own personal needs you will have to take into consideration your age, state of health, occupation and the amount of time you have available. To help you make your choice we have set out below the pros and cons of different types of exercise activity. But remember that regular exercise of any kind takes time and effort, and having embarked on a course of exercise you must be positive and persevere. Start any exercise program slowly and carefully, only gradually increasing the effort you make.

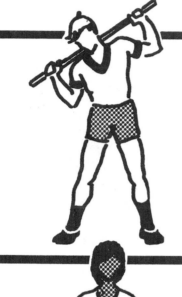

Isometric exercises

These are exercises without movement. The muscles are put into a state of static contraction of maximum or near maximum force against the resistance of other muscles or an immovable object. There is no movement at the joints. (Also see pp. 226–233.) Isometrics are an effective means of increasing muscle strength. They are quick (the entire body can be exercised in only 90 seconds), and can be done in the home, the office, on a bus or almost anywhere else.

Isometrics do not, however, give any exercise to the CR system, nor aid muscular endurance. They should, therefore, always be performed as part of a broader program of exercise.

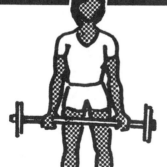

Isotonic exercises

These are exercises with movements in which the body works against its own, or against external, weights. This type of exercise includes calisthenics, but the term is more usually used to refer to weight training or bodybuilding exercises (pp. 234–245), in which the muscles contract with movement against progressively heavier weights. This causes the muscles to increase in size, strength and endurance. Weights can be varied to suit the individual, making this type of exercise suitable for everyone. Isotonic exercises should be performed together with stretching exercises to loosen the muscles, and with a CR exercise — running is excellent — to exercise the heart and lungs.

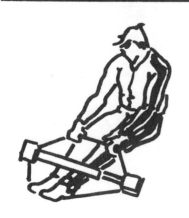

Isokinetic exercises

Isokinetic or resistance exercises combine the principles of both isometric and isotonic exercises. They involve the use of equipment that controls the amount of resistance relative to the degree of exertion; resistance increases as muscle pressure is increased. A bullworker (p. 237) is perhaps the best-known example of an isokinetic exerciser. It is an excellent way of increasing the size and strength of muscles.

This type of exercise has little or no CR value, however, and should be done in conjunction with aerobic and stretching exercises.

Meditative methods

Meditative methods of exercise are not primarily exercises at all, but physical paths to help you to approach spiritual enlightenment and union with the supreme consciousness.

The different forms — such as yoga (pp. 256–269), K'ai Men and T'ai Chi (pp. 246–255) — are all related to a far wider philosophy. Their practice is, however, very good for muscular tone, overall flexibility, internal functions and for relieving stress.

They have little or no CR value, but are an excellent addition to an aerobic exercise program (see p. 20).

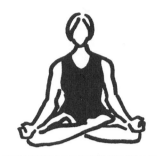

Sports

The effectiveness of sport as a means of exercise varies from sport to sport (see pp. 202–215). Benefits range from the complete fitness obtainable through gymnastics and some of the combat sports, to the very limited physical benefits to be derived from golf or bowling. Conditions vary from dependence on teammates or equipment to considerable self-sufficiency, and from indoor courts to mountain forests.

The great variety of sports means that there is a sport for everyone, whatever his age and wherever he lives. All types of sport can increase the incentive for and enjoyment of exercise, but perhaps the greatest attraction of sport is its contribution to social contact and integration.

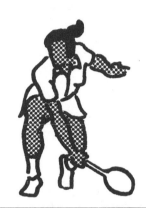

Heat treatments

Saunas, steam baths, rubberized sweatsuits and similar devices (p. 83) do not improve fitness or maintain it.

Their use may result in a temporary loss of weight by causing the body to lose water through sweating, but this is regained as soon as the water is replaced by drinking.

Saunas and steam baths (but not sweatsuits) do help to relax the muscles and to tone and deeply cleanse the skin. They can also help to relax the nervous system and to relieve tension. As far as exercise is concerned, however, they have no effect whatsoever, and prove only that there is no easy way to fitness.

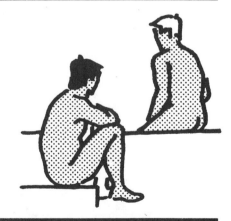

Massage

This refers to the systematic manipulation of the soft tissues of the body (pp. 118–119). It does not aid fitness or provide exercise in any way, other than to help remove "obstacles," such as muscle injury, etc.

Effects of massage are that it relaxes the muscles, reduces mental tension, improves the flow of blood and lymph, stretches muscle fibers, and can be very enjoyable.

All forms of massage, including Shiatsu and other forms of acupuncture and Oriental massage, are forms of physical therapy, not exercise.

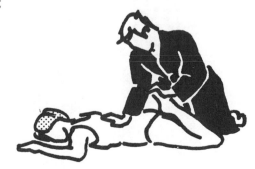

©DIAGRAM

TYPES OF PROGRAM

When choosing a form or system of exercise you should aim at as fine a balance of mobility, strength, endurance, and heart and lung exercises as possible. But make sure your choice is based on developing the heart and lungs — the circulatory-respiratory (CR) system — as this is the precondition for all other forms of fitness, as well as for good health and the prevention of heart disease.

Aerobic means "with air" and refers to any highly active exercise, performed in the open air, which increases the oxygen needs of the body and so exercises the CR system. Perhaps best known is the system devised by Dr Kenneth Cooper and described in his book, *Aerobics*. This calls for progressively harder performances in running, walking, swimming, cycling, stationary running or selected sports. During the 1970s running and jogging became the most popular of all aerobic activities. We include an aerobic program backed by the US President's Council (pages 320–329). The major criticism of aerobics as a means of getting fit, is that they do not form a total fitness program and, except for swimming, do not promote mobility or general strength. Aerobic exercises should therefore be performed with other types of exercise.

Aerobic exercises
Examples of activities giving good aerobic exercise are described on the following pages.
1 Walking (p. 206)
2 Jogging and running (pp. 206, 320–329)
3 Jumping /skipping (pp. 190–195)
4 Cross-country skiing (pp. 207 , 217)
5 Swimming (pp. 206, 216, 295)
6 Team sports (pp. 206, 223)

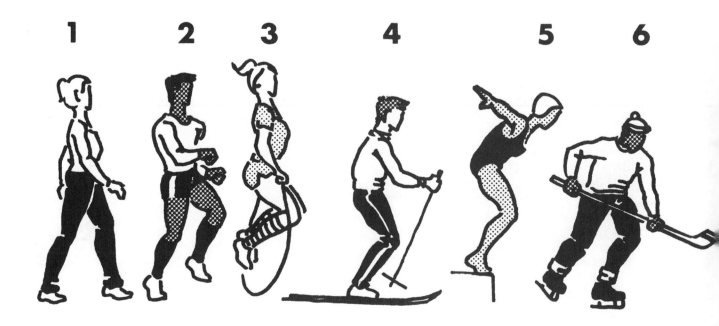

1 2 3 4 5 6

Pulse-rated CR programs are similar to aerobic systems but their emphasis is on maintaining a certain amount of effort (as measured by your heart rate) for a certain period of time rather than over a particular distance. Programs of this type are able to take more account of individual differences than other aerobic programs, but they should still be performed with other types of exercise.

Calisthenic exercises are systems of rhythmic movements aimed at developing mobility and strength. They can tone up nearly all the muscle groups, using little equipment, with a minimum of cost, and can be performed almost anywhere. They have little or no CR value, however, and should be supplemented with some type of aerobic exercise.

Total fitness programs combine CR exercises with others for muscular strength, endurance and flexibility. They therefore combine the best of both aerobic and calisthenic systems without their disadvantages. Another recommendation is that after the basic CR exercise you can choose to concentrate on specific areas to suit your own particular needs, for example weight training for strength. Examples of total programs are those backed by the British (pp. 282–291) and American (pp. 292–319) governments.

Calisthenic exercises
Included in this book are various calisthenic exercises designed for persons with the following special needs.
7 Reducing (pp. 80–89)
8 Posture (pp. 90–101)
9 Back pain (pp. 102–113)
10 Relaxation (pp. 114–125)
11 Pregnancy (pp. 126–137)
12 After forty (pp. 138–155)
13 After sixty (pp. 156–161)

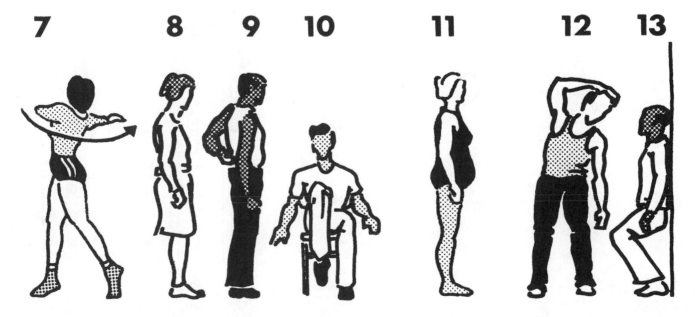

7   **8**   **9**   **10**   **11**   **12**   **13**

©DIAGRAM

MEETING YOUR NEEDS

The effects of exercise depend upon five factors: your personal level of fitness, the type of exercise that you choose, and the intensity, duration and frequency of your exercise activity.

Fitness The basis of all fitness is the circulatory-respiratory (CR) system. Whatever exercise you do, its effect on overall fitness depends on how hard the CR system works — as measured by heart rate, or pulse — and how soon it returns to normal. A medical check-up is recommended before starting an exercise program.

Type There is a type of exercise to suit everybody.

Intensity Check your fitness level (pp. 76–77) and then see the diagram below.

Duration An aerobic exercise should be carried out at the appropriate level for at least 15–20 minutes. It should be preceded by a 5-minute warming-up period and followed by a cooling-down period of similar duration (pp. 320–329). Any non-CR exercises (such as weight training) should be done first, or after a rest period.

Frequency Start with three times weekly, and as your fitness improves build this up to every other day or as often as six times weekly if you wish.

Exercise intensity
The diagram shows the maximum heart rates for people of different ages, and the level to which people of different ages and fitness ratings should raise their heart rate during exercise.

a Maximum heart rates.

b Heart rate training zone for people with a high fitness rating — heart rate raised to 90% of the maximum.

c Zone for people with a medium fitness rating — heart rate raised to 80% of the maximum.
(For example, a moderately fit 40-year-old man should maintain a heart rate of 143–155 beats per minute during training.)

d Zone for people with a low fitness rating — heart rate raised to 70% of the maximum.

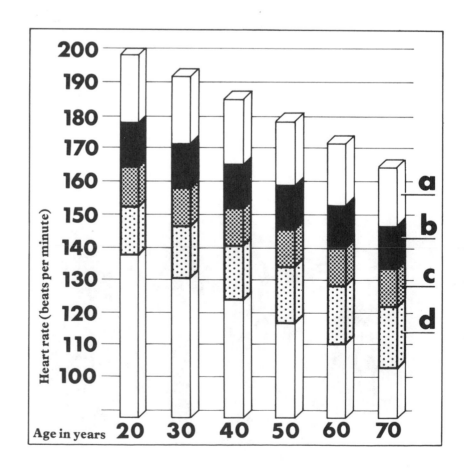

When to exercise

Choose a time that suits your personal routine and body rhythm best. If possible, allow yourself time for a recuperation period after you finish.

Morning exercise necessitates a long warming-up period to arouse the body from sleep, but it can be an excellent way to wake up. It also has the advantage of leaving the rest of the day free.

Noon exercise is good for city workers with nearby facilities. It breaks up the day, leaves the evening free, can prevent afternoon tiredness and boredom, and helps dieting. Exercising before a meal can help you to reduce, diverting blood from the digestive tract and so relieving feelings of hunger.

Evening exercise is often said to be best of all, as it rids the body of the day's tension and relaxes it for sleep.

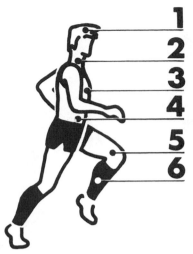

Warning signs

Stop exercising and see your doctor if you experience:
1 dizziness, lightheadedness, loss of coordination, confusion, cold sweat, glassy stare, pallor, blueness, fainting;
2 irregular or racing pulse, very slow pulse after training, fluttering, pumping or palpitations in the chest, pain or pressure in the arm or throat.

Rest if you suffer from any of the following, and see your doctor if they persist:
3 rapid heart rate some time after exercise, extreme breathlessness, nausea or vomiting after exercise, prolonged fatigue;
4 side stitch (cramp of the diaphragm);
5 pain in the joints;
6 muscle strain.

Age limits

The diagram shows probable age limits for sports, but personal constitution and abilities must also be considered.

Performance deteriorates as a result of the aging process, usually starting in the twenties. The older person is more subject to sprains, strains, muscle and tendon rupture and, if unused to exercise, to heart attacks—so do take care.

Decline in CR performance

During middle age the CR system deteriorates at the rate of 1% per year. Compared with 25 years as the optimal age for physical activity, you can expect by the following ages to have slowed down by the amounts given below.

Age 35: 3% reduction
Age 45: 10.4% reduction
Age 55: 21.4% reduction
Age 60: 28% reduction
Age 65: 35.3% reduction
Age 70: 42.7% reduction

Age in years

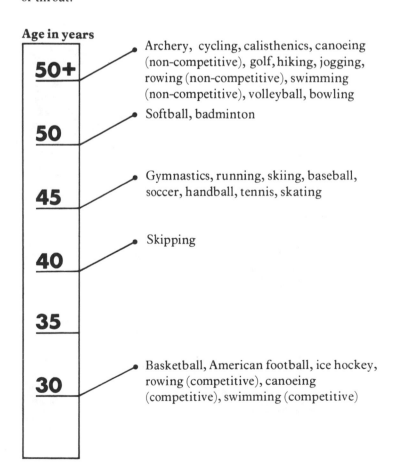

50+ Archery, cycling, calisthenics, canoeing (non-competitive), golf, hiking, jogging, rowing (non-competitive), swimming (non-competitive), volleyball, bowling

50 Softball, badminton

45 Gymnastics, running, skiing, baseball, soccer, handball, tennis, skating

40 Skipping

35

30 Basketball, American football, ice hockey, rowing (competitive), canoeing (competitive), swimming (competitive)

Chapter 2   A FIT BODY

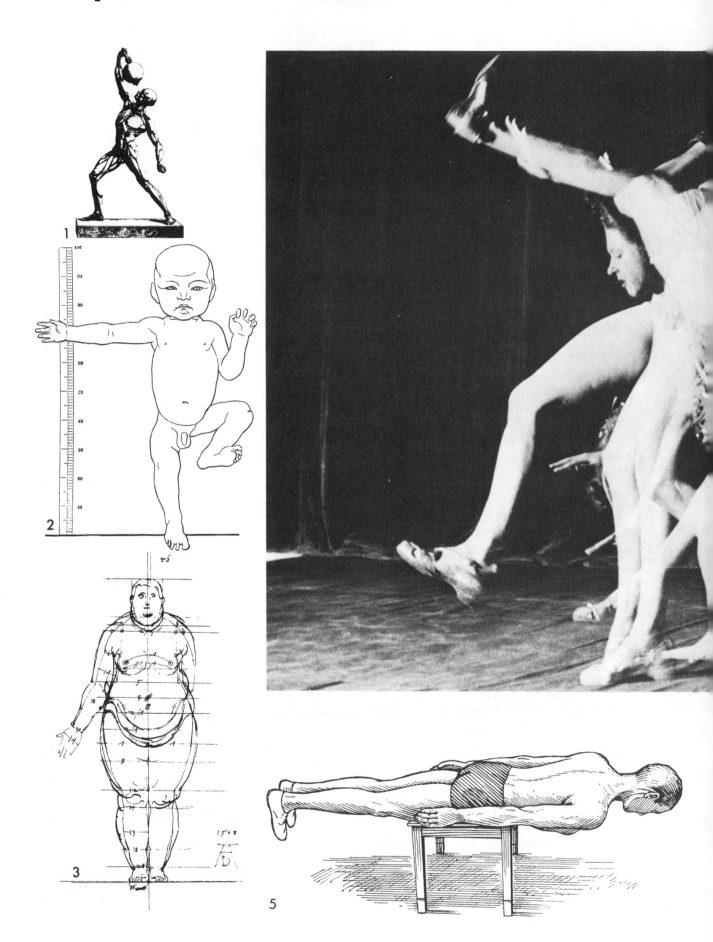

1

2

3

5

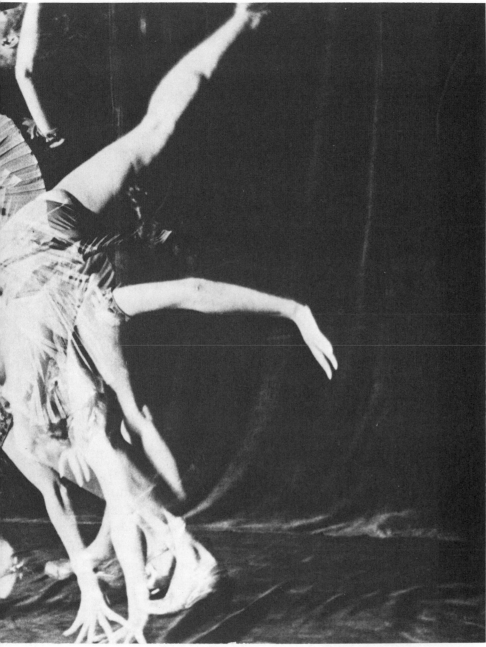

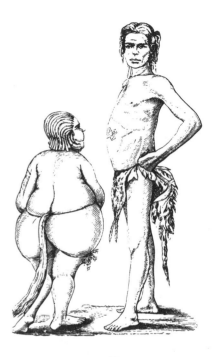

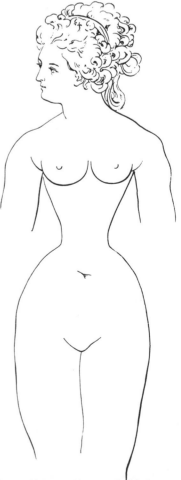

1, 2, 6, 7 *Der Mensche* by Dr Ranke
(Leipzig 1887)
3 *The Anthropometric System* by Albrecht
Dürer (1507)
4 Acrobatic dancers (Radio Times Hulton
Picture Library)
5 *Postural and Relaxation Training* by
John H. C. Colson (Heinemann, London
1956)

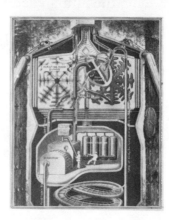

THE BODY MACHINE

Since William Harvey discovered, in the early 1600s, that the heart pumps blood around the body, men have increasingly come to look upon the human body as a machine. For we now realize that—like any truck or car—the body has support, locomotion, fuel, waste and control systems. Like any vehicle, the human body also has measurable efficiency, strength and power determining the limits of its physical performance. This view of man as mechanism finds various expressions in the world today.

In athletics, doctors conduct studies to assess the likely limit of human strength, speed, endurance and so on. In international athletics, men and women are seen as products to be continually improved upon. Just as designers seek to build industrial plant with ever greater output, so coaches train top athletes to try to run and swim faster, jump higher and farther, and lift greater weights than anyone before them. Some athletes even resort to drugs to stimulate their muscles to perform almost literally superhuman feats. All this reflects the altered nature of athletics contests. The original Olympic Games of ancient Greece were competitions between individuals. But sponsorship by nations makes today's Olympics peaceful wars between the major powers. Some countries invest hugely in time and money in Olympic training to help their athletes win more events and break more records than the athletes of rival countries.

The new view of the body as a machine also plays its part in daily life. From factory production line to lunar module, work situations increasingly involve complex technology. Largely for reasons of cost effectiveness, designers plan technology as far as possible to match the form and function of the human bodies that must operate it. Looked at in this way, man is one kind of machine working others in a man-machine system.

And that is not all. For new man-made machines and tools are even helping to work man. Where certain faults develop in the human body, doctors can repair them with the aid of spare-part surgery — replacing damaged bones, joints, lengths of gut or blood vessel, even heart valves and pumps, and also kidneys with artificial substitutes of metal, nylon or plastic.

Most of us never need an artificial pacemaker, never work with complex modern factory equipment, seldom even run a race. But we are all "machines" whose health and fitness hinges on the proper working of our body systems.

Here and on subsequent pages we look briefly at the workings of these various body systems.

A The skeleton — the human chassis — provides support. Bones, joints and tendons serve as wheels, gears, transmission.

B The muscles provide the body with engines that operate levers in the limbs and trunk.

C The circulatory system carries the blood that feeds these engines with the fuel and oxygen required to keep them working, and removes the wastes produced by their activity.

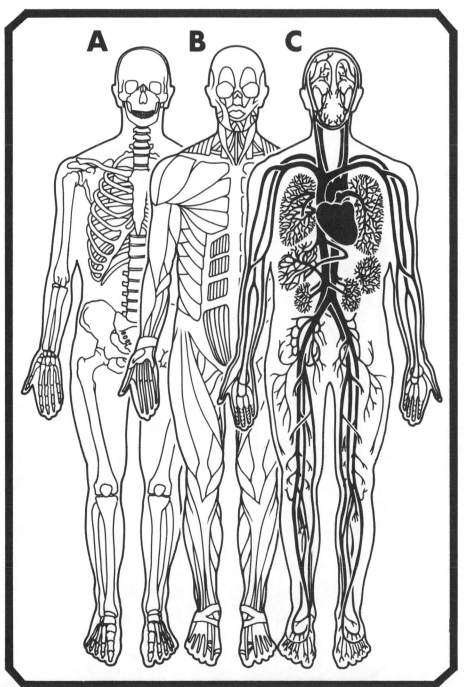

A   B   C

Systems of the body machine
Illustrated here are three of our body systems:
A The skeletal system, with its 206 variously shaped bones (for details see p. 30).
B The musculatory system, made up of over 600 muscles of different sizes and shapes (see p. 36).
C The circulatory system, powered by the heart which drives the blood through a vast network of arteries, capillaries, and veins (see p. 40).

The body machine

D The respiratory system supplies the body with oxygen.
E The digestive system absorbs and breaks down food to provide the body with fuel. It also eliminates undigested substances in food.
F The urinary system gets rid of processed wastes.
G The lymphatic system bathes, nourishes and protects cells from infection.
H The nervous system, together with
I the endocrine system, controls the operations of the various body systems.

Systems of the body machine
D The respiratory system, which includes nasal passages, windpipe and lungs (for details see p. 42).
E The digestive system, from the mouth to the anus, including the stomach and the small and large intestines (see p. 44).
F The urinary system, comprising a pair of kidneys, two tubes called ureters linking the kidneys with the bladder, the bladder, and another tube called the urethra. In a male the urethra leads to the tip of the penis; in a female to an opening in front of the vagina.

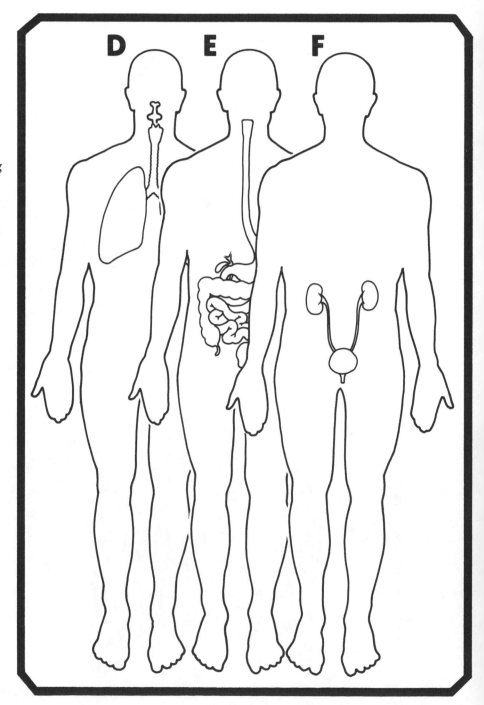

Not illustrated here are the reproductive organs: in males the penis and testes; in females, the ovaries and breasts. Enabling man to multiply himself, these organs set him distinctively apart from the machines he makes and in so many other ways resembles.

How we use our bodies affects our very lives. If we let our machinery run down we become unfit. If we keep at peak efficiency we enjoy fuller lives and may live longer. This chapter probes the human machine more closely — especially those systems we can most readily control.

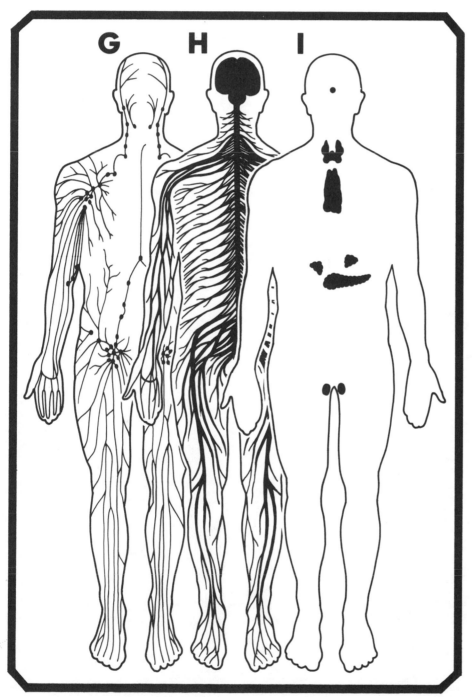

Systems of the body machine

G The lymphatic system, made up of lymph glands, or nodes, where the watery fluid known as lymph is manufactured, and a network of lymph vessels to carry the fluid around the body.

H The nervous system, made up of three different units. The central nervous system (brain and spinal cord), the peripheral nervous system (nerve connections to all parts of the body), and the autonomous nervous system (nerve centers alongside the spine.

I The endocrine system, made up of the following glands: pituitary, thyroid, parathyroids, thymus, pancreas, adrenals, and sex glands (testes and ovaries).

THE SKELETON

The skeleton supports the body; protects vital internal organs; makes it possible to sit, stand, walk and run; stores certain useful minerals; and (in the bone marrow) manufactures blood. All this is feasible partly because the adult body's 206 bones are variously shaped. Ribs, limb bones and collarbones are long bones that act as levers. Bones of the skull, the breastbone, shoulder blades and hip bones are flat and largely serve as shields. Wrist, vertebrae (spinal bones) and weight-bearing bones in the feet are short and strong.

The skeletal system
Shown on the diagrams are bones from all parts of the body (**A**), and different types of vertebrae making up the spine (**B**).

A Names of bones
1 Skull
2 Clavicle
3 Sternum
4 Scapula
5 Humerus
6 Vertebral column
7 Radius
8 Ulna
9 Pelvis
10 Carpals
11 Metacarpals
12 Phalanges
13 Femur
14 Patella
15 Tibia
16 Fibula
17 Tarsals
18 Metatarsals
19 Phalanges

B Types of vertebra
1 Cervical
2 Thoracic
3 Lumbar
4 Sacral
5 Coccygeal

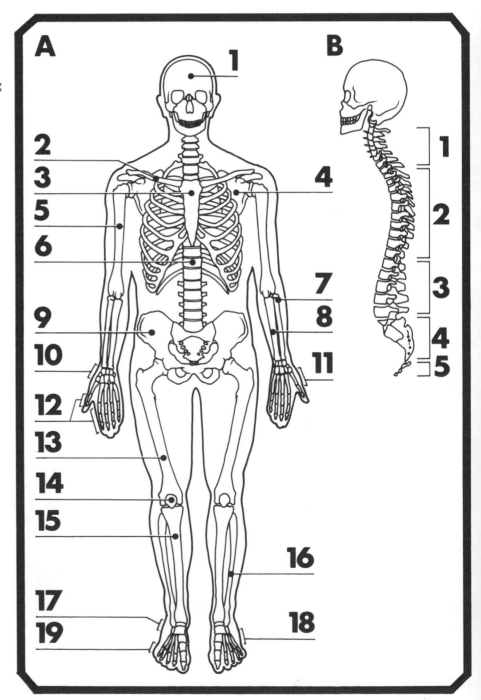

Bodily support, protection and locomotion also depend upon how the body's framework is arranged. When you stand, the weight of the upper body travels down through bones in the torso to others in the thighs, legs and feet. When you stand and move with the lines of thrust acting through the middle of the joints that link these bones, you maintain balanced posture (see page 93) and efficient muscle action. Let us now look at groups of bones in turn.

Skull Its 22 bones make up a movable jaw, and a rigid shell that forms the face and guards the brain.

Backbone This sheathes the spinal cord and forms an S-shaped column designed to bear man's weight when erect. The upper 24 of its 33 vertebrae are flexible. Seven cervical (neck) vertebrae support the head and help support the shoulders, arms and upper chest. Next come 12 thoracic (chest) vertebrae. Below these are five lumbar (lower back) vertebrae, then the sacrum (five fused vertebrae supporting all body weight above) and the coccyx (four fused vertebrae, the vestige of a tail). The backbone "pillar" supports the bony frameworks of the chest and shoulder girdles.

Chest The chest or ribcage is a cage of ribs curving forward from the backbone toward the sternum (breastbone). The upper seven pairs of ribs are called true ribs because they connect directly with the breastbone. Pairs 8 to 10 — the "false ribs" — join the seventh rib before this meets the breastbone. Pairs 11 and 12 — the "floating ribs" — end short. Ribs and breastbone together protect the heart and lungs and, by moving rhythmically up and down, make breathing possible.

Shoulder girdles These comprise clavicles (collarbones), which hold the shoulders clear of the chest, and scapulae (shoulder blades), which hang down at the back of the chest. Anchoring the arms, the shoulder girdles hang across the top of the chest, supported by the backbone via the head and neck.

Arms Each arm has 30 bones, 27 of them in the hands alone. The upper arm has a single bone (humerus); the forearm has two bones (radius and ulna).

Lower limbs feature hip, thigh, leg and feet bones. Hip bones, sacrum and coccyx comprise the pelvis, a bony girdle that transfers the weight of the trunk via the hip joints to the thigh bones (femurs), then via the knees to the shin bones (tibias and fibulas), and on to the tarsal, metatarsal and phalangeal bones of the feet. Their bony arches bear the entire body's weight.

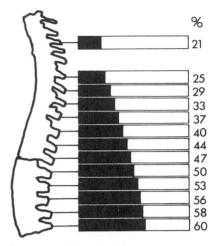

Support of body weight
The diagram shows the % of total body weight supported at the 12 thoracic and 5 lumbar vertebra.

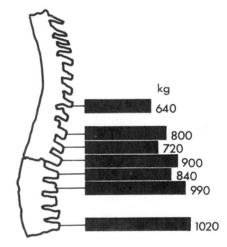

Breaking load
The diagram shows the breaking load for the vertebrae of a 21-year-old.

JOINTS

Bones could not work together to transmit body weight and move the body unless they were in some way linked. Linkage occurs through joints and ligaments. Joints are the places where bone meets bone. Some are movable, some immovable. Immovable joints cushion bones against breakage caused by blows. Movable joints allow bones to move smoothly against each other without damage due to grating. Bones are linked at joints by ligaments: bands of flexible tissue. Torn or overstretched ligaments cause sprains. Bone displacement at a joint is dislocation.

Main flexibility points
1 Ankles
2 Knees
3 Hip joints
4 Where spine joins pelvis
5 Where arm joins shoulder girdle

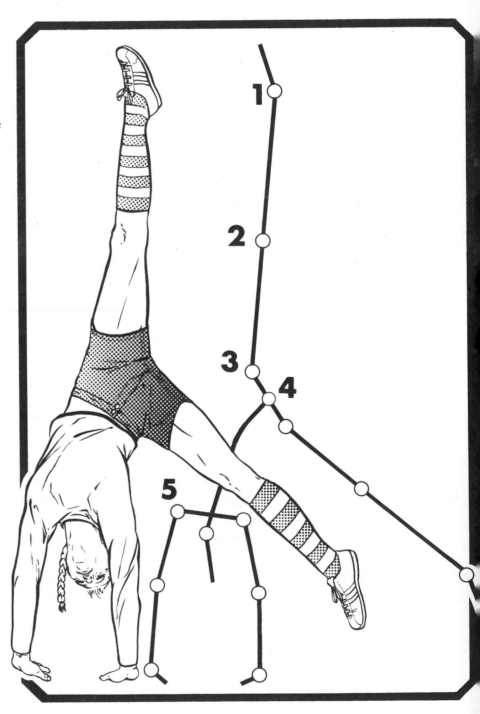

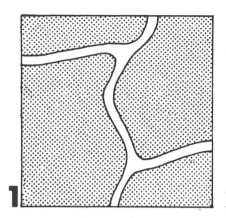

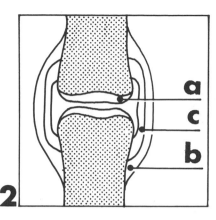

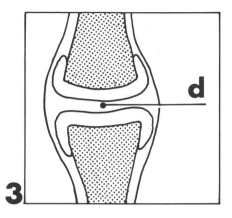

Main types of joint

1 Fibrous joints These include the skull bones' zig-zag sutures buffered by fibrous strands, but fused in old age. In syndesmosis rough-edged bones are bound together by a ligament. Certain paired bones (fibula and tibia; radius and ulna) are linked by a wide band known as an inter-osseus membrane.

2 Synovial joints like those of elbow, ankle, shoulder, have bone ends crowned by smooth articular cartilage (**a**). Ends touch across a joint cavity, enclosed by a fibrous joint capsule (**b**) consisting of strong ligaments to hold opposing bones in place. A fatty, smooth and slippery synovial membrane (**c**) lines the capsule and lubricates joint surfaces with sticky fluid.

3 Cartilaginous joints include those between the vertebrae and the front halves of the pelvis. The cartilage-capped bone-ends in such a joint are separated by a thick fibrocartilage cushion or plate (**d**). Such plates form the disks between vertebrae. The movement of one cartilaginous joint is slight, but the combined movements of several joints in the spine can be substantial.

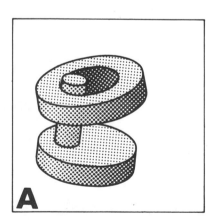

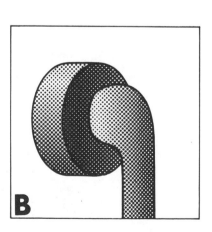

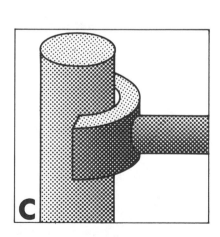

Types of movement

Different types of joint have different types and ranges of movement. Fibrous joints, as in the skull, are immobile. Cartilaginous joints permit the backbone to bend and extend. But synovial joints have the greatest range of movement. All are capable of a gliding movement of one surface across another. Many are pivot, ball-and-socket or hinge joints. A pivot joint (**A**) where the skull sits on the spine enables you to turn your head. A pivot joint in the forearm's radius bone enables you to turn your hand palm up or down. The ball-and-socket joints (**B**) of hip and shoulder have the greatest range of all. In such joints the rounded head of one bone fits into the cup-shaped end of another so that movement may occur forward, backward, outward and inward. Hinge joints (**C**) allow movement only in one direction. They occur in ankles, elbows, toes and fingers. Synovial joints also include the saddle-shaped joint of the thumb. They allow movement in two directions. Joints that permit considerable movement nonetheless keep the bony system reasonably rigid.

Joints

TESTS

Trunk movements

Try these tests to show the variety of movements allowed by joints in your trunk. They will show the backbone working as a universal joint.

(Use caution with these and other tests unless you do them regularly as part of a planned exercise program.)

1a Stand with your knees slightly bent.

1b Bend forward. This action flexes the vertebrae and hip joints.

1c Bend backward, thrusting your hips forward and head back.

2a, b Standing square-hipped, thrust your left arm down as if to grasp a heavy weight. Repeat this action with your right arm. These movements bend your backbone sideways.

3a, b Standing square-hipped, swing your trunk around to the left as though you were trying to see something behind you. Then swing to the right.

4a, b, c Standing square-hipped, and keeping your head, neck and upper backbone stiffly in line, make clockwise circling movements with your head by pivoting from your lower back. Do the same thing in a counter-clockwise direction.

Head movements

Neck joints act as a kind of universal joint.

5a, b, c Nod your head forward, then tilt it back. The joint between head and first neck vertebra makes this possible.

6a, b Rotate your head left then right. This involves the joint between the first two vertebrae.

7a, b, c Tilt your head sideways. This involves your whole neck.

8a, b, c Rotate your head clockwise then counterclockwise.

1a 1b 1c 2a 2b 3a 3b 4a 4b 4c

5a 5b 5c 6a 6b 7a 7b 7c 8a 8b 8c

TESTS

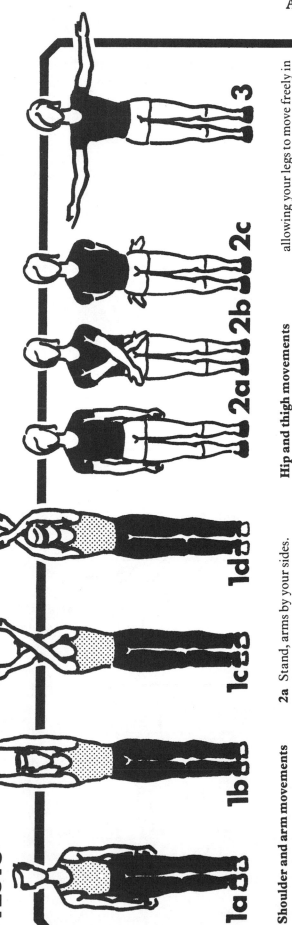

1a **1b** **1c** **1d**

2a **2b** **2c**

3

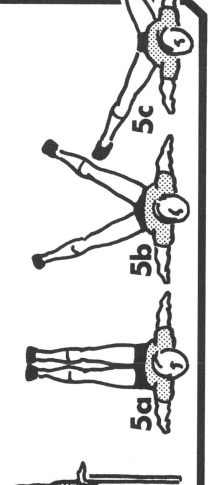

5a **5b** **5c**

4a **4b** **4c** **4d**

Shoulder and arm movements
Shoulder joints get most use of all
and are potentially the most free.
They let the arms hang, swing
forward, backward and sideways,
and rotate.
1a Stand with your arms by your
sides.
1b Lift your arms straight up.
1c Cross your arms in front of
your face.
1d Then cross your arms behind
your neck.

2a Stand, arms by your sides.
2b Cross your arms in front of
your chest.
2c Cross your arms behind your
back. Then, with your arms still
behind your back, clasp hands and
thrust both arms backward.
3 Stretch both arms sideways and
rotate them in their shoulder
sockets by turning hands palm up
and down. Lastly, make giant
circles with both arms.

Hip and thigh movements
The big ball-and-socket joints
where thighs meet hips rank
second in the body for both size
and range. Because they support
the body's weight yet also allow the
hips to move, these joints endure
considerable strain, and slight
damage to them can badly hamper
movement and affect joints low
down in the back.
The tests below show that hip
joints act as universal joints,
allowing your legs to move freely in
any direction.
4a Stand on one leg, supported by
a wall or table. First swing your
other leg sideways.
4b Then swing it forward and in.
4c Next swing it across in front of
your supporting leg, and then
behind it.
4d Then rotate your leg.
5a Lie down with buttocks
touching a wall and legs raised.
5b, c Open your legs wide apart.

©DIAGRAM

MUSCLES

Muscles are the body's engines. They move limbs, drive blood around the body, force food through the digestive tract. Muscles make up much of the body's weight: 40% in men, 30% in women. There are more than 600, differing in size, shape and type according to the work they do.
The three main muscle types are skeletal, cardiac and smooth. Skeletal muscles move the head, trunk and limbs. Cardiac muscle operates the heart. Smooth muscles work the stomach, intestines and blood vessels. Smooth muscles are sometimes called involuntary, because we can't control

The musculatory system
A Back view
1 Triceps
2 Trapezius
3 Deltoid
4 Erector spinae
5 Latissimus dorsi
6 Gluteals (gluteus maximus, gluteus minimus)
7 Extensor group
8 Hamstrings (semimembranosus, semitendinosus, biceps)
9 Gastrocnemius
10 Achilles tendon
11 Flexor group

B Front view
1 Pectorals
2 Biceps
3 Flexor group
4 External oblique
5 Rectus abdominis
6 Adductors (longus, brevis, magnus)
7 Quadriceps femoris (vastus lateralis, intermedius, medialis, rectus femoris)
8 Sartorius
9 Extensor group
10 Tibialis anterior

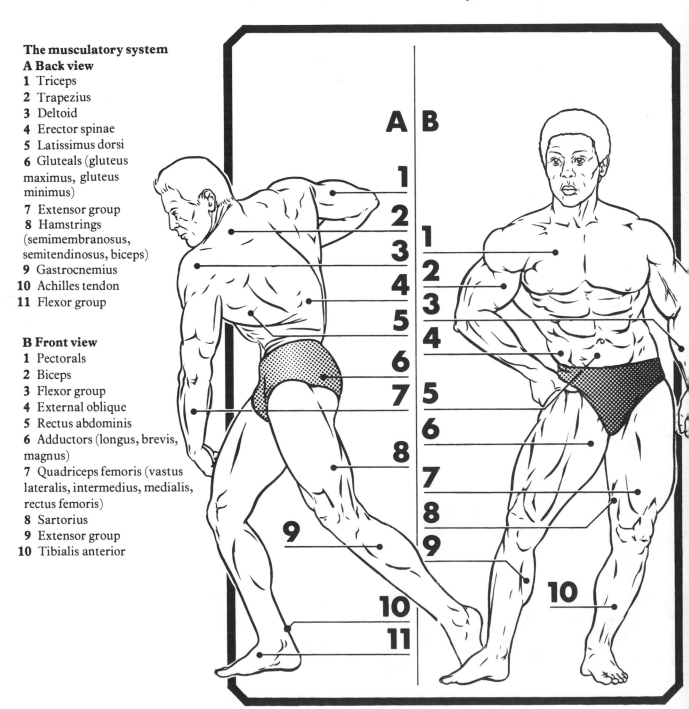

them: they work automatically. Skeletal muscles are called voluntary muscles, because they usually obey our will. Cardiac muscle tissue shares some features of both the other kinds. Here we concentrate on skeletal muscles — the ones that operate our joints and greatly affect the body's strength, power and even shape.

Much of the face, neck, chest, abdomen and limbs consists of skeletal muscles. They range in size from tiny eye muscles to big strong thigh muscles. All consist of long, slim fibers bound in bundles. They have a striped appearance if seen beneath a microscope, and thus are called striate or striated muscles. One muscle may be attached to two bones directly or by tough white cords of tissue known as tendons. When a muscle receives an electric signal from a nerve it contracts. In muscles known as flexors, contraction bends joints and pulls limbs toward the body. In muscles called extensors, contraction straightens joints and moves limbs away from the body.

All muscles can only pull or squeeze and relax. They cannot push. Thus to and fro movements of limbs, jaws or eyes are only possible because muscles work in synchronized pairs; when one contracts the one opposing it relaxes.

Skeletal muscles can be grouped in four ways by how they work. Prime movers cause active movement when they contract. Antagonists oppose prime movers. Fixation muscles steady one part (e.g. a shoulder blade) as a base for movement caused by other muscles. Synergists work with prime movers to fix joints and prevent unwanted movements.

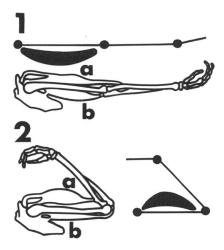

Prime movers and antagonists
1 To extend the elbow, the biceps muscle (**a**) relaxes and the triceps muscle (**b**) contracts. In this movement the triceps is a prime mover and the biceps an antagonist.
2 To flex (bend) the elbow, the biceps muscle (**a**) contracts and the triceps (**b**) relaxes. Here the biceps is a prime mover and the triceps is an antagonist.

Body levers
Each set of muscles, bones and joint works as a lever. In physics a lever is "a rigid rod moving about a fixed point." This fixed point, called a fulcrum, is drawn in our diagrams as a triangle and labeled F. Joints provide the body's fulcra. There are three different types, or orders, of levers, and all are found in the human body.
1 **Levers of the first order** Here the fulcrum (F) is between the point of resistance, or weight (W), and the muscle power (P) causing the movement. Nodding the head is this type of lever.
2 **Levers of the second order** Here W is between F and P, as in the walking movement of the foot.
3 **Levers of the third order** Here P is between F and W. Most of the body levers are of this type. One example is raising the forearm by bending the elbow.

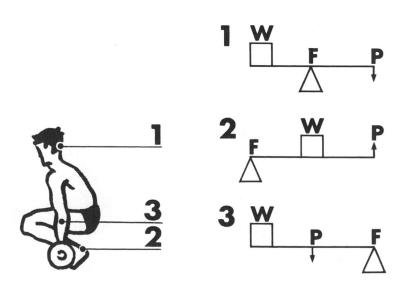

Muscles

Muscular strength

Muscular strength depends upon the working of a muscle's motor units. Each consists of a group of muscle fibers triggered by a nerve cell. The more motor units that are activated and the faster they "fire," the more a muscle contracts and the greater its tension. The greater its tension, the greater its strength.

1a Isotonic or dynamic strength is muscular strength needed to move a resistance through the full or almost full range for the joint involved. The action of a weight lifter provides our example. Isotonic strength is measured by the weight resistance moved.

1b Isometric or static strength is the greatest tension produced by a muscle keeping a joint fixed in one position. In an isometric exercise (see p. 226) we can push against the pressure of another person, or can oppose two parts of our own body.

Muscular endurance

Muscular endurance depends upon how well a muscle or group of muscles persists in contraction.

2a Isotonic or dynamic endurance involves the repeated movements of a limb against a resistance. Jogging and cycling involve this kind of endurance. It can be measured by how many times limb muscles continue isotonic contractions against a measured resistance.

2b Isometric or static endurance involves holding a limb in a certain position; the longer the position is held the greater the muscular static endurance.

Muscular power

Muscular strength and endurance should not be confused with muscular power. Power is the rate at which work is done. Thus muscular power is the speed with which a muscle contracts in order to move a joint or resist an opposing force.

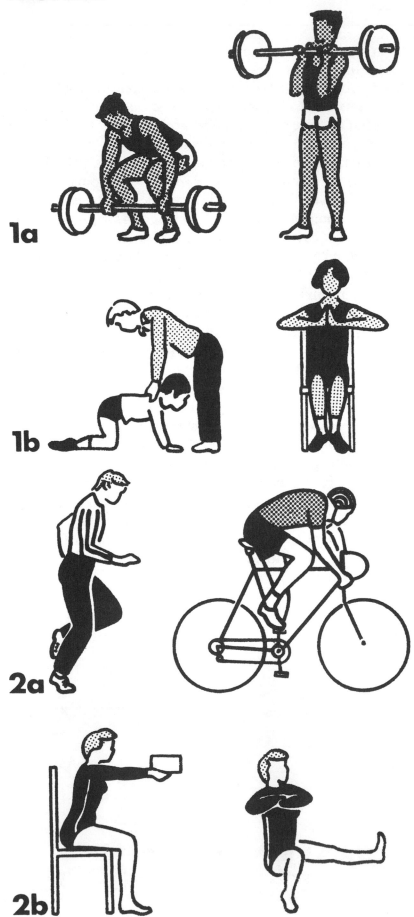

1a

1b

2a

2b

Applying muscle force

Bones, joints and muscles combine to operate as levers capable of moving the body's limbs and other loads. But some parts of the body are stronger than others. For instance, legs exert more force than arms. Then, too, laboratory studies show that some muscle groups exert more force if applied in one way rather than another.

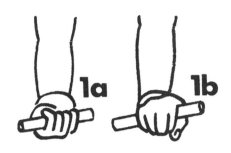

Using hands

1a If you need to make an inward rotating movement of the hand involving force, you exert more force if you start with the palm of the hand facing up.
1b If you need to make an outward rotating movement of the hand, you can exert more force if you start with the palm of the hand facing down.

Applying force while seated

2a If you sit in a seat that cannot move and push a lever with your hands, they exert the greatest force when your elbow forms an angle of 150–160° and if the hand grip you are holding is about 28in (70cm) from the back of the seat.
2b If you exert a pulling force while seated, your pull is most forceful when your arm is fully stretched.
2c If you push against a foot pedal while seated, you exert the greatest force if your knee makes an angle of 160° and your ankle makes an angle of 120°. Pushing with the leg from 165° may create a thrust as great as 700lb (318kg). This is 11.7 times greater than the thrust achieved from only 90°.

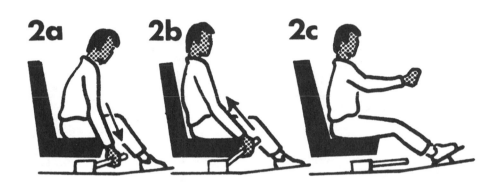

Using arms

3a If you need to push an object away by straightening your arm, you can exert more force if you start with your elbow fully bent instead of partly bent.
3b The bending force exerted by an arm is greatest when the elbow forms an angle of 90°. Incidentally, a standing man with his elbow at 90° increases the weight his arm can lift by one-third if he holds his hand palm up instead of down.

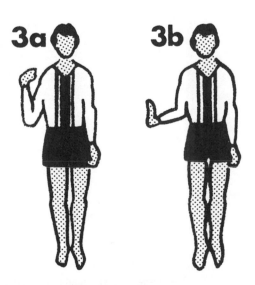

©DIAGRAM

CIRCULATION

Blood, a complex fluid, takes oxygen and nutrients to muscles and other organs, and removes local body wastes. Blood courses around the body in a closed system of tubes called blood vessels. The heart pumps oxygen-rich blood out through vessels called arteries. These branch into tiny capillaries, which yield up oxygen and nutrients before they reunite as veins. Veins return blood to the heart, which sends it to the lungs where it loses carbon dioxide and gains oxygen. Thus purified and enriched, blood returns to the heart for recycling.

Circulatory system
The illustration shows the heart and the major arteries and veins taking blood to and from muscles involved in exercise.

1 Carotid artery
2 Jugular vein
3 Subclavian vein
4 Subclavian artery
5 Cephalic vein
6 Aorta
7 Basilic vein
8 Heart
9 Brachial artery
10 Inferior vena cava
11 Iliac artery
12 Femoral artery
13 Saphenous vein

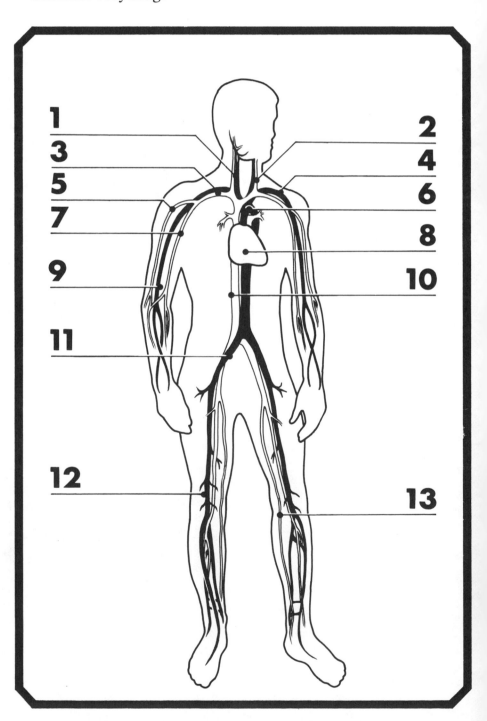

1 The heart-lung system

The heart (**a**) is two pairs of pumps separated by a wall of muscle. Each pair comprises two chambers linked by a valve. One pair of pumps (**a1**) receives blood from the body (**b**) and sends it to the lungs (**c**) where carbon dioxide waste is exchanged for oxygen. The other pair of pumps (**a2**) receives oxygenated blood and sends it on around the body.

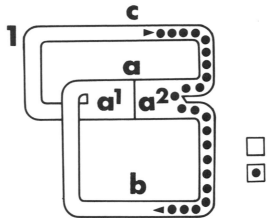

☐ Deoxygenated blood

⊡ Oxygenated blood

2

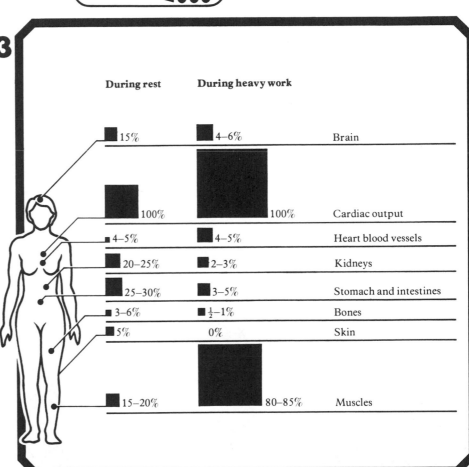

	Untrained person	Trained person
a Stroke volume	60 / 100	100 / 150
b Heart rate	85 / 198	64 / 185
c Cardiac output	5 / 18	6 / 28

☐ When resting

■ During maximum effort

3

	During rest	During heavy work	
	15%	4–6%	Brain
	100%	100%	Cardiac output
	4–5%	4–5%	Heart blood vessels
	20–25%	2–3%	Kidneys
	25–30%	3–5%	Stomach and intestines
	3–6%	½–1%	Bones
	5%	0%	Skin
	15–20%	80–85%	Muscles

2 Effectiveness of the heart

This is indicated by stroke volume, heart rate and cardiac output. Stroke volume (**a**) is the volume of blood (shown in milliliters) pumped out by one contraction (beat). Heart rate (**b**) is the number of contractions per minute. Cardiac output (**c**) is the quantity of blood (shown in liters) pumped out in 1 minute. Effective hearts beat slowly to expel a lot of blood.

3 Blood flow to body parts

The diagram compares blood flow to different parts of the body when at rest and during heavy physical activity. The amount of blood each part receives varies with its need to get oxygen and nutrients and to lose wastes. During rest, most of the blood flow goes to internal organs dealing with digesting food, filtering out body wastes, and so on. During exercise, the flow is largely diverted to the muscles.

This happens because arteries to organs with smaller and less urgent needs contract and let through less blood.

At the same time, during exercise the amount of blood flowing through the body in a given time increases sharply. This happens because heart rate and stroke volume both increase. The result may be cardiac output five times greater than at rest.

THE RESPIRATORY SYSTEM

Muscle contraction and other processes occurring in our bodies depend on chemical reactions in the body cells. Energy-producing chemical reactions depend in turn upon a rich supply of oxygen. The body gets the oxygen it needs from the surrounding air. It does this by means of a respiratory system that includes nasal cavities, windpipe (trachea) and lungs located in the chest and worked like bellows. When signals sent down from the brain expand the chest cavity, air flows into the lungs through linked air passages. Entering the body through the nose, where it is

Respiratory system
Identified on the illustration are parts making up the respiratory system.
1 Nasal cavities
2 Pharynx
3 Larynx
4 Trachea
5 Bronchus
6 Bronchiole
7 Lung

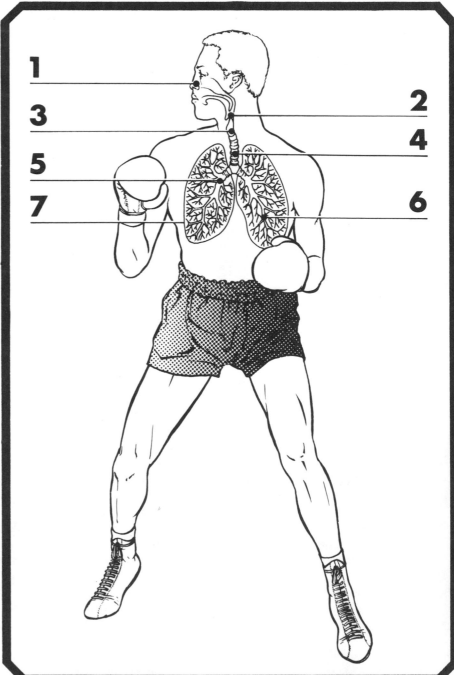

Bronchiole and alveoli
The diagram shows a bronchiole (**a**) to which alveoli (**b**) are connected by alveolar ducts (**c**).

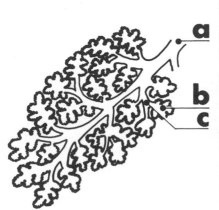

warmed and moistened, air flows on down into the pharynx and larynx, and through the trachea, a broad tube stiffened with up to 20 rings of cartilage. This "tree trunk" divides into two major branches called bronchi. Each leads to a lung, where it divides and subdivides into smaller branches called bronchioles. Bronchioles lead on to tiny cup-like air sacs or alveoli. About 600 million of them cluster around the bronchioles. The right lung has three major alveolar clusters, or lobes. The left lung has two lobes. All told this system gives the lungs at least 600sq.ft (56sq.m) of surface where oxygen may be absorbed by a mesh of tiny blood vessels called capillaries embedded in the alveolar walls. Besides absorbing oxygen, lungs expel waste carbon dioxide and some waste water from the body.

The rate at which a person breathes varies with his oxygen needs. These depend very much on body size and level of bodily activity. Thus resting adults breathe 14 to 20 times a minute, but children and adults exerted by activity breathe faster. By breathing as hard as possible out and then in you may draw in eight times as much new air as enters lungs with normal, quiet breathing.

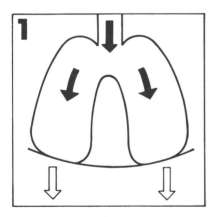

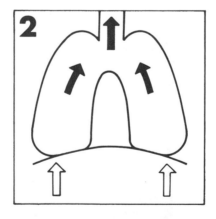

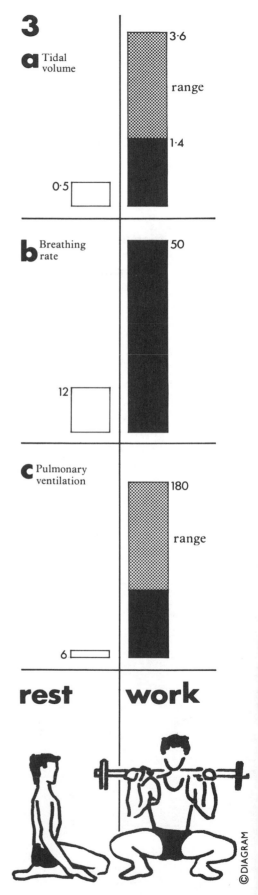

Breathing in and out

1 Breathing in occurs as muscles pull the ribs up and out and the diaphragm (a dome-like muscle) moves down. These movements reduce air pressure in the lungs, and air flows in to fill the partial vacuum.

2 Breathing out occurs as the diaphragm moves up and rib muscles relax, allowing ribs to move down and in. Ribs and diaphragm force air from lungs.

The work of the lungs

3 We compare three aspects at rest and during hard muscular work. Tidal volume (**a**) is the volume of air inhaled in one breath (in liters). Breathing rate (**b**) is breaths per minute. Pulmonary ventilation (**c**) is the amount of air breathed in per minute (in liters). Performance depends on health and size of lungs and the force of the respiratory muscles.

DIGESTION AND ENERGY

The food we eat is broken down inside us into simple substances that travel through the blood to build new body cells and provide the energy to fuel our muscles. The first stages in this process happen in the 30ft (9m) long tube of the digestive tract. This runs from the mouth to the anus. Inside the mouth, food is chewed into small pieces, mixed with saliva and formed into a rounded ball, called a bolus. Swallowing sends the bolus down the esophagus (gullet) to the stomach. This elastic, double-ended bag churns food into even smaller pieces, mixes it with gastric juice and

Digestive system
Parts forming the digestive system are identified on the illustration.
1 Mouth
2 Esophagus
3 Stomach
4 Gall bladder
5 Pancreas
6 Duodenum
7 Small intestine
8 Large intestine
9 Appendix
10 Rectum
11 Anus

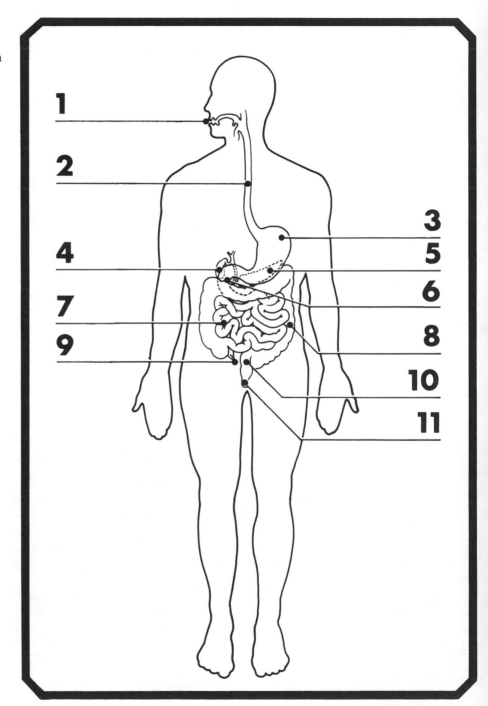

disinfects it with hydrochloric acid. Here, too, fat is melted down by heat.

From the stomach, food passes into the small intestine. Its first part, the duodenum, mixes food with pancreatic and intestinal juices and with bile from the gall bladder. Then here, and in the remaining 21ft (6.4m) of the small intestine, most of the useful elements in food are absorbed through the intestinal walls into the blood and lymph streams.

The 6ft (1.8m) long large intestine absorbs water and stores roughage such as bran that cannot be digested but is vital for the digestive system's healthy working. Bacteria convert such wastes into feces which leave the body through the anus.

Meanwhile, from the simple molecules of digested fats, proteins and carbohydrates, the body builds its own fat, proteins and carbohydrates. For instance, glucose is stored in the liver as glycogen — a kind of starch — or elsewhere as fat. Fat and glycogen are rich in energy. It is the burning of such food material with oxygen that yields energy to keep you alive and to work your muscles.

Digestion and energy

A Oxygen enters the body via the nose, food via the mouth.

B Oxygen enters blood via the lungs. Digested nutrients enter blood via stomach and intestines.

C Oxygen and nutrients are both carried around the body in arteries and capillaries.

D Cells absorb nutrients and oxygen and their stored energy is released by structures called mitochondria.

Energy release occurs in muscles in two major steps. Anaerobic respiration (**E**) yields energy by producing pyruvic acid and lactic acid from glycogen or glucose without aid from oxygen. Aerobic respiration (**F**) uses oxygen to release energy from pyruvic acid, removes waste lactic acid, and yields water and carbon dioxide wastes.

G Energy is stored in special molecules and then released.

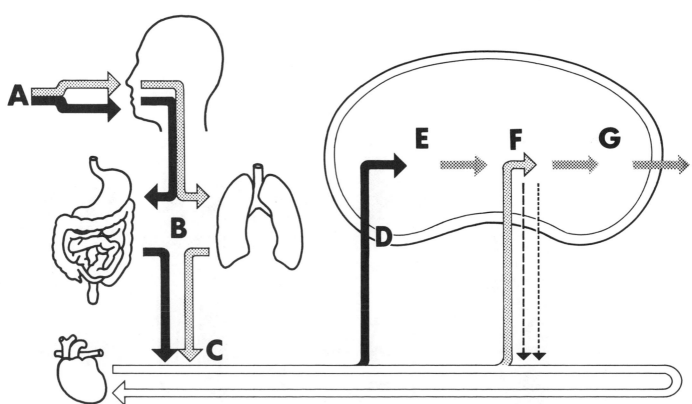

©DIAGRAM

ENERGY NEEDS

Food is the fuel that builds and energizes bodies. It comes in three main forms: as proteins, carbohydrates and fats. Proteins are vital for the growth and repair of the body. The main sources of proteins are meat, fish, eggs, dairy produce, beans, peas, grains and nuts. Plant proteins individually lack certain substances needed by the body. Carbohydrates and fats supply energy. Carbohydrates include sugars, starch (stored food in plants), and glycogen (equivalent to starch but found in animals). Bread, potatoes, rice, wheat, sugar, honey, vegetables, fruit, jam, liver, milk, eggs and cheese are rich in carbohydrates. Fats are our most concentrated source of energy. They include butter, margarine, lard and cooking oils, and occur in meat, fish, eggs and cream.

Our body also needs tiny quantities of minerals and vitamins. A varied diet provides enough of these. The amount of food a person needs varies with age, sex, size, activity, climate and the energy content of foods consumed. Nutritionists measure this in kilocalories (often commonly known simply as Calories). One kilocalorie is the heat needed to raise the temperature of 1 kilogram of water by 1 degree centigrade.

Energy needs by age

The diagram shows typical daily energy needs, in Calories, of males and females from age 7 to adulthood, from which time needs decline with age. (Note that some nutritionists favor rather different figures.)

Every minute of the day people use energy to maintain body functions or as fuel for physical exercise. Children have high Calorie requirements in relation to their size, because energy is also needed for growth. For the first 10 years or so, boys and girls of the same age have similar needs. But changes at puberty bring differences in growth rate, body size, and activity patterns. From then on, males need more Calories per day than females. Even sedentary men need more than women doing comparable work.

	1	**2**	**3**	**4**
Age	7–9	12–15	15–18	18–35
Female*	2100	2300	2300	2200
Male*	2100	2800	3000	2700

*Daily Calorie needs

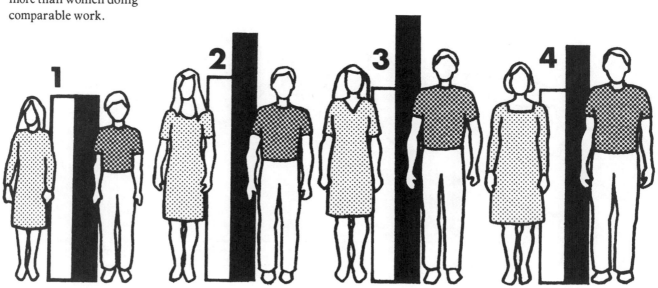

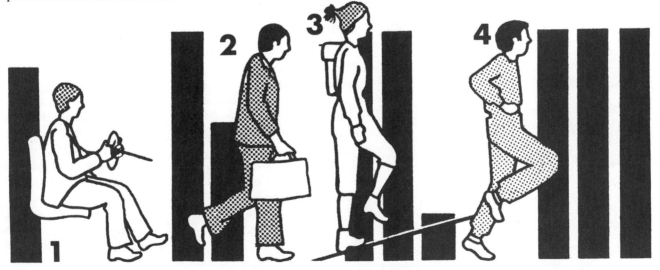

Energy consumed by women

Women use less energy than men because they weigh less and possess more body fat to trap heat. This means they need less energy to stay warm.

An average woman uses up about 1400 Calories a day — as much as two-thirds of her total daily needs — in order to maintain basic life processes. A further 600 to 800 Calories a day should probably be plenty to provide the energy needed for all her other activities at work and during recreation. Given here are examples of hourly energy consumption for some of the most common everyday activities.

1 A women lying asleep uses up about 55 Calories an hour.

2 A seated woman uses about 70 Calories an hour, or about one-quarter more than when she lies asleep.

3 A standing woman consumes about 100 Calories an hour, or nearly twice as many as when she lies asleep.

4 A woman climbing a slope needs 360 Calories an hour, more than three times as many as a woman standing still. If she climbs stairs she is likely to need still more.

Energy consumed by men

An average man uses up about 1650 Calories a day just for basic life processes such as heartbeat, breathing, digestion and excretion. His work or other daily activities will use up at least 600 extra Calories and about 2400 more if his job involves hard manual labor. Included here are examples of hourly energy consumption. In each case men tend to use more energy than women who perform the same activity. This is mainly because men's bodies are larger than women's and thus more energy is needed to operate them.

1 A seated man driving a car "burns up" Calories at the rate of 170 per hour. (This is nearly twice the quantity consumed by simply sitting.)

2 A walking man requires about 320 Calories per hour; almost twice the energy required to drive a car.

3 A man climbing a hill uses about 440 Calories an hour, or nearly half as many again as a man walking on level ground.

4 A running man consumes some 600 Calories an hour, or nearly twice as many as a man who simply walks on level ground.

REACHING THE LIMITS

However powerfully heart and lungs feed nutrients and oxygen to muscles, there are limits to your body's energy output. If oxygen demand outstrips supply, muscles can at first work anaerobically (without oxygen). But as wastes accumulate, you incur an oxygen debt and muscle fatigue that halt activity until oxygen clears the wastes. Thus panting and resting are needed for recovery after brief but intense anaerobic exercise like sprinting. But jogging can be kept up longer, because such lower level activity is aerobic: oxygen supply balances demand.

1

Factor increase possible

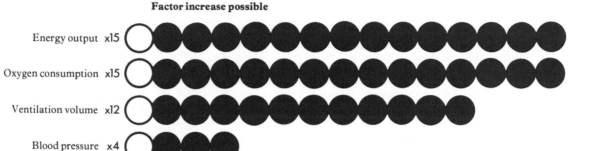

Energy output x15	
Oxygen consumption x15	
Ventilation volume x12	
Blood pressure x4	
Heart rate x3	

1 Response to exercise
The diagram shows the limits of some of the body's responses to the demands of heavy exercise. Total energy output depends largely on the blood and oxygen supply to muscles, and on muscle volume or diameter. Also, unless he loses weight, no one can expend more energy than that provided in the food he eats.

2 Oxygen supply and demand
Before exercise begins, oxygen supply is low — but adequate for oxygen demand. As mild, aerobic exercise begins, oxygen demand increases — but supply keeps pace. When a person switches to heavy, anaerobic exercise, oxygen demand outstrips supply — and he is forced to stop until raised respiration and heart rates return to normal.

2

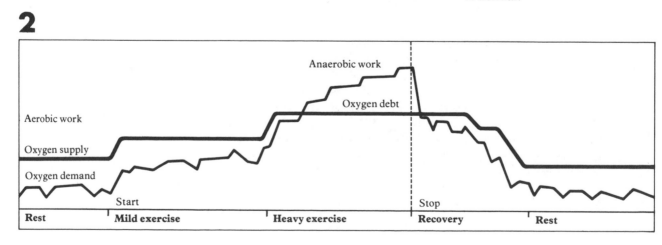

Anaerobic work

Oxygen debt

Aerobic work

Oxygen supply

Oxygen demand

Start

Stop

| Rest | Mild exercise | Heavy exercise | Recovery | Rest |

3

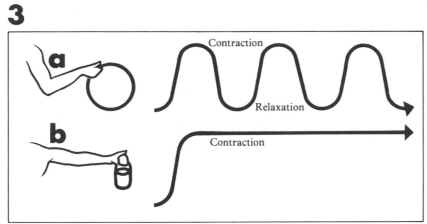

4

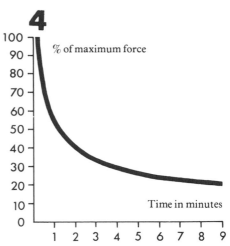

3 Comparison of dynamic (a) and static (b) muscular work

a When a hand cranks a wheel, muscles alternately contract and relax. As muscles contract, the chemical energy in glucose is converted into mechanical energy and lactic acid waste. (The upward curve shows an increase in expended energy.) As muscles relax, less mechanical energy is expended, but more blood reaches the muscles, bringing oxygen that changes lactic acid back to glucose to help fuel the next muscular contraction.

b When an arm supports a load in one position, muscles remain contracted to maintain a level of energy expenditure. But contraction expels blood from muscles, reducing oxygen supply, increasing lactic acid build up and hastening fatigue.

4 Muscular force and duration

The graph shows the relation between the force applied by a muscle (as a % of the maximum) and the time (in minutes) for which it can operate. The greater the force, the lower the blood supply, and the shorter the time the force can be maintained. But a force just under 20% of the maximum can be maintained for many minutes.

5

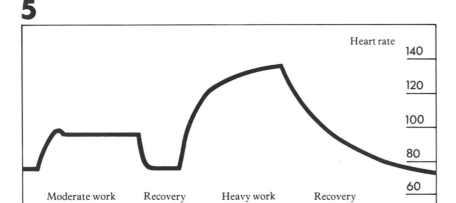

6

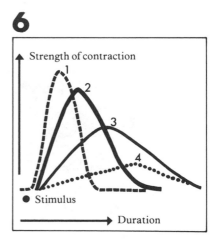

5 Work and recovery

The diagram shows how two kinds of work affect heart rate and the time needed to recover afterward. A spell of moderate work raises heart rate relatively slightly. After moderate work, heart rate soon drops to normal and the body needs only a brief period for recovery.

A spell of heavy work of similar duration raises heart rate sharply. After heavy work heart rate is slow to drop to normal. The body needs a long period for full recovery. Thus the heavier the work, the longer the rest needed afterward. For greatest output and least fatigue, someone performing work that consumes 7 Calories per minute should operate in spells of 10 minutes, separated by 7-minute periods of rest.

6 Fatigue and performance

The diagram shows the results of four successive tests on a frog's muscle. In response to a stimulus, the muscle contracted as shown. Hump heights show strength of contraction; hump lengths the time taken. Continued activity reduced the strength of contraction but increased duration and also the time taken to start contracting.

BODY HEAT

Chemical activity in muscles and internal organs produces heat. This must be dispersed or body temperature will rise dangerously high.

Most heat is lost through the skin: by radiation, convection, perspiration and sweating. Radiation and convection are high when heat makes blood vessels near the skin dilate. Perspiration is continuous: about 17oz (0.5kg) of water is lost daily by this evaporation from the skin. In sweating, millions of sweat glands in the skin release water containing salt and chemical wastes. Sweating is triggered (via the

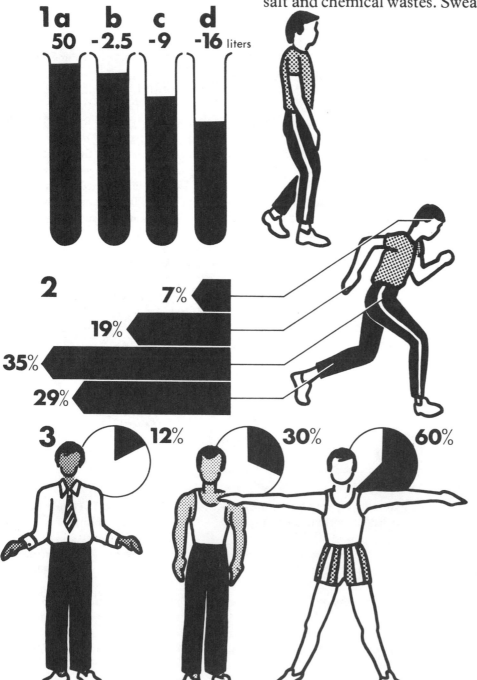

1a b c d
50 -2.5 -9 -16 liters

2
7%
19%
35%
29%

3
12% 30% 60%

1 Water loss through sweating
Before exercise, a man's body may hold 50l (13.2 US gal) of water (**a**). Sportsmen active through the day may sweat out 2.5l (0.7 US gal) in one hour (**b**), although much higher losses have been measured in laboratory tests. Other figures show the likely amounts of water lost by a sportsman after 5 hours (**c**), and by the days end (**d**).

2 Heat loss from different parts through sweating
More than one-third of the total heat loss comes from the trunk, closely followed by the legs and feet. Arms and hands rank third. The head is fourth. Palms of the hands and soles of the feet lose water three times faster than other parts, but are affected more by nervous factors than rise in body temperature.

3 Clothing and sweating
Heat loss increases as more of the body is exposed to the air. A man in pants and a shirt with long, buttoned sleeves is only 12% exposed. In pants and undershirt he more than doubles his exposed area. This in turn is doubled if he wears shorts not pants, for limbs and head account for more than half the total heat lost by sweating.

nervous system) by a slight rise in body temperature. A healthy man can safely lose over $\frac{1}{2}$ US gallon (2l) of sweat hourly for a while, and up to $2\frac{1}{2}$ US gallons (10l) for 8 hours. In vigorous exercise, especially in hot climates, well-being depends largely on the ability to sweat effectively. This is not always possible. People in a hot, very humid atmosphere, or who are overdressed in non-porous, non-absorbent clothing find that sweat does not evaporate to cool their bodies. For a while skin temperature may safely rise 57°F (15°C) above the body's inner or core temperature. But continued overheating damages the brain's vital centers, and wrecks the heat-regulating mechanism. Body temperature soars and the victim dies of heat stroke, in coma or convulsions.

Too much unimpeded sweating can be as bad as too little. Its major risks are dehydration and loss of salt. Salt-deficient blood causes excessive muscular contraction and cramping pain. If sweating is prolonged, drinking more water than you lose prevents dehydration. To prevent cramp, take $\frac{1}{4}-\frac{3}{4}$oz (7–21g) of extra salt per day, preferably in tablet form. To relieve cramp, gradually stretch the affected muscle.

4 Effects of dehydration
Described below are the progressive effects on the body of dehydration, caused by sweating away an increasing proportion of total body water without replacing it by drinking. People doing heavy work in high temperatures are likeliest to suffer dehydration and ensuing heat exhaustion. Loss of 30% of body water is reckoned fatal.

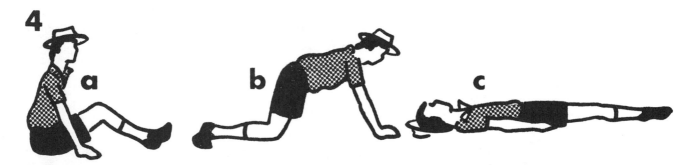

a A person losing body water equal to 1–5% of total body weight:
feels thirsty;
is vaguely uncomfortable;
moves economically;
loses appetite;
has a flushed skin;
becomes impatient;
feels sleepy;
has a rapid pulse;
has a raised rectal temperature.

b A person losing water equal to 6–10% of total body weight:
feels dizzy;
has a headache;
is short of breath;
feels tingling in arms and legs;
has reduced blood volume;
has more concentrated blood;
cannot salivate;
turns bluish;
speaks indistinctly;
cannot walk.

c A person losing water equal to 11–20% of total body weight:
is delirious;
suffers spasms in the limbs;
has a swollen tongue;
cannot swallow;
goes deaf;
sees only dimly;
has shriveled skin;
urinates painfully;
loses feeling in the skin;
cannot urinate at all.

HUMAN EFFICIENCY

An automobile engine converts only about 20% of the chemical energy in gasoline into mechanical energy to drive the wheels. The rest is lost as heat. In the same way a human body may convert only a small part of the chemical energy in food into mechanical energy that has measurable effect. Most of the rest is converted into heat energy, much of which is wasted. Thus the human body is a living engine with an efficiency which we can measure as the difference between the energy that is consumed and the energy that is produced in useful work.

But human efficiency varies with the kind of activity involved and the way in which this is performed. If the activity involves static stress, for example shoveling while stooped, efficiency can be as low as 3%. This is because much of the muscular energy expended goes to keep the body stooped. But if all the mechanical energy used has a measurable effect (in walking up a slope for instance), efficiency can be as high as 30%. Efficiency in certain tasks can be improved by changing tools. Tests showed that just by changing one type of saw for another, a man halved the time needed to cut a given quantity of wood and more than halved the energy in Calories required. Resting to reduce time lost by fatigue, and using muscles to exploit their strength in the most effective way also influence efficiency (see pages 39 and 49).

In a more general sense, the body's continuing efficiency depends on using muscles, joints and bones in the ways for which these were designed. Poor posture can cause stress in certain parts of the body. In time this causes discomfort or injury and curbs performance.

Relative efficiency
Shown below is the relative efficiency of the human body in four activities; figures show the highest energy expended, as percentages of energy consumed. In weight lifting (**a**) efficiency is low, because much energy is used to maintain the body in a static posture. Driving (**b**) is slightly more efficient because relatively more effort goes into the measurable movement of turning a wheel. Cycling (**c**) is almost twice as efficient as driving, and walking on a flat surface (**d**) is more efficient still. In these last two cases almost all muscular activity is channeled to useful effect.
Other activities that are more than 20% efficient include cranking; climbing stairs; pulling and pushing a cart; and walking up a gentle slope.

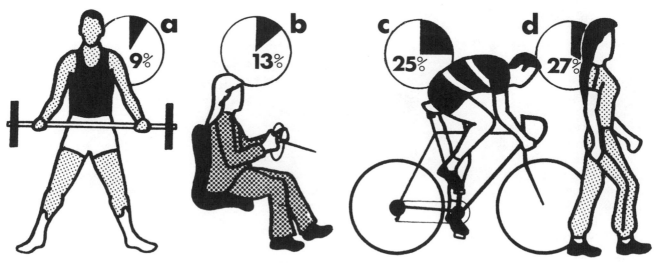

a 9% b 13% c 25% d 27%

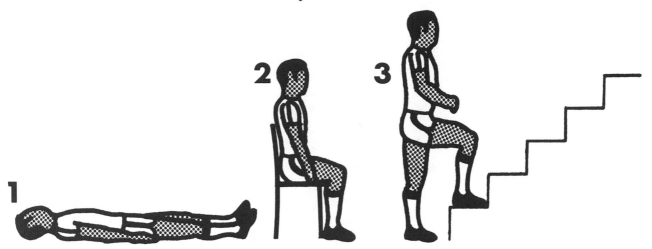

Efficient body use

Using your body efficiently involves transmitting its weight so that the line of thrust runs centrally through the joints. Balanced posture means that muscles use energy economically. Unbalanced posture wastes energy and sets up stresses that strain tissues and cause pain.

1 To rest, lie on your back with head, torso, arms and legs evenly supported so that muscles can properly relax. Lying in a twisted posture, with arm or leg dangling, stretches muscles for an undesirably long time.

2 To sit, keep your trunk upright above its supporting base: the thighs. Knees should be bent as shown and feet placed flat on the floor. When the parts of the body are balanced in this way, muscles use less force than if the body is unbalanced. But change position now and then. (Make sure you use a chair with back and seat that do not cut into your back and thighs.)

3 To climb stairs, put a foot on the next step, and shift your weight to balance over that foot. Thrust the knees and hips forward. Raise the body up and forward as you place the other foot upon a step. Descend stairs in similar fashion.

4 To walk, hold your body balanced a little forward. Movement forward should involve a smooth extension from the ball of the foot thrusting back on the ground, to the big toe, and then to the knee, hip, torso and head. Meanwhile the other lower limb leads forward in the sequence hip, knee, ankle, toes. To shift your weight onto the leading foot, put the center of the heel down first, transferring weight to the outside half of the foot, then the ball of the foot, before you push off once more with the big toe. Keep both feet parallel; hips and knees balanced; and arms swinging to counterbalance the legs.

5 To run, keep your center of gravity ahead of your supporting base; extend hips, knees, ankles, toes; and swing arms to balance.

6 To run fast, start with short, fast steps, then lengthen your stride. Land on the ball of the foot. Drive the legs and arms straight ahead with an easy swinging rhythm.

7 To make a standing jump, put the feet apart, bend the knees and hips, and swing the arms back as the body bends forward. Extend hips, knees and ankles. Push off with the toes as you swing the arms forward and up, and extend your back. Reach, stretch, and accelerate as you leap. Give at the toes, ankles, knees and hips as you land, and thrust arms forward for balance.

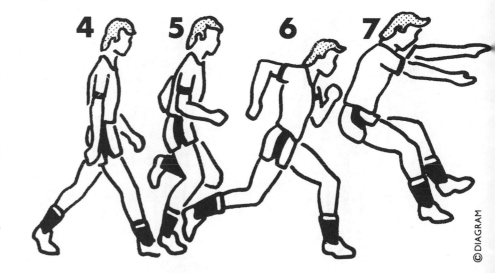

©DIAGRAM

BODY TYPES

The way the human body works limits the physical feats that any person can perform. But different people have different capabilities. Among those of the same sex and age one major reason for such differences lies in shape and size. In the 1940s the American psychologist W. H. Sheldon devised somatotyping ("body typing") — a system for grading body types in terms of three tendencies: endomorphy, mesomorphy, and ectomorphy. Endomorphy is a tendency to soft roundness; mesomorphy, a tendency to muscularity; ectomorphy, a tendency to linearity. Research has shown that people of one somatotype may be better at some activities than other people. In general terms, mesomorphs and meso-ectomorphs rank highly in strength, endurance, power, agility and body support. Ectomorphs display endurance, agility and good body support. Meso-endomorphs reveal strength, power and agility. Endomorphs perform poorly in all five categories. Range of joint movement tends to be great among ectomorphs because they have long, slim muscles, lax ligaments and small joints. Then, too, size, weight and strength tend to go together. Large mesomorphs tend to have stronger muscles than other people. But differences in quality and quantity of

Plotting somatotype scores
A person is given a score from 1 to 7 for the variables endomorphy, mesomorphy and ectomorphy. These scores are then plotted on a shield, each corner of which represents one of these variables. Here we plot:
A extreme endomorph (score 711);
B extreme mesomorph (171);
C extreme ectomorph (117);
D an average man (444).

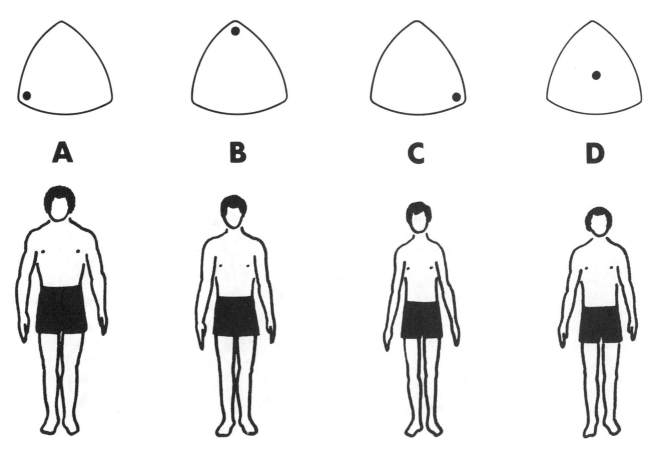

A **B** **C** **D**

muscle tissue can mean differences in strength among individuals of the same size. Less powerful bodies may prove more efficient in exerting a force for a long time. One finding suggests physique has no bearing on the ability to exercise. Moreover, slim people stand up best to swiftly fatiguing exercise, while people of average build do best at moderate exercise taken to the point of fatigue.

Studies of Olympic athletes showed that heavy athletes tended to be mesomorphs; track athletes, ectomorphic but muscular; swimmers, meso-endomorphic; weight throwers and weight lifters, meso-endomorphic; agile athletes, gymnasts and tumblers, meso-ectomorphic. Other studies revealed sprinters as short and muscular; throwers, tall and heavy; hurdlers, long-legged; basketball players, ectomorphic; American footballers, wrestlers and baseball players, mesomorphs and average types.

Sheldon's system assumes that our somatotype never changes. Some experts believe that somatotype can be altered a little by exercise in puberty. But all agree that by age 16 or 17 we are stuck with what we are.

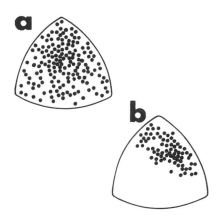

Somatotype samples
Shields on which many people's somatotypes are plotted allow us to make some interesting comparisons.
a A shield for US students shows a wide scatter, with some concentration around the center.
b A shield for Olympic track and field athletes shows a marked bias toward mesomorphy and ectomorphy.

Examples of physiques
1 A typical weight lifter or shot putter, taller and heavier than other athletes, with arms big relative to legs.
2 A modern high jumper, more muscular and less ectomorphic than earlier high jumpers.
3 A traditional high jumper, with legs long relative to body.
4 An average man.

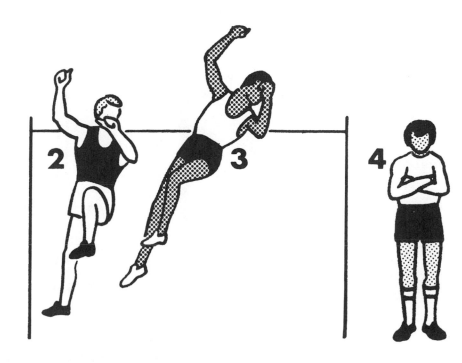

©DIAGRAM

MEN AND WOMEN

Men tend to be larger, heavier, and more muscular than women. These differences contribute to differences in physical performance, as seen in Olympic records. As this book was written, women's record times for running were 9% slower than men's over 100 meters; 12% slower over 3000 meters. In freestyle swimming the lag was 12% for 100 meters; 8% for 1500 meters. In high and long jumping the female "shortfalls" were respectively 14% and 21%. In discus throw and shot put, women's records were close to men's, but gained with far lighter missiles. In the javelin

The average man and woman compared for size

The average man (**A**) is just over 5ft 9in (175cm) tall. He weighs almost 162lb (73.5kg). His chest is 38¾in (98cm) round, his waist 31¼in (81cm), his hips are 37¾in (96cm). The maximum weight he reaches is about 172lb (78kg) and that is between the ages of 35 and 54.

The average woman (**B**) is almost 5ft 3¾in (162cm) tall. She weighs almost 135lb (61.2kg). Her bust is 35½in (89cm), her waist 29¼in (74cm). Hips are 38in (96cm). The maximum weight she reaches is about 152lb (69kg) and that is between the ages of 55 and 64. These figures are for people in the USA. Of course average men and women — people with all these measurements — are rare. Most people are taller, shorter, heavier, lighter, fatter or thinner than those shown here.

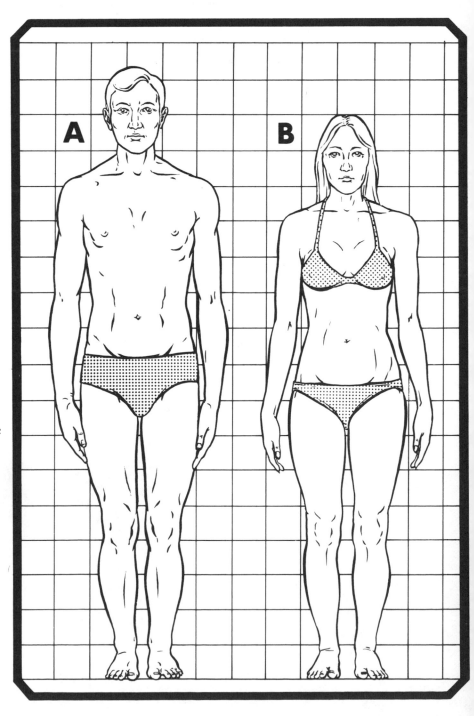

event the women's javelin was three-quarters as heavy as the men's but the longest female throw fell short of the male record by 27%.

Differences in physical performance between the sexes explain why women compete separately from men in most events, and why few women take up "heavy" sports like wrestling or football. But because women's bodies are more flexible than men's, women are unrivaled in those gymnastic exercises that stress agility and grace.

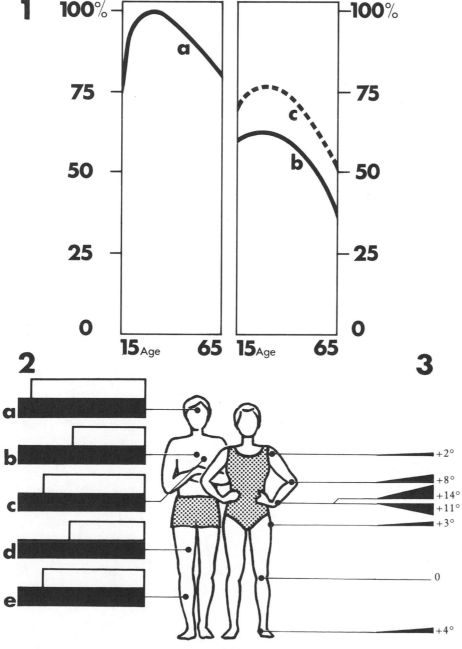

1 Strength

The graphs compare average muscle strength for men (**a**), actual average muscle strength for women (**b**), and the theoretical performance of women if they were the same size as men (**c**). The curves show the percentage of maximum strength at ages from 15 to 65.

Although women are about two-thirds as strong as men, their relative strength varies with different groups of muscles. Women's forearm flexors have only just over half the strength of men's. But hip flexors and extensors and lower leg flexors are four-fifths as strong as men's.

2 Body content

Here we compare characteristics of a typical male and female. Female characteristics (white bars) are shown as a percentage of the male's: brain weight (**a**), lung capacity at age 25 (**b**), heart weight (**c**), skin surface area (**d**), volume of blood (**e**).

3 Flexibility

The number given for each indicated joint shows on average how many degrees more a woman can move that joint than can a man. Movement of the shoulder is backward; of the elbow is to bend and straighten; of the wrist is to raise to level (14°) and then bend; of the knee is to bend and stretch. Only the knee joint is as flexible in men as in women.

EFFECTS OF AGING

Age, as well as somatotype and sex, deeply influences body form, size and ability.

A growth spurt sets in with puberty. Girls stop growing at about 16, boys at 18 or later. Full stature and full muscular strength come by 20 or soon after. Adults tend to gain weight in middle age but, through the aging process, lose weight and height by their sixties. Strength and other faculties also diminish with age. (See also p. 138.)

These changes to the body produce measurable changes in physical performance. By their teens, children show much

Signs of aging
Outward changes
As illustrated, the aging body after maturity loses height; gains, then loses weight; and acquires a jutting chin, curved spine, pigeon chest, stiff joints, wrinkled skin, and gray hair. These outward changes and a drop in physical ability reflect inward changes.

Lungs
Lung tissue and chest wall grow less elastic.
Alveoli hold less air.
Vital capacity (amount of air breathed in and out of lungs with one breath) diminishes.
Pulmonary ventilation (air breathed in per minute) declines.

Blood supply
Heart can handle less oxygen per minute.
Peak heart rate is reduced.
Heart weight and volume rise.
Blood pressure rises.

Muscles, joints and bones
Muscles lose strength, size, weight and shape.
Joints become worn and lose ease of articulation
Bones lose calcium and become brittle.

Fat
Percentage of body fat increases during middle age.

Temperature control
Heat tolerance declines.
Heat stroke is likelier.
Temperature returns to normal slowly after heat exposure.

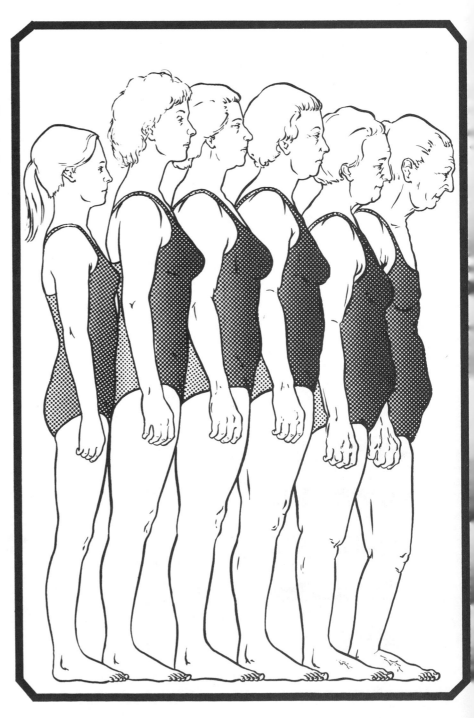

improved power and bodily coordination. Some swimmers, ice skaters and girl gymnasts reach their peak before 20. Studies of past US Olympic contestants gave median ages in the twenties for 23 of 27 listed sporting categories. Only in three was the median age above 30. Generally speaking, the early twenties are best for physically demanding sports, the late twenties and early thirties for sports where experience counts more than strength. But trained athletes can persist with certain sports indefinitely — a few even into their eighties and nineties. (See also page 23.)

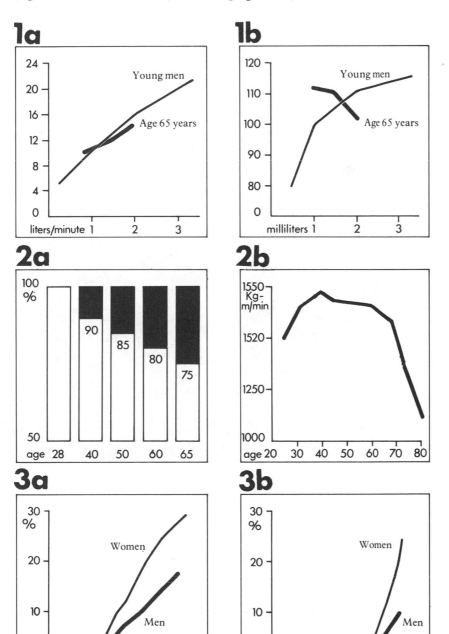

1 Heart-lung performance
Graphs compare cardiac output (**a**) and stroke volume (**b**) in men aged 65 and in young men. The higher a line, the greater the cardiac output (liters/minute) and stroke volume (milliliters); the farther a line extends right, the more oxygen is consumed (liters/minute). In the old, stroke volume drops as effort increases; cardiac output peaks with less work.

2 Muscle strength
a The diagram shows the % decline in overall muscular strength from the maximum reached in the late 20s to age 65.
b The graph compares the medium cranking rates (kg-m/min) of men aged 25 to 80. Arm and shoulder strength peaks between 30 and 40, stays on a plateau until 60, but then drops sharply from 65 onward.

3 Bone loss and fractures
Aging is associated with a progressive deterioration of the bones. Graph (**a**) shows the % decrease in bone material and minerals for men and women from their 30s onward. This decrease is more marked in women than in men. A similar pattern is seen in graph (**b**) which shows the % increase in fractures in men and women over a similar period.

Chapter 3   RATING YOUR FITNESS

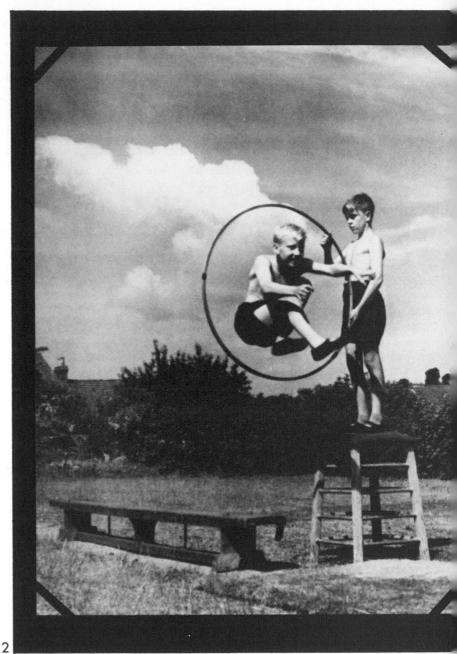

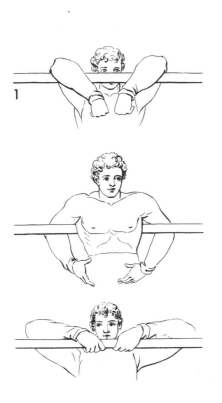

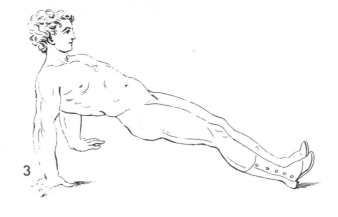

1, 3 *Gymnastic Exercises* by Capt. P. H.
Clias (London 1825)
2 *Planning the Programme: Physical
Education in the Primary School* (London
1953; reproduced by permission of the
Controller of Her Majesty's Stationery
Office)
4 *Gymnastik und Tanz* by R. von Laban
(Germany 1926)
5 *Home Gymnastics for the Well and the
Sick* by E. Angerstein (USA 1889)

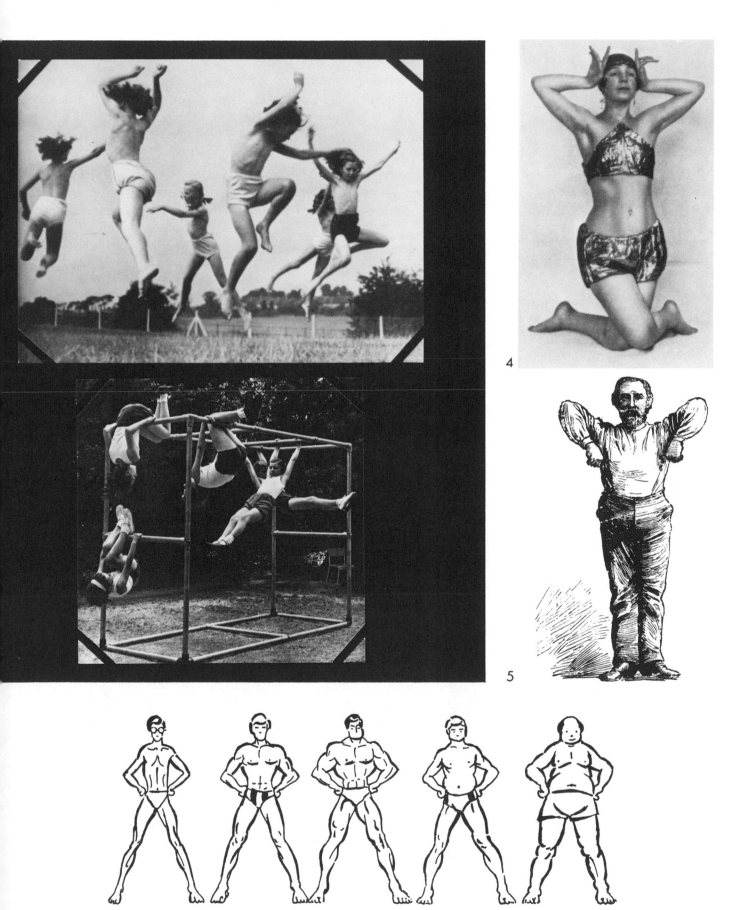

4

5

WHAT IS FITNESS?

Fitness has been defined by the US President's Council on Physical Fitness and Sports as "the ability to carry out daily tasks efficiently with enough energy left over to enjoy leisure time pursuits and to meet unforeseen emergencies." Fitness is not the same as health. Olympic athletes can be ill, and you can be in perfect health but be unable to run or swim only a few hundred yards.

There are two major aspects to your level of fitness. Your potential or realizable fitness is determined by your physiological make-up: health, body type, age, sex and other

What is fitness?
Fitness is the ability to perform physical tasks with the minimum of effort. This means that fitness is associated with efficiency. The fitter you are, the more efficiently your body works, and this increase in efficiency affects the whole of your organism. It can combat depression, indolence and illness, foster an active, positive attitude toward all aspects of life, and lead to greater mental clarity.

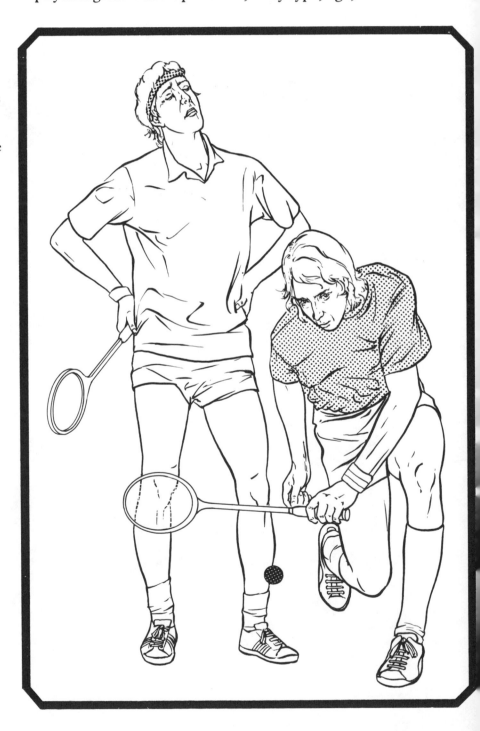

inherited factors. Your actual or realizable fitness is the degree to which that potential has been fulfilled and developed or harmed by your life-style and activities. Fitness is a relative concept. A certain level of realized fitness is necessary for everyone to prevent the deterioration of their organic functions and to keep their bodies working properly and efficiently (see pages 26–59). Beyond that it depends upon the requirements of your daily life or personal preference: a lumberjack or a professional footballer, for example, needs to be fitter than an office worker or a student.

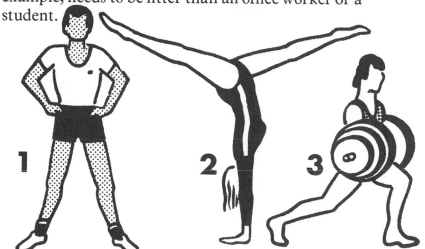

Components of fitness
Your realized fitness depends upon five major factors.
1 Body composition: the fat content of the body, your body shape and proportions, and your weight to size ratio.
2 Flexibility: the range of movements at each joint. This is determined by the mobility of the muscles, tendons and ligaments that control it.

3 Muscular strength: the maximum force a muscle, or muscle group, can apply in one contraction. This is closely related to muscular power, the ability for explosive movement.
4 Muscular endurance: the length of time particular muscles can continue to perform a certain task — the number of repetitions of a movement or sequence.

5 Cardio-vascular and respiratory (CR) fitness: how well the heart and lungs can supply the active muscles with oxygen and remove the waste products. This is the primary factor in overall fitness.
Other factors Fitness is also affected by your motor abilities — your coordination, balance, agility, reaction time, speed of movement, and power.

Body efficiency
This diagram compares the efficiency of the human body with different types of machine. Efficiency is the amount of energy you get out (work) for a set amount of energy you put in (fuel). (Note the difference between a fit and an unfit body.)

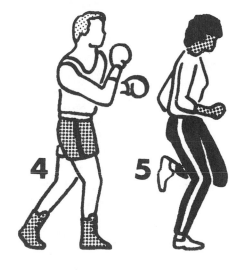

Electric motor (80%)

Steam turbine

Gas (petrol) motor

Steam engine

Human body

☐ Normal efficiency
▨ Normal variation
▦ Efficiency with fitness

©DIAGRAM

FITNESS AND UNFITNESS

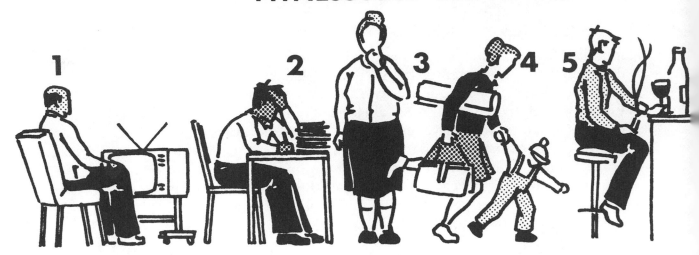

Causes of unfitness

1 Inactivity is the primary cause of unfitness, especially in the modern, automatic world with all its labor-saving devices. Without activity the body tissues atrophy (waste) and physical capacity declines.

2 Stress wastes the body's physical and mental resources, draining the energy necessary for efficient activity (see p. 114).

3 Overeating leads to excessive consumption of energy for the rate of activity. This extra energy is stored as fat.

4 Straining your system, i.e. being overactive for your realizable fitness, leads to a general "running down" of the abilities of body and mind.

5 Self-destructive habits such as smoking, drinking too much, drugs, and a dissipated life-style — bad diet, insufficient sleep, insufficient medical care — can all destroy the health and fitness of your body.

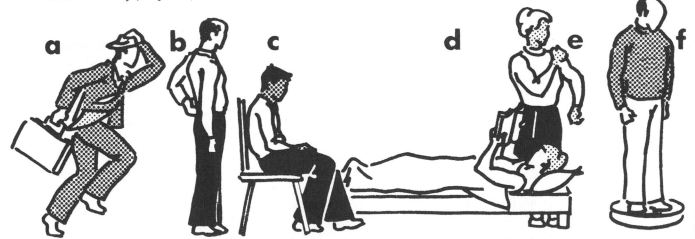

Signs of unfitness

In addition to a general feeling of being run down, that everything is too much trouble, and a constant avoidance of physical effort, you may experience the following particular signs of being unfit.

a Breathlessness and a pounding heart after short bursts of exercise, such as running to catch a bus.

b Backache because of insufficient support from weak muscles of the back and abdomen.

c Bad posture through laziness, fatigue or a lack of physical awareness of your body.

d Sleeping problems because mental activity is unbalanced by physical activity or simply because insufficient energy is used to feel properly tired.

e Aching muscles after activities like walking upstairs or carrying shopping.

f Overweight with too high a percentage of body fat.

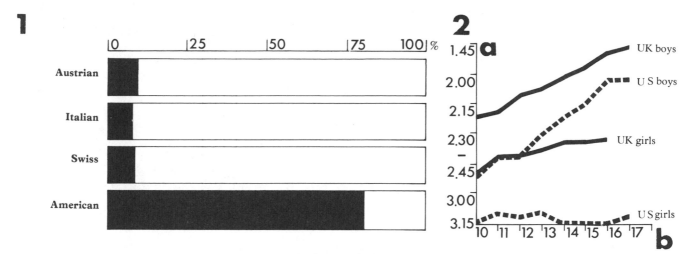

1

2a

b

Levels of fitness
These are often difficult to ascertain because different countries use different tests, making it difficult to compare results. National levels of fitness are related to a country's standard of living, as shown by the general use of automatic and labor-saving devices, food consumption per head, and overall physical awareness.

1 In 1954 Kraus and Hirschland used the same six tests on 678 Austrian children, 1036 Italian, 1156 Swiss and 4264 American children to test their minimum muscular fitness. The diagram shows the percentage of the tests failed by the children of the different countries. These results led in the USA to the establishment of the President's Council on Physical Fitness.

2 In a test carried out in the mid-1960s, Campbell and Pohndorf compared the performance of American and British boys and girls. The graph shows the results for a 600yd (548m) walk/run:
a time, in minutes and seconds;
b age in years.

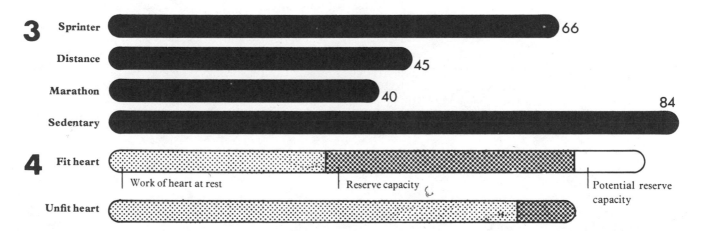

3 Sprinter 66 / Distance 45 / Marathon 40 / Sedentary 84

4 Fit heart — Work of heart at rest — Reserve capacity — Potential reserve capacity

Unfit heart

The unfit heart
During exercise the heart pumps more blood around the body to meet the increased oxygen needs of the muscles (see p. 41).
Exercise makes a heart larger and stronger. Because it pumps more blood with each stroke, a fit heart beats more slowly than an unexercised one. Being less efficient, an unfit heart has a much smaller reserve capacity to cope with physical activity, and needs much longer to return to normal after it has been exerted.
3 The diagram compares the resting pulse rates of different types of runner and of a typical sedentary individual. Rates are expressed in beats per minute.
4 The diagram compares the heart rate and reserve capacities of a fit heart and an unfit heart. (Note that the increased size and strength of the fit heart gives it an extra potential capacity as well as that gained from a slower heart rate, see also p. 13.)

BODY SHAPE

The shape of your body depends upon your posture, somatotype, distribution of body tissues, age and sex. Your somatotype (see page 54) will determine outline and general proportions, but the distribution of fat and muscle on top of that is a result of your life-style — in general, a man's chest should be at least 5in (12.5cm) larger than his waist, a woman's 10in (25cm) larger. Age also affects tissue distribution. Check your shape in a mirror without holding yourself in. Do you look good, or, more to the point, would you like to look better?

General body shape

Within the limits of skeletal shape and somatotype it is possible to control your own body shape. Diet and exercise will affect almost every muscle and tone up the entire body. This checklist will help you pinpoint any areas that need attention.

Remember, however, that body shape is only an indication of fitness. If you smoke heavily, for instance, you may have very little fat on your body but be extremely unfit. Moreover, the fact that you may have large hips, short legs or thin shoulders does not mean that you should want to change them, or that you are not, or cannot, be as fit as someone with the classic athletic figure. The look of your

body should always be secondary to its feel; a fit and healthy body will also be attractive.

When you check your body shape, concentrate on the soft tissues — the muscle, fat and skin — as these can be changed, whereas the bone cannot. For instance, a "bowlegged" look may be caused by an underdevelopment of the leg muscles, which can be changed by exercise, or by a curved femur, which exercise will not change. Body shapes differ with each person and with particular needs. Here we give only very broad and general outlines to give you an indication of what the average body should be like if it is being properly used.

A Feet
A1 Ankles should be straight and slender, not thick or crooked.
A2 Body weight should be carried on the ball of the foot near the big toe, not on the heel or the outer edge of the foot.
A3 Feet should be straight and parallel to each other.

B Legs
B1 Thighs should be firm, tapered and hard when flexed; not heavy.
B2 Knees should be straight, transferring your weight straight down through the balls of your feet; not knock-kneed, pushed back or covered with soft tissue.
B3 Lower legs (below the knees) should taper fairly evenly toward the ankles, without pronounced curving or heavy, thick calves.

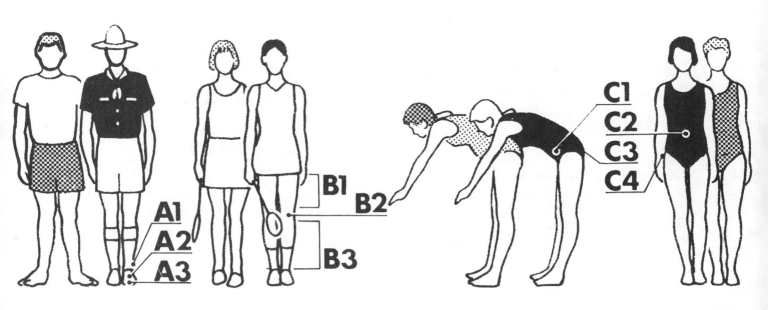

Footprints

Feet tell a great deal about posture, weight and mobility. Look at your wet footprints.

a Arches high and weight properly supported on the ball of the foot; mobility high.

b Slightly flat feet with weight too near the center of the foot; reduced mobility.

c Flat feet with no arches; low mobility.

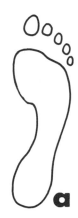
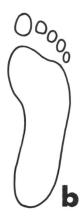
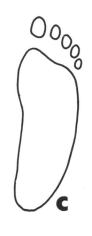

C Lower body

C1 When bending forward your abdomen should be tight and flat, not protruding or pushed out.

C2 Abdomen should be flat, with a discernible groove down the middle through the navel. It should not protrude or be soft and rounded.

C3 Buttocks should be tight and small, not soft and highly rounded or flabby and hanging.

C4 Hips should be slender, not broad and fat (relative to the size of your pelvis, of course).

D Upper body

D1 Shoulders should be straightened by using the muscles in the middle back, not by pulling up or back at their tips.

D2 You should stand with your back straight, your muscles relaxed but visible; not stooped forward or bent back.

D3 Shoulders should hang relaxed, square and slightly tapered, not pulled forward, up or back.

E Head and neck

E1 Head should be held straight and balanced on the neck, not bent to the side, front or back. You should use mainly the muscles at the back of the neck for its movement.

E2 Neck should be even and slender, not too skinny or bulging with fat.

E3 Neck should not be hollow and skinny near the collarbone, nor have a double chin or an over-prominent Adam's apple.

F Arms

F1 Arms should be raised from the shoulder when you raise them straight to body height; you should not raise them by pulling up the hand or the elbow.

F2 Elbows should be held straight and relaxed, not bent forward or pulled back with tense triceps.

F3 Arms should not be flabby, thick at the wrist or too thin. The upper arm should taper to the elbow; the lower arm taper from the elbow to the wrist.

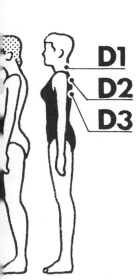
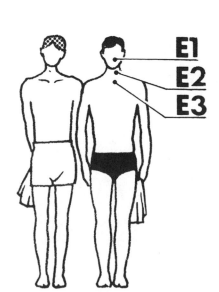
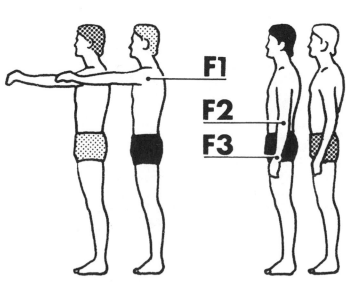

FITNESS AND WEIGHT

Weight relative to height is an important aspect of fitness. People who are overweight run a greater risk of suffering from a variety of physical disorders (see p. 80). They are also likely to find exercising more difficult — although failure to take sufficient exercise will only make matters worse. Factors affecting weight are sex, age, height, frame size, hormonal activity, diet and exercise level. Insurance companies have drawn up tables giving desirable weights for men and women of different heights and frame sizes. Such tables are a useful guide for assessing whether or not

Desirable weights

It is not easy to say what any one person should weigh. Tables showing "average" or "typical" weights are not very helpful, since in a society where more people are overweight than underweight, the average weight for a particular height is likely to be too high to be healthy.

The diagram included here (and the more detailed chart on p. 81) is a better guide, showing "desirable" weights for men and women of different heights and frame sizes at age 25. It is based on the research of US insurance companies.

A study of the graph shows the importance of height as a determining factor, and also how weight is affected by frame size and sex. For example, the desirable weight of a woman of 5ft 6in (167cm) with a small frame (**a**) is 127lb (57.6kg), compared with 146lb (66.2kg) for a large-framed woman (**b**) of similar height. A man of 5ft 6in with a small frame (**c**) has a desirable weight of 132lb (59.9kg), compared with 151lb (68.5kg) if he had a large frame (**d**).

Probably the best time to weigh yourself is in the morning, before breakfast. Make sure your weight is evenly distributed on the scales. (If you think you may be overweight, also see the section on reducing, pp. 80–89.)

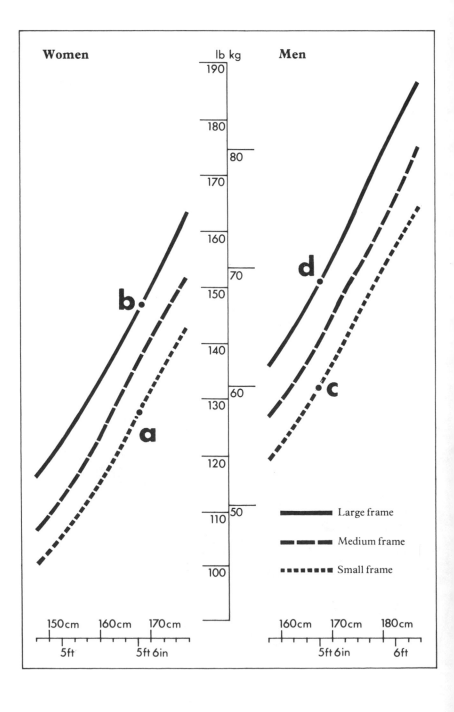

Large frame

Medium frame

Small frame

you are overweight — although looking at yourself in a mirror or pinching your flesh may be even more effective! More important than actual weight is the amount of useless fat that you carry around. In an adult male, 15% of his body weight should be made up of fat — certainly not more than 20%. In an adult female, 19% fat is the ideal and 30% the absolute maximum. Dieting is really the only way to lose excess fat. Exercise may help to some extent by consuming extra Calories, but its main contribution is to make the figure look trimmer by improving body proportions.

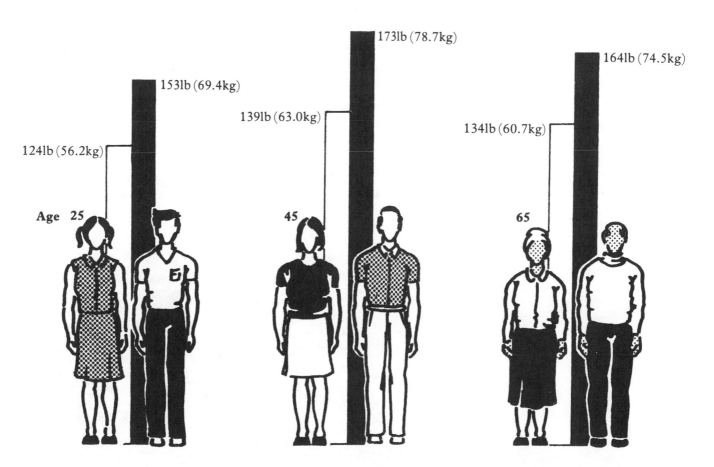

Age and weight
The diagram shows the effect of age on body weight. It compares the desirable weight at age 25 of a man and woman of average height and medium build, with their likely weights at ages 45 and 65. It is usual for persons of both sexes to put on weight steadily between the ages of 25 and 45 or 50, after which time weight progressively declines.

Increase in weight is usually due to an accumulation of fat, although this is sometimes masked by a lightening of the bones and wasting of the muscles. Thus although excess weight diminishes in the fifties and sixties, the thickness of the subcutaneous fat layer remains unaltered or even increases; weight loss is due to atrophy of lean tissue rather than to loss of fat.

Testing for overweight
Weighing yourself is not the only test for overweight. Try some of the methods described on p. 81.

© DIAGRAM

FLEXIBILITY

Flexibility refers to a joint's range of movement. It depends upon the tissues of the joint, and also upon the tendons and muscles that surround it (see page 32). Flexibility is not something that is lost only with age, as anyone who has had a knee in plaster will know! Unless a joint is stretched, the tissues soon lose their elasticity and become stiff. This stiffness can cause the joints to ache, as for example in backache, especially when, for some reason, they may be stretched beyond their normal limit.

Flexibility can be improved with either passive or active exercises. In passive exercises, the joints are flexed so that the muscles are stretched as far as possible and then held in this position for about one minute. Active exercises are bobbing or bouncing movements. Either type should be practiced four or five times a day for best effect, but take care, as some flexibility exercises are now being criticized as potentially damaging to the unfit. In most cases, any exercise activity, especially swimming, will produce enough flexibility, although some activities, for example weight training, require extra work. Make allowance for your body type and shape — the longer your legs, the harder you will find it to touch your toes! — and do not overdo things.

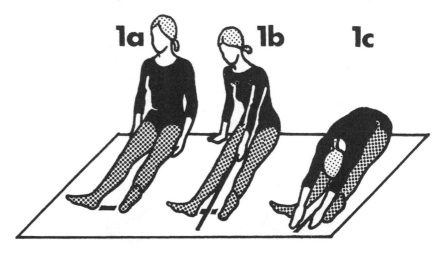

1 Test for lower back and back of thighs This test will allow you to measure your improvement.
1a After stretching exercises, sit on the floor with your legs straight out in front, heels about 5in (12·5cm) apart, touching a fixed piece of tape.
1b Place a yard or meter rule between your legs, with the 15in (38cm) mark at the near edge of the tape and with the lower measurements toward you.
1c Without jerking, reach as far forward as you can. Repeat 3 times and record your best score.

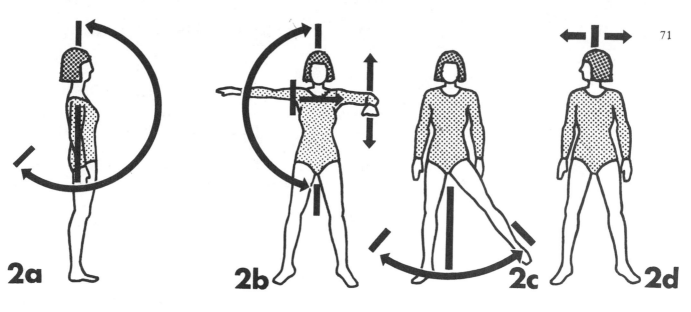

2a **2b** **2c** **2d**

2 Tests for shoulders, elbows, hips and neck

Compare your performance with the average.

2a Keeping your arm straight from the shoulder, it should reach 180° forward, and 45° backward.

2b With your arm held out straight to the side, it should move through 180° (straight up to straight down) and 40° across your front. If you bend your elbow with your arm out to the side, the forearm should point straight up and down without raising or lowering the upper arm.

2c Keeping your leg straight, it should go to 45° out to the side and 40° across your front.

2d Your head should rotate 90° to each side.

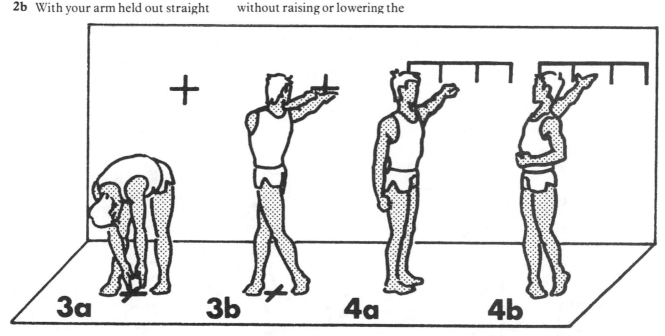

3a **3b** **4a** **4b**

3 Test for dynamic flexibility

This test measures dynamic flexibility — flexibility in repeated rapid movements. First mark a wall at shoulder height and then make a mark on the ground in front of it.

3a Stand with your back to the mark and your feet a shoulder-width apart at either side of the mark on the ground. Now bend down to touch the mark on the ground with both hands.

3b Straighten up and twist to the right to touch the mark on the wall. Touch the mark on the ground again, and then rise and twist to the left to touch the mark on the wall. Repeat as often as possible in 20 seconds.

4 Test for extent flexibility

This measures the range of movement in one action. First mark a horizontal 3ft (1m) scale at shoulder height on a wall, numbers reading left to right.

4a Left side facing the wall, stand an arm's length (fist clenched) away from it, in line with the 12in (30cm) mark.

4b Twist clockwise to touch the wall with your right hand, your arm extended, palm down and fingers stretched. Record furthest point held for 2 seconds. (If left-handed, reverse instructions.)

© DIAGRAM

MUSCULAR STRENGTH

Muscular strength is the amount of force that a muscle, or group of muscles, exerts during one contraction. It is closely related to muscular endurance (see page 74), but is measured in terms of "how much?" rather than "how many?" A weight lifter needs a great amount of strength, whereas a swimmer or gymnast needs greater muscular endurance.

A certain amount of strength is necessary for the performance of any sport or exercise, and strength development, as part of a training program, will improve results in almost any such activity. Strength is developed by the "overload" principle — using increasingly heavy resistances or weights in order to increase gradually the force (and usually the size) of the muscles involved. Exercises for increasing strength may be isotonic, isometric or isokinetic (see page 18); most effective in this respect being isotonic weight training (see page 234).

In general, the development of muscle strength is emphasized by high-resistance, low-repetition exercises, whereas muscular endurance is favored by lower-resistance, higher-repetition exercises — although, of course, any desired personal balance of strength and endurance can be achieved by a carefully planned individual program.

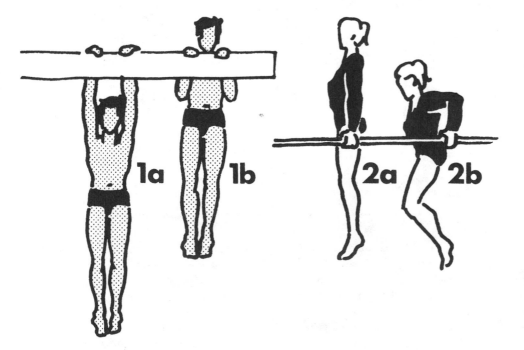

Strength tests using bars
These exercises test the strength of the whole body, not only your arms. For men, 5 repetitions of each is average, 10 good, 20 or more very good. Most women will do less well.

1a Using an overgrasp (backs of hands facing you), hang from a high bar, with your arms straight and your feet off the ground.

1b Pull yourself up so that your chin is level with the bar. Hold for a moment and then lower yourself again until your arms are straight. Repeat.

2a "Dips" use lower parallel bars (the backs of two sturdy, straight-backed chairs will do). Stand between the bars, holding one with each hand. Lift your feet off the ground and push up until your arms are straight.

2b Lower yourself until your elbows form right angles. Then straighten your arms to repeat.

Home strength test

These exercises test all the key muscle groups. Only a minimum level of fitness is needed to do them all. Failure indicates a serious weakness; regular repetitions will bring improvement.

1 Abdominal and psoas muscles

(The psoas muscles connect spine and thighs.)

1a Lie flat on your back, feet together, hands behind your head. Ask a friend to hold your feet down, or hook them under a bar.

1b Keeping your back relaxed, roll up into a sitting position.

2 Abdominal muscles

2a As in 1a, but with your knees bent and feet flat on the ground.

2b Keeping your hands behind your neck and without helping yourself with your arms, use your stomach muscles to roll up into a sitting position.

3 Psoas and lower abdomen

3a Lie as in 1a.

3b Keeping your feet together and legs straight, raise your heels 10in (25cm) off the ground and hold for 10 seconds.

4 Upper back muscles

4a Lie facedown with your hands behind your head and a pillow under your hips and abdomen. Ask a friend to hold your feet down.

4b Raise your head, chest and shoulders off the ground and hold for 10 seconds.

5 Lower back muscles

5a Lie as in 4a, but with your arms under your face and your friend holding your chest down.

5b Keeping your legs and feet straight, raise them from the ground and hold for 10 seconds.

6 Chest, shoulders, triceps

6a Lie facedown, legs straight, toes tucked under, hands (palms down, fingers forward) under your shoulders.

6b Keeping your body and legs straight, push your body up by straightening your elbows.

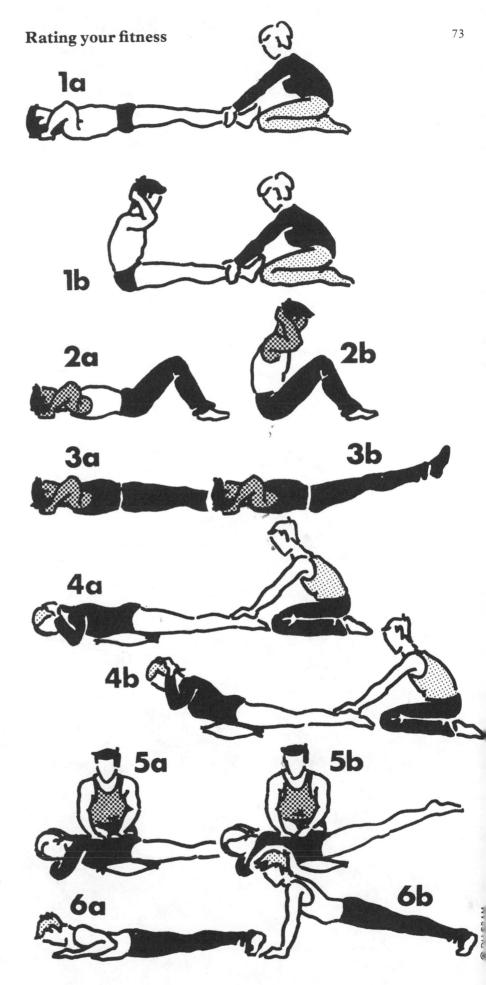

MUSCULAR ENDURANCE

Muscular endurance is the ability of a muscle, or group of muscles, to continue a certain activity over a period of time without muscular fatigue. As a measure of your ability to perform over a period of time it is also a measure of your work capacity. It is closely related to muscle strength (p. 72) and muscle power (the maximum force exerted in one explosive movement) and also to circulatory and respiratory (CR) fitness. Muscle groups of the same power and strength may have different degrees of endurance. There are two forms of muscular endurance: isometric and isotonic. Isometric endurance is the ability to sustain a static muscle contraction of maximum, or near maximum strength — as in the isometric exercises included in this book (pp. 226–233), and also in isokinetic "bullworker" exercises (p. 237). Isotonic endurance is a measure of a muscle's ability to continue to lift and lower a submaximal load through a full movement.

A certain amount of strength is necessary for endurance, but muscle-strengthening exercises, such as weight training, tend to harden the muscles, whereas endurance exercises, such as distance swimming, tend to relax them.

Muscle power
This is the maximum amount of force that a muscle, or group of muscles, can exert in one explosive movement. Good tests are overhand throwing, and jumping from a standing position.

1 Overhand throw Stand behind a mark and throw a softball as far as you can.
Men should achieve 180–200ft (55–61m); women 70–100ft (21–30m).

2 Standing broad jump Stand behind a line, with your feet comfortably apart. Swinging your arms for momentum, jump forward to land with both feet together. Measure from the starting line to the part of your foot nearest to it on landing.
Men should be able to jump 7–8ft (2.1–2.4m); women 5–6ft (1.5–1.8m).

Rating your fitness

Muscle endurance

This is the ability of a muscle, or group of muscles, to continue performing a particular action. It can be tested with sit-ups, squat thrusts and push-ups.

3 Sit-ups This exercise tests a major group of muscles which, though often neglected, are extremely important.

3a Lie flat on your back, with your feet together, hands on top of your thighs, and fingers straight. Ask a friend to hold your ankles.

3b Use your stomach muscles to pull your upper body upward and then lean forward to touch your knees with your fingers. See how many times you can repeat the exercise, and look at the chart to assess your performance.

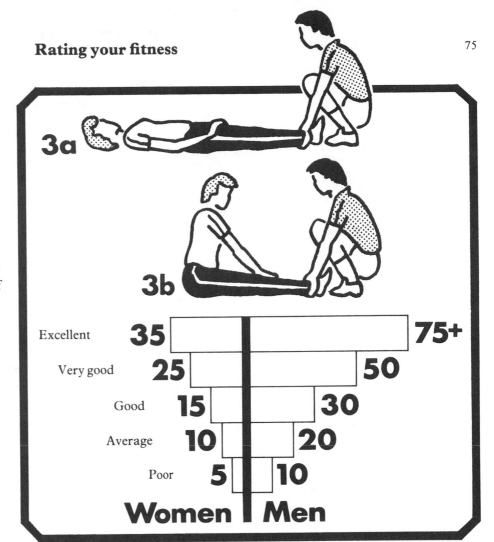

	Women	Men
Excellent	35	75+
Very good	25	50
Good	15	30
Average	10	20
Poor	5	10

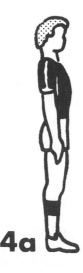
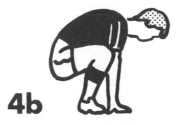
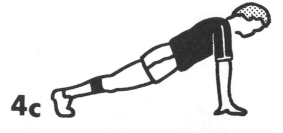
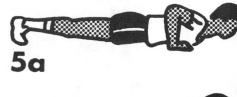
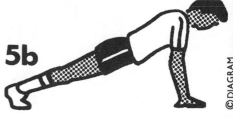

4 Squat thrusts These test the endurance of many muscle groups.
4a Stand up straight.
4b Bend your knees and lean forward to put your palms flat on the ground.
4c Supporting yourself on your straight arms, kick your legs back to adopt the position shown. Return to position 4b, then stand up straight. Can you do this 10 times without stopping?

5 Push-ups are another good test.
5a Lie facedown, legs straight and together, toes tucked under, hands (palms down and fingers forward) under your shoulders.
5b Keeping your body and legs straight, push up from the ground by straightening your elbows. Lower your body and repeat. For men 10 is good, 20 average, 30 very good; for women 3–5 is average, 10 good, 15 very good.

©DIAGRAM

CR FITNESS

Circulatory-respiratory (CR) endurance is the basis of work capacity. Muscles need oxygen to release energy from food (see page 44), and the major limiting factor upon their work capacity (as long as the muscles themselves are fit and strong) is the rate at which oxygen is received. This is affected by the size of the lungs, the speed with which the oxygen enters the blood, the speed with which the blood can carry oxygen to the muscles, and the speed with which the muscles can get rid of their waste products. CR fitness therefore depends upon the efficiency of the lungs and the cardio-vascular system. Strong and enduring muscles are obviously necessary for any activity that is going to cause maximum changes in the CR rate, but their role in this respect is secondary.

CR fitness is easily measured using the number of heart beats (the pulse rate) per minute. The more efficient your CR system, the less furiously it has to work during exercise, and the quicker it can return to normal afterward. All aerobic forms of exercise, such as running or swimming, and aerobic fitness programs, such as that devised in the USA by the President's Council on Physical Fitness (see page 320), concentrate on improving the fitness of the CR system.

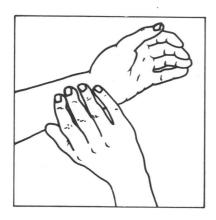

Taking your pulse
Taking your pulse after exertion is the best way of measuring CR fitness. To take your pulse, turn your left hand palm up and then place the first three fingers of your right hand on your left wrist, as shown. Count the number of beats for either 15 or 30 seconds, and then multiply by four or two respectively to find your rate per minute.

Tecumseh step test
Comparative CR fitness can be measured by means of the Tecumseh step test. This test is considered safe for persons aged 10–69 (unless in poor health). It involves stepping onto and off an 8in (20cm) bench for 3 minutes at a rate of 24 steps per minute.
a Stand facing the bench;
b put your left foot on it;
c bring your right foot alongside;
d step down with your left foot;
e step down with your right foot, and then repeat.
Wait exactly 1 minute after the exercise and take your pulse. Then use the table below to check your rating.

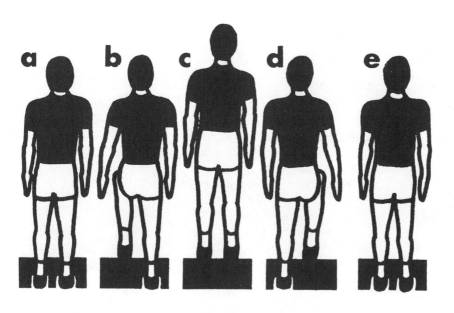

	Men	Women
Excellent	–68	–76
Good	68–79	76–85
About average	80–89	86–94
Below average	90–99	95–109
Very poor	100+	110+

CR fitness affects agility and speed. Agility is the speed with which you can change body position or direction. Speed is the rapidity with which a movement or movements can be performed. Both of them also depend upon strength and endurance. Step tests, like the Tecumseh step test described here, are an excellent means of testing CR fitness.
All-round fitness can be tested with a battery test — a series of exercises designed to test different aspects of fitness; probably most popular is the test devised by the American Association for Health, Physical Education and Recreation(AAHPER).

	Age	Time
Men	13–19	9 min 41 sec–10 min 48 sec
	20–29	10 min 46 sec–12 min 00 sec
	30–39	11 min 01 sec–12 min 30 sec
	40–49	11 min 31 sec–13 min 00 sec
	50–59	12 min 31 sec–14 min 30 sec
	60+	14 min 00 sec–16 min 15 sec
Women	13–19	12 min 30 sec–14 min 30 sec
	20–29	13 min 31 sec–15 min 54 sec
	30–39	14 min 31 sec–16 min 30 sec
	40–49	15 min 56 sec–17 min 30 sec
	50–59	16 min 31 sec–19 min 00 sec
	60+	17 min 31 sec–19 min 30 sec

AAHPER test
This excellent all-round test consists of pull-ups (**1**), sit-ups (**2**), shuttle run (**3**), standing broad jump (**4**), 50yd (45m) dash (**5**), softball throw (**6**) and 600yd (550m) run/walk (**7**).

The table below shows good (**a**) and moderate (**b**) fitness levels for men and women, based on 75% and 50% performance levels of college men and women.

1½ mile run/walk test
Given above are Kenneth Cooper's "good" fitness ratings for a 1½ mile (2.4km) run/walk — times in minutes and seconds for men and women of different ages. Do not attempt this test unless you have been participating in a CR fitness program for at least 3 months.

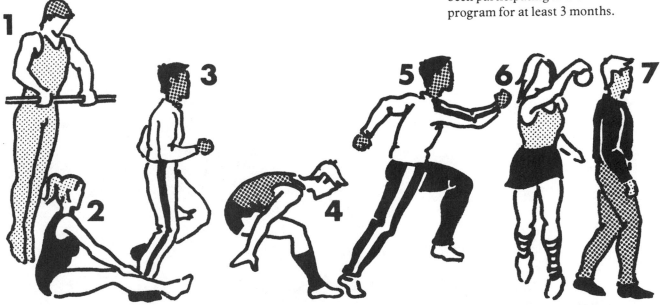

	1 Pull-ups*	**2** Sit-ups	**3** Shuttle run	**4** Standing broad jump	**5** 50yd dash	**6** Softball throw	**7** 600yd run/walk
Men (a)	8	61	9.4sec	7ft 8in	6.5sec	206ft (62.6m)	1min 44sec
Men (b)	6	47	9.7sec	7ft 3in	6.8sec	184ft (56.1m)	1min 52sec
Women (a)	28	27	11.0sec	5ft 10in	7.9sec	86ft (26.2m)	2min 41sec
Women (b)	20	20	11.6sec	5ft 4in	8.4sec	70ft (21.3m)	2min 58sec

*Modified for women

Chapter 4

EXERCISES FOR SPECIAL NEEDS

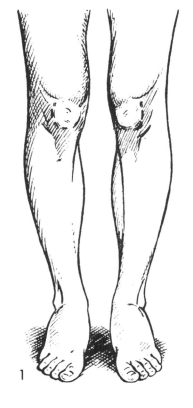

1

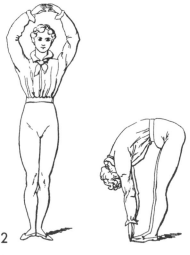

2

3

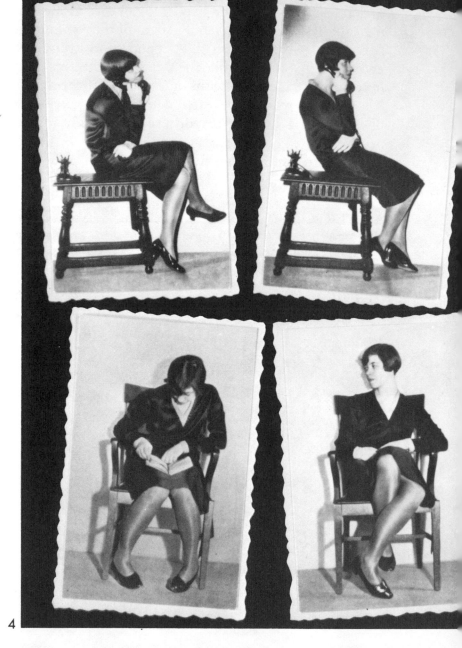

4

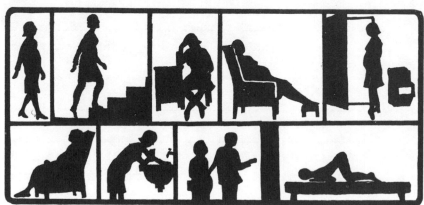

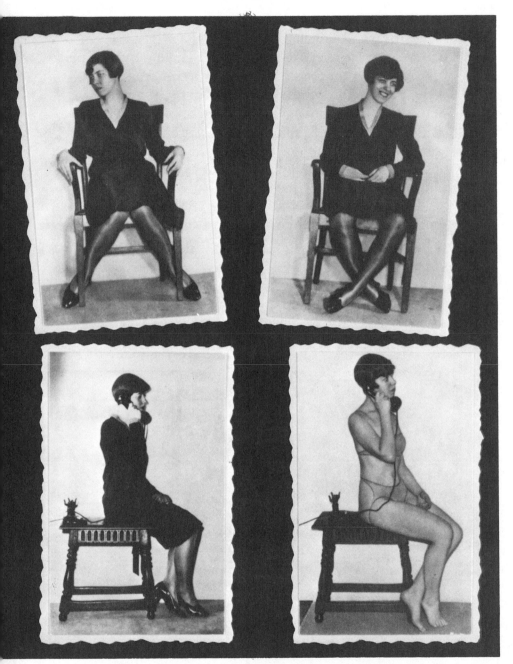

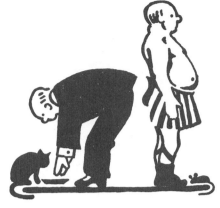

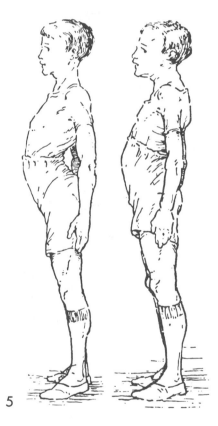

5

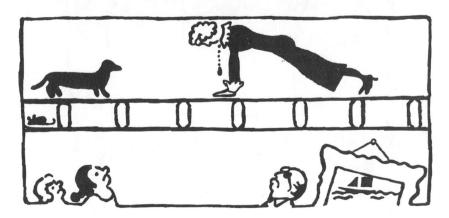

1 *Postural and Relaxation Training* by John H. C. Colson (Heinemann, London 1956)
2 *Walker's Manly Exercises* (London 1834)
3 *Home Gymnastics for the Well and the Sick* by E. Angerstein (USA 1889)
4 *Its Up To You* by Bess M. Mensendieck (USA 1931)
5 *Syllabus of Physical Education* (Board of Education, UK 1919)

REDUCING

Obesity Doctors define obesity as "excessive generalized depositing and storing of fat under the skin." It is not necessarily the same as overweight, which may only mean that you weigh more than the accepted average for your height and age. This may result from such things as unusually heavy bones or well-developed muscles.

Calories A Calorie is a unit of heat, producing energy. The amount of energy a food contains is measured by the number of Calories it holds. Any Calories you do not use through activity are stored in the body as fat.

Consequences of obesity
Bodily changes
A Double chin
B Flabby upper arms
C Drooping breasts in women
D Bulging stomach
E Fatty deposits on thighs
F Flat feet

Increased disease risks
1 Respiratory disease
2 Heart disease, high blood pressure, atherosclerosis
3 Cirrhosis of the liver
4 Diabetes
5 Kidney disease
6 Inflammation of the gall bladder
7 Hernias
8 Arthritis
9 Varicose veins
Obesity can also lead to conception and pregnancy problems, higher rates of mortality and shorter life expectancy.

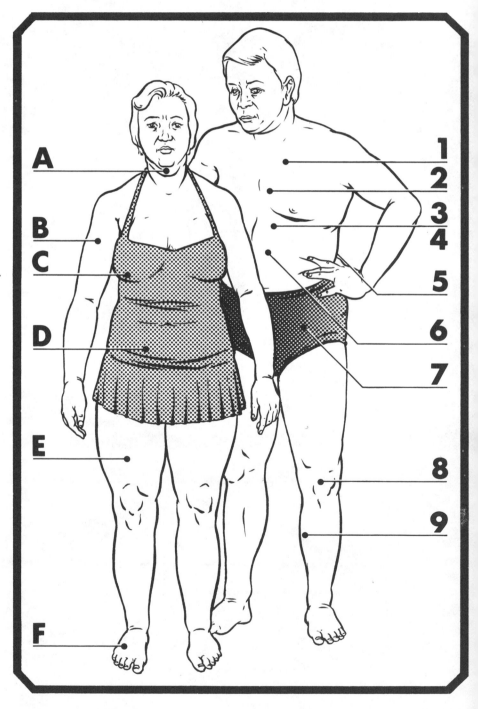

Testing for overweight
Overweight can be tested for in the following ways.
1 Look at your body profile in a mirror, and don't pull in your stomach. Do you have any bulges, and do you look much fatter than you used to?

2 Pinch your upper arm, thigh or midriff and see whether there is more than 1in (2.5cm) of flesh between your thumb and forefinger.
3 Measure yourself with a tape. Have your measurements increased appreciably?
4 Compare your weight with a

desirable weight table like that included here. When weighing yourself always use the same scales, weigh yourself at the same time of day, wear clothes of similar weight, and stand on the same place on the scales, with your weight evenly distributed.

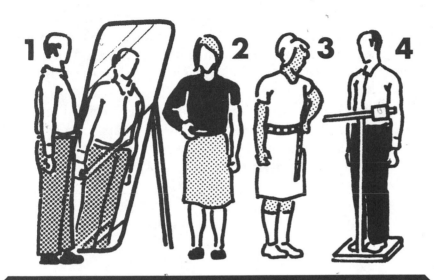

	Height		Weight					
			Small frame		Medium frame		Large frame	
	ft in	(cm)	lb	(kg)	lb	(kg)	(lb)	(kg)
Men	5 2	(157)	119	(53.9)	127	(57.6)	136	(61.7)
	5 3	(160)	122	(55.3)	130	(58.9)	140	(63.5)
	5 4	(162)	125	(56.7)	133	(60.3)	143	(64.9)
	5 5	(165)	128	(58.0)	136	(61.7)	147	(66.6)
	5 6	(167)	132	(59.9)	140	(63.5)	151	(68.5)
	5 7	(170)	136	(61.7)	145	(65.8)	156	(70.8)
	5 8	(172)	140	(63.5)	149	(67.6)	160	(72.6)
	5 9	(175)	145	(65.8)	153	(69.4)	164	(74.4)
	5 10	(177)	149	(67.6)	157	(71.2)	169	(76.7)
	5 11	(180)	153	(69.4)	162	(73.5)	174	(78.9)
	6 0	(183)	157	(71.2)	166	(75.3)	178	(80.7)
	6 1	(186)	161	(73.0)	171	(77.6)	183	(83.0)
	6 2	(188)	165	(74.9)	176	(79.8)	188	(85.2)
Women	4 10	(147)	100	(45.4)	107	(48.5)	117	(53.0)
	4 11	(149)	103	(46.7)	110	(49.9)	120	(54.4)
	5 0	(152)	106	(48.8)	113	(51.3)	123	(55.8)
	5 1	(154)	109	(49.4)	116	(52.6)	126	(57.1)
	5 2	(157)	112	(50.8)	120	(54.4)	130	(58.9)
	5 3	(160)	115	(52.1)	124	(56.2)	134	(60.8)
	5 4	(162)	119	(53.9)	128	(58.0)	138	(62.6)
	5 5	(165)	123	(56.0)	132	(59.9)	142	(64.4)
	5 6	(167)	127	(57.6)	136	(61.7)	146	(66.2)
	5 7	(170)	131	(59.4)	140	(63.5)	150	(68.0)
	5 8	(172)	135	(61.2)	144	(65.3)	154	(69.9)
	5 9	(175)	139	(63.1)	148	(67.1)	159	(72.1)
	5 10	(177)	143	(64.9)	152	(68.9)	164	(74.4)

Desirable weight table
Given here are desirable weights for men and women of different heights and body sizes at age 25. The table is based on statistics collected by US insurance companies. Older people can expect to exceed these weights, perhaps by 10–20lb (4.5–9kg), but should avoid gains beyond this. Weights given are without clothes; heights without shoes.

Reducing

Reducing Only if your energy input is less than your energy output will you get thinner. A Calorie-controlled diet enables you to see how much energy you are putting into your body. This should be compared with the amount of energy you expend in daily activities. But if you want to lose weight, do be sensible. Remember that the reason to reduce is to be healthier. Consult your doctor before embarking on any drastic diet, and never reduce your Calorie intake to below 800 per day.

In anorexia nervosa, a serious disorder mainly affecting adolescent women, the sufferer takes dieting to such extremes that severe emaciation and even death will result if the condition remains untreated. At the opposite extreme is compulsive eating. Here, the sufferer becomes psychologically addicted to food, perhaps using it to relieve feelings of depression, loneliness, frustration or boredom. Severe cases usually need medical help, although sometimes compulsive eaters can solve their own problem, for example by physical activity when the craving for food begins, by avoiding being alone, and by making sure that there are only low-Calorie snacks in the home.

Active reducing aids
These help you reduce by requiring you to perform some type of physical exercise. This exercise burns up extra Calories and so helps reduce surplus fat supplies. It also helps to tone up flabby muscles and to give your body a firm, trim shape. But remember that the only real way to reduce is to eat less; exercise is an aid to reducing, not a substitute for dieting.
1 Roller to trim your figure.
2 Trim cycle, used for pedaling movements while lying on the ground.
3 Rowing machine (see p. 197).
4 Bullworker (see p. 237).
5 Cycling machine (see p. 197).

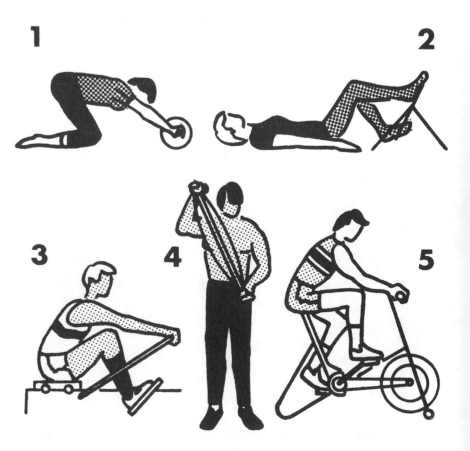

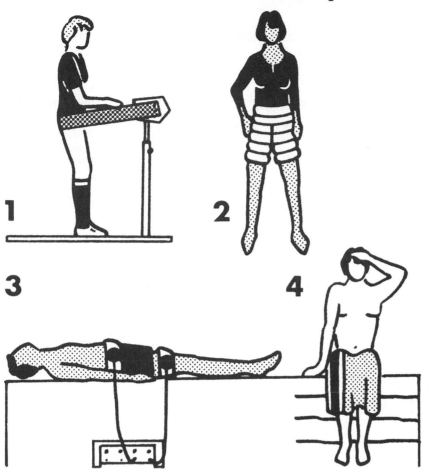

1

2

3

4

Passive reducing aids
A selection of passive reducing aids is now widely available, appealing largely to people vainly seeking an easy answer to their weight problems.
1 Vibrator belts do not burn up Calories and there is no evidence to show that they break down fat tissue, although their effect can be relaxing.
2 Reducing garments cause weight loss through loss of water in sweating, but drinking puts the weight back.
3 Artificial exercisers cause muscle contraction by electrical stimulation. If your muscles are particularly flabby they may improve muscle tone, but they do not cause weight loss or improve fitness.
4 Saunas and Turkish baths; like reducing garments, these cause only temporary weight loss through sweating.

Help with reducing In this book we concentrate mainly on figure control through simple home exercises. Some people may also seek outside help for their weight problems. Health or beauty farms will take over responsibility for a dieter's lack of self-discipline, but only at a price. At them your Calorie intake will be matched up with your output, and your body toned up with massage, saunas and exercises. You will lose some, but not usually a lot, of weight, and there will still be the problem of weight-watching after your stay. Reducing or weight-watching clubs are cheaper and will help you over a longer period. They also provide the encouragement and competition of fellow sufferers. Commercial reducing clinics, like health farms, are expensive and do little which, with the will to succeed, you couldn't do yourself. Even doctors can't usually do much if you won't help yourself. They will prescribe a diet, recommend exercise, perhaps prescribe some pills, but in most cases the treatment is up to you. A doctor's advice and treatment are, of course, essential when obesity has some underlying physical cause.

Reducing

EXERCISES

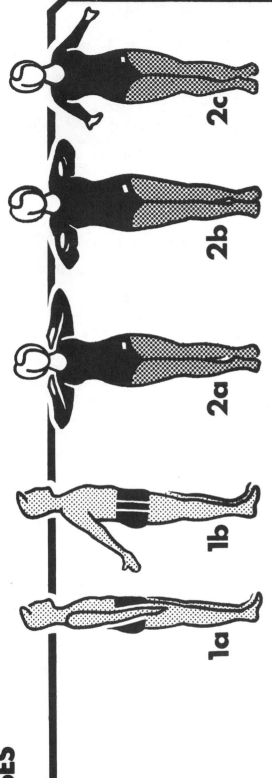

2c

2b

2a

1b

1a

Neck and shoulder exercises

1a Stand erect with your feet together, stomach well in and your arms at your sides.

1b Swing your arms back and twist them so that the palms face out and the thumbs point directly behind you. Return to starting position. Repeat 10 or more times.

2a Stand erect with your feet together, your stomach well in, your hands under your chin, and your elbows at shoulder level.

2b Keeping your arms horizontal and your elbows bent, draw your elbows back as far as you can behind your shoulders. Return to your starting position.

2c Stretch your arms straight back as far as they will go, turning the palms outward. Return to starting position. Repeat 8–10 times, alternating instructions 2b and 2c.

3a Sit with your back straight, your shoulders relaxed, hands on your lap, and your head erect.

3b Lower your chin to your chest.

3c Raise your head and then, opening your mouth, let your head fall back to touch your shoulders. Keeping your head back, close and open your mouth twice. Return to starting position. Repeat 4–8 times.

4a,b Start as in 3a. Keeping your chin parallel to the ground, turn your head slowly from side to side to look over each shoulder.

5a Sit as in 3a but with your head down.

5b Keeping your shoulders still, raise your chin over your right shoulder and then roll your head back as far as you can.

5c Bring your chin back over your left shoulder to return to the starting position. Repeat several times in alternate directions.

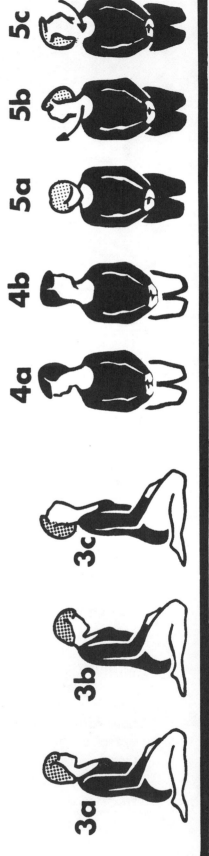

3a　**3b**　**3c**

4a　**4b**

5a　**5b**　**5c**

EXERCISES

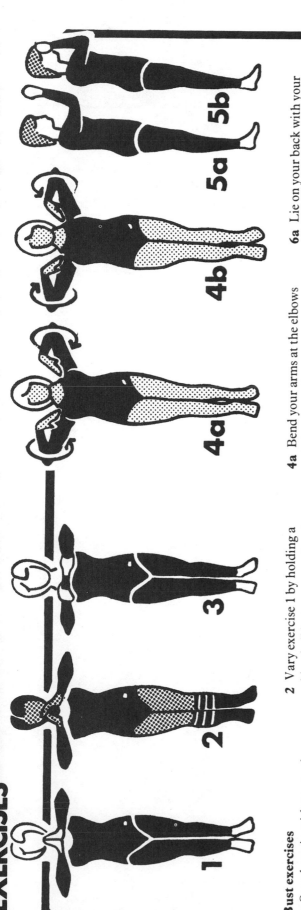

Bust exercises

1 Stand, or sit, with your palms together, fingers pointing up, hands about 8in (20cm) in front of your chest, and elbows level with your shoulders. Breathe in. Then, breathing out slowly, press your hands together for a few seconds. Then lower your arms and relax before a further 3 repetitions.

2 Vary exercise 1 by holding a rubber ball between your hands.

3 Fold your arms a few inches in front of you, gripping the inside of your left arm just above the wrist with your right hand, and gripping your right arm in the same way with your left hand. Keeping your elbows level with your shoulders, push your elbows sharply inward. Repeat 5 times.

4a Bend your arms at the elbows and place your fingertips on your shoulders. Rotate your elbows forward 5 times.

4b Rotate your elbows another 5 times backward.

5a Stand with your elbows forward, on a level with your shoulders, and your forearms raised.

5b Pull your hands slowly toward you, pretending you are holding a bar. Repeat 5 times.

6a Lie on your back with your knees slightly bent, your arms stretched out to the sides, and a book in each hand.

6b Keeping your arms straight, slowly raise your hands to bring the books together. Then slowly lower them again. Repeat up to 20 times.

7a Lie facedown on the floor, with your hands under your shoulders and your fingers pointing inward.

7b Raise your upper body but not your pelvis from the ground. Then lower it again. Repeat 5 times.

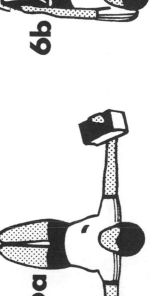
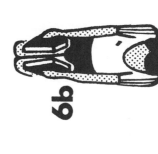
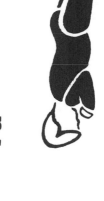
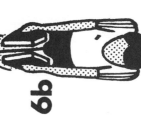
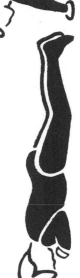

©DIAGRAM

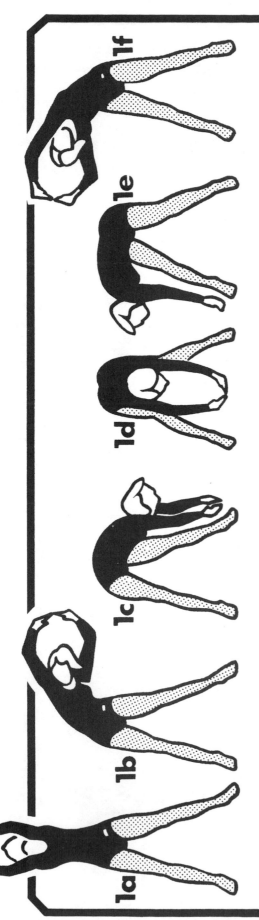

1a

1b

1c

1d

1e

1f

Waist and stomach exercises

1a Stand with your feet well apart and your hands clasped above your head. Look up and stretch toward the ceiling.

1b Keeping your hands together, lean as far as possible to the left.

1c Without bending your knees, drop down to try and touch the floor by your left foot.

1d Touch the floor between your feet.

1e Touch the floor by your right foot.

1f Swing upward, leaning as far as possible to the right. Repeat the whole exercise 3 times.

2a Lie on your back with your arms out at right angles, palms down. Raise both your knees toward your chest.

2b Keeping your knees and ankles together and your hands and shoulders pressed firmly to the floor, roll your knees over to touch the floor first on one side and then on the other. Repeat 15–30 times.

2a

2b

3a Stand with your feet apart and your arms by your sides.

3b Swivel on the balls of your feet and raise your left heel as you swing your arms up and round to face right from the waist. Repeat alternately to left and right, 6 times to each.

4a Stand with your feet apart and your arms stretched forward.

4b Swivel on the balls of your feet to swing round to the right, leading with your right arm and folding your left arm across your chest. Repeat 6 times alternately to left and right.

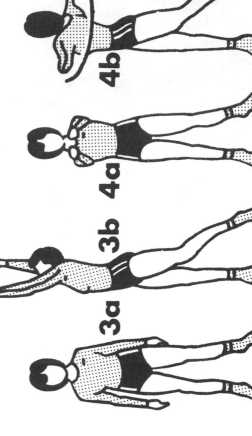

3a

3b

4a

4b

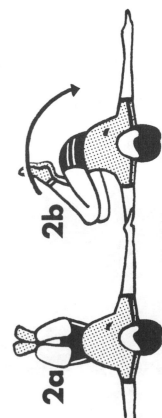

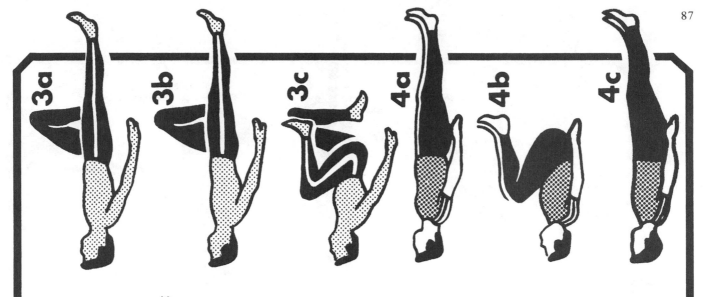

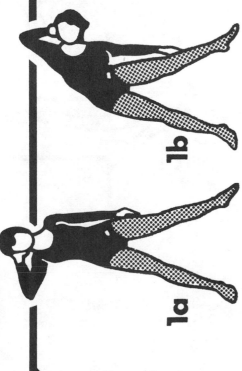

Waist and stomach exercises

1a Stand with your feet apart, your left arm at your side, and your right arm bent so that the palm of your right hand is against your right ear.

1b Push on your right ear and slide your left arm down your left leg to bend as far as you can. Straighten up and bend to the left. Reverse arm positions to repeat to the other side. Repeat the exercise 10 times alternately to right and left.

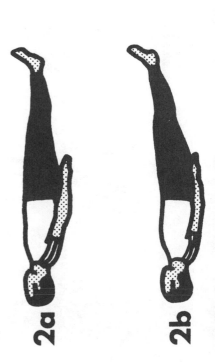

2a Lie flat on your back with your legs straight, feet together, arms by your sides, and palms down.

2b Keeping your legs straight and pressing your hands down on the floor, raise your feet a few inches off the ground. Hold this position and then slowly lower your feet back to the ground.

3a Lie flat on your back with your left leg bent, your right leg stretched straight forward, your arms lying loosely by your sides, and your palms up.

3b Keeping your right leg straight, raise your right foot a few inches off the ground.

3c Bend your right knee and bring it back toward your chest. Then straighten your leg out again and hold your right foot a few inches off the ground before lowering it. Repeat with alternate legs, 6 times each.

4a Lie flat on your back with your palms facedown under your buttocks.

4b Bend both knees and draw them back toward your chest.

4c Swing your legs back toward the ground, straightening your knees. When your feet are a few inches off the ground, hold this position for a moment before lowering your feet completely. Repeat with alternate legs, 5 or more times each.

EXERCISES

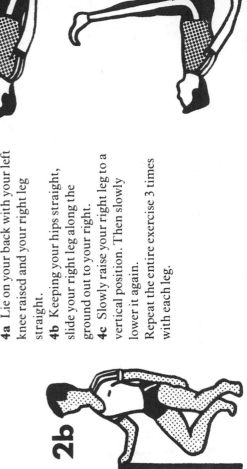

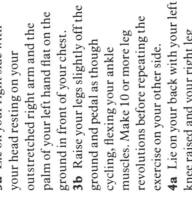

Leg exercises

1a With your right hand out to the side to hold onto a table or chair back for support, stand up straight, with your feet together.
1b Swing your right leg up to the right, keeping your leg straight and with your foot at right angles to your leg.
1c Swing your right leg to the left across in front of your left leg. Continue swinging your right leg from side to side up to about 20 times. Then repeat the exercise with your other leg.

2a With one hand resting on a table or chair for support, stand up straight with your heels together and your toes turned out. Rise onto your toes.
2b Squat down, keeping your back straight and staying on your toes. Stand up again. Then lower your heels. Repeat 10–20 times.

3a Lie on your right side with your head resting on your outstretched right arm and the palm of your left hand flat on the ground in front of your chest.
3b Raise your legs slightly off the ground and pedal as though cycling, flexing your ankle muscles. Make 10 or more leg revolutions before repeating the exercise on your other side.
4a Lie on your back with your left knee raised and your right leg straight.
4b Keeping your hips straight, slide your right leg along the ground out to your right.
4c Slowly raise your right leg to a vertical position. Then slowly lower it again.
Repeat the entire exercise 3 times with each leg.

EXERCISES

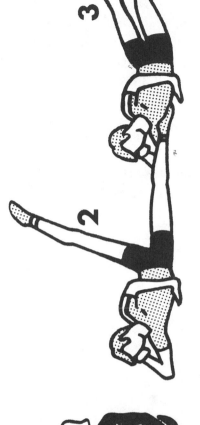

3

2

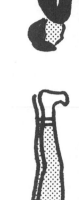

5b

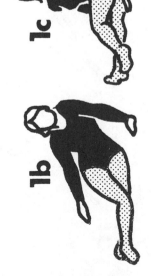

1c

1b

1a

Hip exercises

1a Sit on the ground with your legs straight out in front of you, your right ankle crossed over your left ankle, and your hands by your sides.

1b With your left hand on the ground, roll over on your hips until your right knee touches the ground to your left.

1c Push off with your left hand and roll over to the right, putting

your right hand down and continuing to roll until your right knee touches the ground to your right. Then push off with your right hand and roll back to the left. After 10 repetitions, cross your left ankle over your right ankle and repeat the exercise to touch the ground with your left knee.

2 Lie on your right side with your head raised on your right hand and your left hand on the ground for support. Keeping your left leg straight raise it as high as you can. Lower it and repeat 10 times. Then change sides and raise the other leg.

3 Vary the previous exercise by raising both legs at once.

4a Sit on your left hip bone, with your legs tucked back to the right and your arms stretched out in front of you.

4b Keeping your back straight and your arms in front of you, rise to a kneeling position.

4c Lower yourself onto your right hip bone, with your legs back to the left. Repeat 5 or more times from side to side.

5a Lie on your front with your chin on the floor, your arms at your sides, your legs straight and your toes under.

5b Pushing down with your left hip bone and tightening your buttocks, raise your right leg without bending your knee. Lower your leg again. Repeat 8–10 times with your right leg before repeating with your left leg.

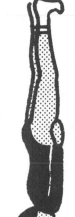

5a

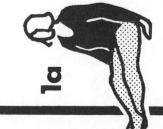

4c

4b

4a

©DIAGRAM

POSTURE

Posture refers to the relative positions of the different parts of the body. Good postures are those that combine the minimum amount of effort to balance the body steadily, with the minimum amount of strain to joints and muscles, so giving maximum efficiency. Bad posture, and the wrong movements that it causes, can damage the joints and muscles and slow or even prevent recovery from injuries, especially in the back. Correct posture also helps to reduce accidents by ensuring greater precision and control of movements.

Variations of posture
Cultural differences can determine the range of postures we are likely to adopt. To sit on the legs for long periods of time, like the Japanese woman (**A**), would be uncomfortable for many Westerners. The Sudanese (**B**), by contrast, is depicted standing on one leg, which would be very unusual and inconvenient for someone from North America or Europe with dirty shoes and high prices for cleaning clothes.

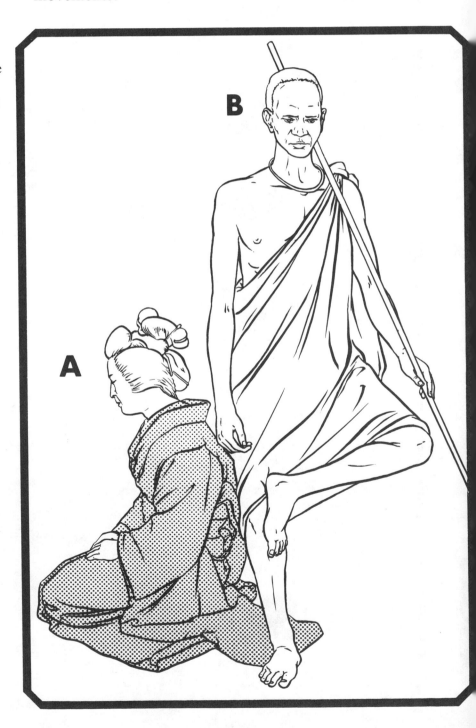

Postural habits and changes of posture are usually unconscious reflexes. To improve your posture, an awareness of how your body is held and used should be developed to avoid unnecessary and dangerous strain. Posture is also an expression of your attitude toward yourself and just as varying moods, such as fear, depression or fatigue, affect posture, so a change in postural habits can affect your outlook and personality — try smiling the next time you're angry, and remember the effect of "pulling yourself together." A person who moves awkwardly wastes an enormous amount of energy, while someone whose body operates harmoniously will have plenty of energy left for leisure activities.

The ability to maintain good posture is dependent, primarily, upon good health — bodily awareness, muscle tone, the suppleness of joints — and environmental conditions. The way a child is handled, and then taught to walk and perform other actions, also affects the postures it uses in later life. It is, therefore, a person's cultural background that decides which postures he uses. Some postures are common to all people, such as standing upright with the arms hanging behind, beside or in front of the body. But research shows that postures also affect and are affected by clothing, housing and other environmental factors. At least 25% of mankind squats at work or rest, which to Westerners may seem primitive or ugly. Chairs are status symbols in many societies; use of them for relaxing is a result of technological developments. (Many bowel problems, however, have have been associated with chairs and the toilet seat, and with the inability of Western man to "squat" properly!)

Occupations can also determine posture. Many coal miners squat easily because they work in coal seams with low ceilings. The "cowboy" squat, with one knee on the ground and the other knee up, results from a lack of seats. In the East it is common to sit cross-legged on the floor for the same reason.

Males and females adopt different postures because of anatomical differences and different social roles. Sitting on the floor with the legs straight ahead and crossed at the ankles, or with the legs folded out to the side, is a primarily feminine posture, as is sitting on the legs and heels. The "cowboy" squat, by contrast, is usually a male position.

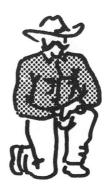

The "cowboy" squat
This semi-kneeling position adopted by African tribesmen, Australian Aborigines, American Indians and crapshooters is known also to have been common in ancient Greece.

Posture

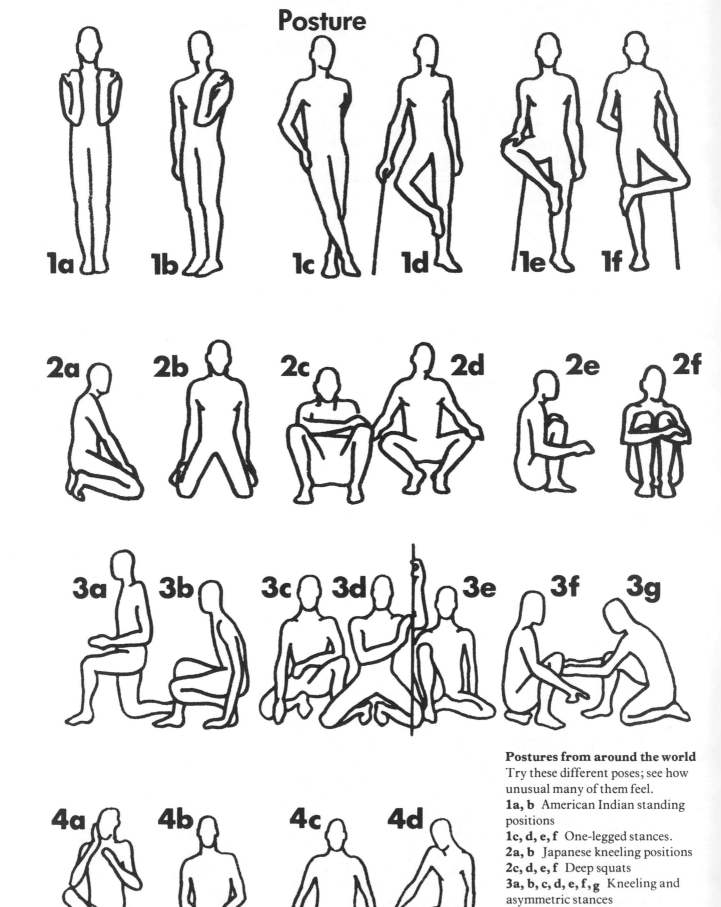

Postures from around the world
Try these different poses; see how unusual many of them feel.
1a, b American Indian standing positions
1c, d, e, f One-legged stances.
2a, b Japanese kneeling positions
2c, d, e, f Deep squats
3a, b, c, d, e, f, g Kneeling and asymmetric stances
4a, b, c, d Cross-legged positions of Asia and America.

Checking your posture Stand sideways in front of a full-length mirror and check your "gravity line" (see below). Feel your head pulled upward and slightly forward. See that your shoulders are relaxed and back; arms hanging loosely with your hands slightly to the front of your thighs. Keep your chest well out; your back straight but not stiff or tense. Hold your hips at the same even level, keeping your buttocks relaxed. Knees should be slightly bent and loose; feet balancing your weight on the balls and outer edges.

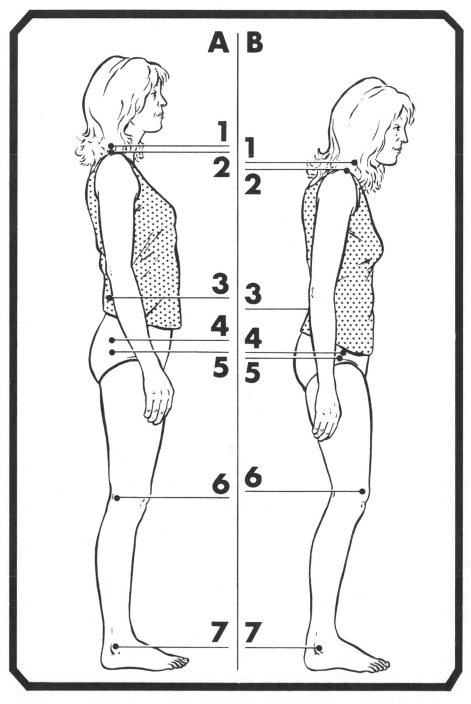

Posture and the gravity line
Illustrated is a person standing with good posture (**A**) and bad posture (**B**). In good posture, the body's centers of gravity are in line with each other; in bad posture they are out of alignment. To stand well, see that all the following points are aligned.
1 Neck
2 Shoulders
3 Lower back
4 Pelvis (the body's main center of gravity)
5 Hip joints
6 Knee joints
7 Ankle joints

©DIAGRAM

Posture

Good posture Balance is the key to good posture. The upright body's center of gravity is in the pelvis, at the second sacral vertebra. To remain upright the center of gravity must be positioned vertically over its base. There are several main sections to the body, each with its own center of gravity (see page 93). A pile of bricks is most stable when the center of gravity of each brick is directly in line with that of the others. So the body is most stable and resilient when the center of gravity of each of its parts is in line with the vertical plane of the body's center of gravity. In this position the groups of muscles around each joint are balanced, each exerting an equal force that is the minimum necessary for maintaining the upright position. The same is true for the upper body when sitting with the legs inactive. The action of the muscles also keeps a joint poised, preventing gravity from squashing it and straining and damaging its inner structure. In good posture, therefore, the force of gravity literally pulls you together. Whatever the circumstances, always try to arrange your posture so that all unsupported parts are balanced.

Bad posture is often the result of a sedentary life, unnatural immediate environment and lack of exercise. These cause poor control and laziness which, in turn, lead to bad posture. In bad posture the weight of each body section falls either in front or behind the body's main center of gravity. The force of gravity then pulls each section down in a separate direction, causing the body to fold — the body is in a state of disequilibrium. The weight of each body section must, therefore, be supported by an unbalanced set of muscles and by the joint tissues. Primarily this causes muscle strain, which results in aching, tense muscles and, ultimately, in muscle spasm. If the neck is out of line, the head is pulled forward, and the trapezius and deep neck muscles must work to keep it upright. This causes aches and tension in the neck and upper back, leading to pain and headaches. If the upper body is out of line, the erector spinae and muscles around the vertebrae must contract, causing backache. They can also pull the vertebrae out of position because of the unequal pressures applied. Bad posture means joints are not protected by the muscles, so they are easily damaged by shocks and strains. Recovery from injuries is also delayed because stress falls directly on damaged tissues.

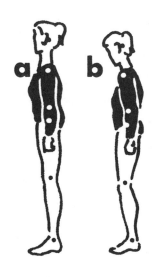

Good and bad posture
The diagram shows how in good posture (**a**) all the body's centers of gravity (shown here as dots) are in alignment. In bad posture (**b**) they are out of alignment, causing muscle strain to keep the body in this unnatural position against the force of gravity.

Application of good posture
Remember your body's centers of gravity and always try to keep your body in balance.

1 When carrying, try to balance loads by using your two hands.

2 When picking up an object from the floor, bend your knees and crouch down so that your back stays nearly upright.

3 The same applies when pulling out a low drawer or putting food in the oven.

4 When sitting, make sure that your pelvis touches the back of the chair and that your spinal curve is maintained but not exaggerated.

5 When kneeling to wash the floor, raise your buttocks so that shoulders and hips support your spine.

Causes and effects of different types of bad posture

a Seat too high, causing strain in the back and neck.

b Seat too far away, straining the arms and back.

c Chair too curved, straining the upper back and neck.

d Slouching posture puts strain on unprotected joints.

e Heels too high, straining backs of legs, buttocks and lower back.

Relieving aches and pains
If you have aches or pains from temporary, unavoidable bad posture, rotate the neck, shoulders, trunk or appropriate joint. This will relax the muscles and ease the joints. If possible, perform some of the exercises described in the following pages.

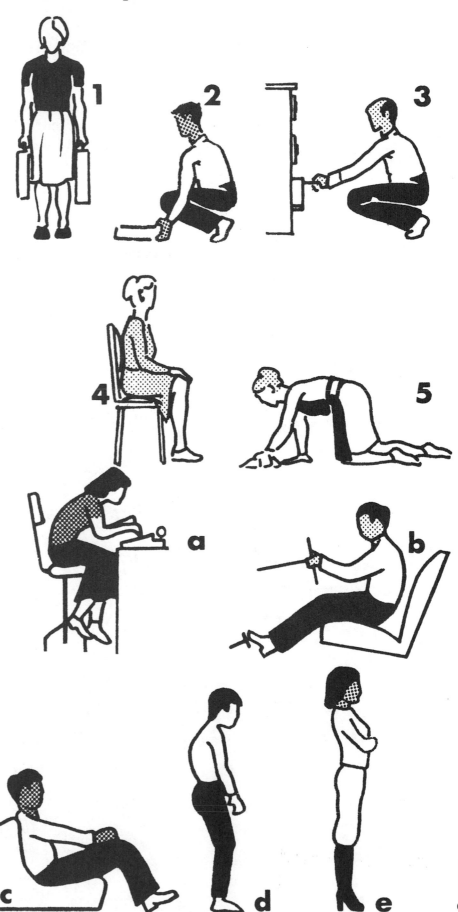

©DIAGRAM

Posture

The Alexander principle
Various theories have proposed the spine as the center of most other physical and mental complaints. The best known of these is the Alexander principle, formulated and developed by Frederick Matthias Alexander, a Tasmanian who spent his working life studying the relationship between the ways we use our bodies and their efficient functioning.

Alexander decided that every individual has the freedom to choose his own posture, and his studies showed that

Posture and the skeleton
The correct symmetry of the body (**A**) is compared here with the distorting effects of bad posture on the entire skeleton (**B**).

Vertebral distortion
Shown here are the ideal position of the neck vertebrae (**a**), and the effects of craning forward (**b**) and overstraightening (**c**).

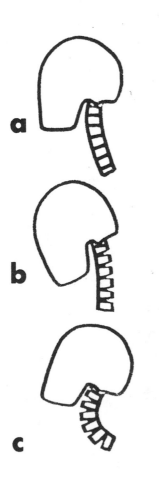

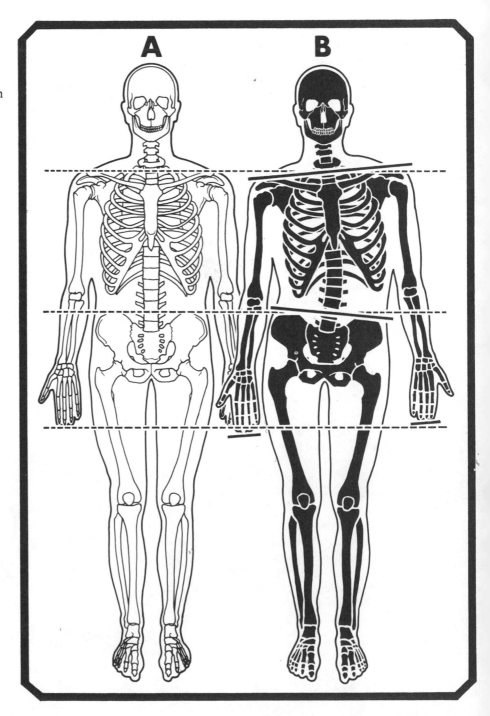

although young children exhibit good posture, most people soon opt for an "easy" slumping pose that requires little effort to maintain. Unfortunately, in most cases this involves severe distortion of the neck vertebrae, either forward, backward or sideways, which leads in turn to related distortion throughout the body. Very quickly the "easy" position becomes the norm. Bone and muscle distortion aggravate one another, and contribute to respiratory and circulatory troubles, pain, inflammation, hypertension, etc. For full mental and physical health, the patient must be reeducated to use his bones and muscles correctly, so that they are well balanced, in movement and in rest, around his spinal cord.

The individual must learn to "inhibit" all adverse muscular reactions to tension, stress or his physical environment. He must then consciously impose a beneficial pattern of use and movement onto his distorted bones and muscles in order to reeducate them. Because all bad posture stems from misuse of the spine, the patient must learn to align his vertebrae correctly until eventually the spine is loosened and fully straightened. The shoulders should be brought outward and forward, and the stomach tucked in; the pelvic girdle should be tipped upward and forward slightly. If the knees are slightly bent, all this will be much easier, and eventually correct posture will become the comfortable norm. The individual must learn to be continually aware of the way in which he is using his body, and he will then be able to maintain a high standard of fitness and health.

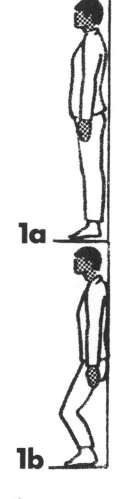

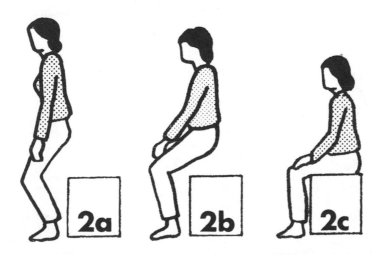

Standing correctly
To correct faulty posture, stand against a wall (**1a**); bend the knees slightly, tip up the pelvis, drop the head and widen the shoulders (**1b**).

Sitting down correctly
To sit down correctly, ensure that the neck and spine are in a straight line (**2a**); bend at the hips and knees (**2b**); and sit without slumping (**2c**).

©DIAGRAM

EXERCISES

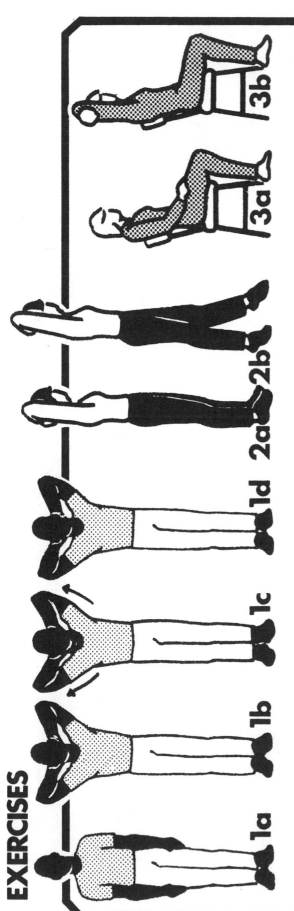

1a 1a
1b 1b
1c 1c
1d 1d
2a 2a
2b 2b
3a 3a
3b 3b

Posture improvement
These exercises will improve habitual bad posture. Remember to relax and use only those muscles necessary for each movement.
1a Stand with correct posture.
1b Clasp your hands behind your neck.
1c Pull your elbows up and back. Hold 3–5 seconds.
1d Relax, then repeat 3 times.

2a Stand with your hands clasped on the back of your head.
2b Rise onto your toes and then push one leg forward, keeping it straight. Count 5. Repeat with the other leg. Repeat 3 times.
3a Sit with correct posture.
3b Keeping your back straight, raise your arms behind your head and touch your elbows with the fingers of the other hand. Count 5. Repeat 3 times.

4a Sit with correct posture on a chair that does not obstruct your shoulders.
4b Clasp forearms behind the chair and pull your shoulders back. Hold 10 seconds. Relax.
5a Sit with correct posture.
5b Keeping your back straight, raise one knee, clasp it and then pull it to your chest without your foot touching the chair. Repeat 3 times for each leg.

6a Sit upright 3–4in (8–10cm) from the back of a chair, with a cushion on your knees.
6b Lift the cushion over your head.
6c Release the cushion and trap it against the back of the chair with your lower back.

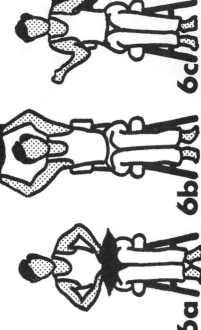

6a 6a
6b 6b
6c 6c

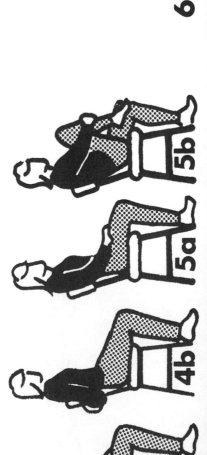

4a 4a
4b 4b
5a 5a
5b 5b

EXERCISES

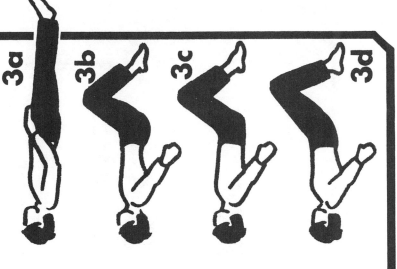

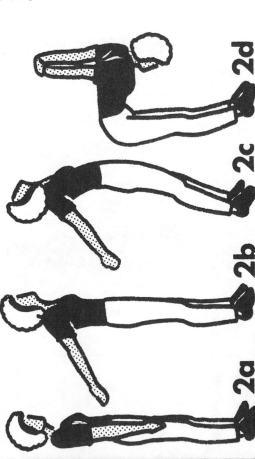

Posture improvement

1a Stand firmly, feet wide apart.
1b Raise your arms forward, keeping them straight.
1c Continue the movement upward and try to brush your ears with your shoulders.
1d Moving slowly and stretching, complete a backward circle with your arms. Repeat 5–10 times.

2a Stand with correct posture.
2b Move your arms out backward as far as you can without straining. Clasp your hands and straighten your arms.
2c Bend gently backward without strain. Count 5.
2d Bend as far forward as possible from the waist, holding your arms up over your back. Count 5.

Slowly straighten up and relax. Repeat 3 times.
3a Lie flat on the floor and relax.
3b Place your arms out to the sides, palms down. Raise your knees. Arch your back, keeping your buttocks on the floor.
3c Press your spine flat down on the floor.
3d Tighten your buttocks and raise them off the floor, keeping your arms and shoulders pressed down. Repeat 3 times.

EXERCISES

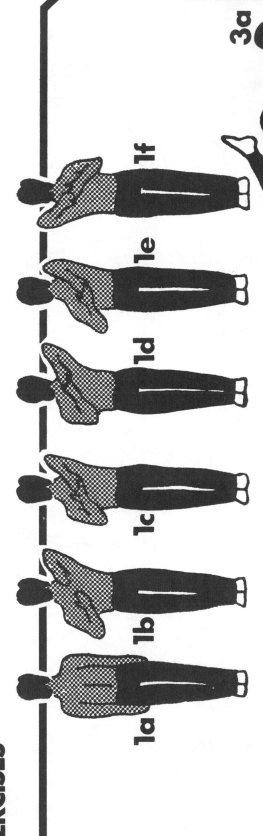

1a **1b** **1c** **1d** **1e** **1f**

Posture improvement
1a Stand with correct posture.
1b Put your hands behind your back, with one elbow up and the other down as illustrated.
1c Lock your fingers or, if you are unable to do this, hold a cloth between your hands.
1d Gently pull up with your higher arm. Count 5. Relax.
1e Gently pull down with your lower arm. Count 5. Relax.
1f Change arms and repeat. Repeat 3 times with your arms in each position.

2a Sit cross-legged on the floor.
2b Stretch your arms out straight behind your back and clasp your hands.
2c Twist your trunk to the right and try to touch your right knee with your head. Count 5. Straighten up slowly.
2d Repeat the twisting movement to the left. Repeat the whole exercise 3 times.

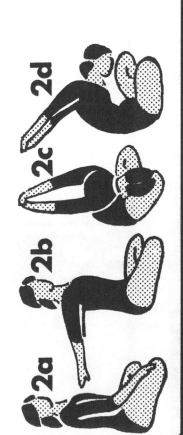

2a **2b** **2c** **2d**

3a Lie facedown on the floor, with your arms by your sides. Keeping your heels together, bend your knees.
3b Reach back and try to hold both feet with your hands.
3c Hold your head up and gently raise your trunk. Count 5.
3d Try to lift your knees off the floor. Repeat the exercise 3 times.
4a Lie flat on your back on the floor, with your hands on your chest. Relax.
4b Raise your head and heels slightly off the floor. Hold for 10 seconds. Repeat 5 times.

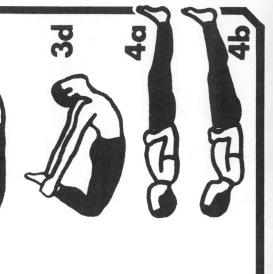

3a **3b** **3c** **3d** **4a** **4b**

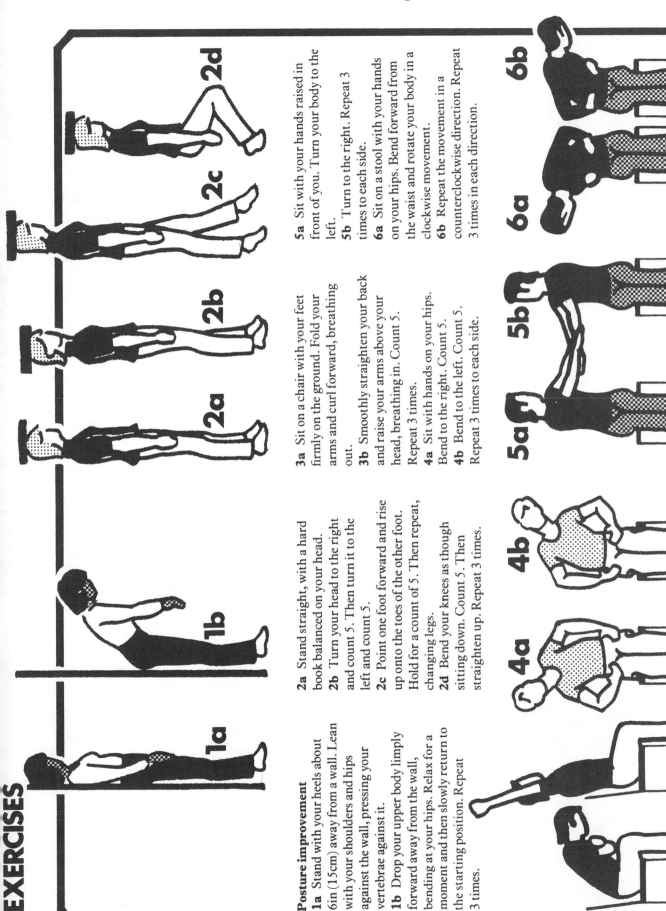

EXERCISES

Posture improvement

1a Stand with your heels about 6in (15cm) away from a wall. Lean with your shoulders and hips against the wall, pressing your vertebrae against it.

1b Drop your upper body limply forward away from the wall, bending at your hips. Relax for a moment and then slowly return to the starting position. Repeat 3 times.

2a Stand straight, with a hard book balanced on your head.

2b Turn your head to the right and count 5. Then turn it to the left and count 5.

2c Point one foot forward and rise up onto the toes of the other foot. Hold for a count of 5. Then repeat, changing legs.

2d Bend your knees as though sitting down. Count 5. Then straighten up. Repeat 3 times.

3a Sit on a chair with your feet firmly on the ground. Fold your arms and curl forward, breathing out.

3b Smoothly straighten your back and raise your arms above your head, breathing in. Count 5. Repeat 3 times.

4a Sit with hands on your hips. Bend to the right. Count 5.

4b Bend to the left. Count 5. Repeat 3 times to each side.

5a Sit with your hands raised in front of you. Turn your body to the left.

5b Turn to the right. Repeat 3 times to each side.

6a Sit on a stool with your hands on your hips. Bend forward from the waist and rotate your body in a clockwise movement.

6b Repeat the movement in a counterclockwise direction. Repeat 3 times in each direction.

©DIAGRAM

BACK PAIN

Virtually everyone suffers from some form of back pain at some time in their lives. The pain may be constant, or intermittent, or it may be caused by specific forms of activity such as climbing stairs or lifting things. It can be agonizing or just nagging, but it is there. This book does not seek to diagnose the cause of your particular pain, nor to prescribe a cure for it — that's a job for your doctor. It does, however, describe the sort of precautions you should take if you have a bad back, and demonstrates some of the helpful exercises you can do to alleviate the pain. Very often, all that is

Muscles and vertebrae
Identified on the diagram are major back muscles (**A**), and the different types of vertebrae that make up the spine (**B**). The number of vertebrae in each region is given in brackets.
A1 Trapezius
A2 Latissimus dorsi
A3 Gluteus maximus
B1 Cervical (7)
B2 Thoracic (12)
B3 Lumbar (5)
B4 Sacral (5)
B5 Coccygeal (4)

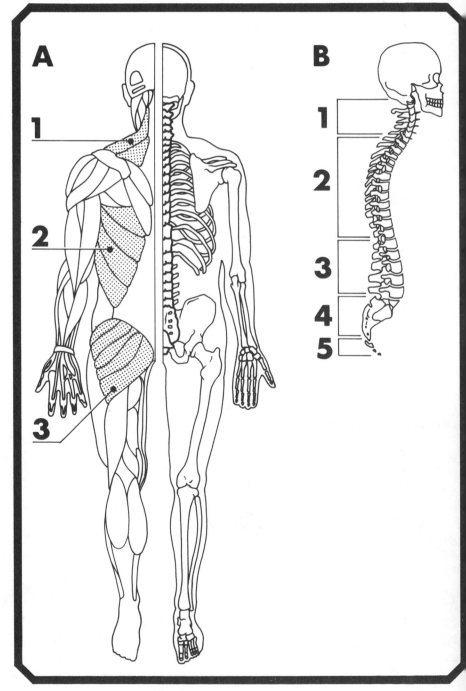

needed for low back pain is exercise of the right sort.
There are many possible causes of back pain. You may have
torn a muscle or ligament, or muscles may be tight when
they should be loose and vice versa. It could be that a bone
has slipped slightly out of place, or is misshapen or worn;
don't forget that the backbone is under constant strain. It
may be that you have curvature of the spine, or even an
infection, so if the pain is persistent it is wise to seek medical
advice.

The backbone, or spine, is made up of a column of bones
called vertebrae, which are held together by ligaments —
bands of tough, flexible tissue. Each vertebra has two bony
arches, with openings that lie directly over each other, and
through the tunnel or canal thus formed passes the spinal
cord. This runs from the brain downward and is one of the
key components of the central nervous system, for from it
come the nerves that control the body's muscles. A pair of
nerves branches off between every vertebra.

There are 33 vertebrae in the spine, and these are classified
into five groups: cervical, thoracic, lumbar, sacral and
coccygeal. The bones in the sacral and coccygeal sections
fuse together in adult life. Each spinal area gives its name to
the nerves that emerge from its own vertebrae. It is not
surprising that this comparatively delicate bony structure,
combined with the sensitive nervous system radiating from
it, should be a potential source of trouble, and it will be seen
that many of the exercises that follow are ostensibly to do
with the muscles and joints but in fact relate closely to the
back.

Some causes of backache are inherited, others are induced,
while others are simply disorders. Lordosis and scoliosis are
disorders that are sometimes inherited. In lordosis there is
an inward arching of the spine; in scoliosis the spine is out
of the straight to one side or the other (also see page 104).
Attention to posture and appropriate exercises will often
alleviate these conditions even in cases where they are
inherited. Induced causes include pregnancy, bad posture and
being overweight. Backache during pregnancy is not to be
wondered at because of the additional strain put on the back
muscles. Similarly, carrying heavy objects imposes burdens
on the back muscles. This, like posture, can be controlled by
the victim, and exercise is valuable in both cases. Backache
through faulty posture may arise from slouching while
sitting or standing, or sometimes from working in wrong
physical conditions — too high or too low a desk or
workbench, for example.

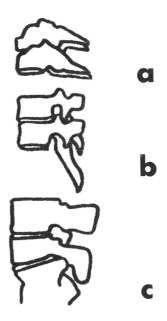

Types of vertebrae
Illustrated here are the
characteristic shapes of three types
of vertebra: cervical (**a**), thoracic
(**b**), and lumbar (**c**).

Back pain

The principal disorders that may cause back pain are "slipped disk," sciatica, lumbago, spondylitis, osteoarthritis and rheumatoid arthritis.

Slipped disk Between each of the 24 movable vertebrae is a ring of cartilage, or disk, and when one of them cracks and pushes out to press on a nerve it can cause acute pain — especially in the large nerve that runs down the back of each thigh, the sciatic nerve.

Sciatica This is the name usually given to inflammation of the sciatic nerve.

Lumbago One of the causes of this very painful affliction — a form of rheumatism — is a spasm of muscles in the lumbar region. This sudden pain, which may prevent the victim from standing up, often occurs after exercise out of doors or in a draft.

Spondylitis This is the inflammation of one or more of the vertebrae, and may result from injury or disease. It causes stiffness in the joints between the vertebrae (spondylosis) and actual deformation (kyphosis).

Osteoarthritis This condition may result from a thinning of the spinal disks, and the growth of small, bony protuberances which may press on the sciatic nerve.

Rheumatoid arthritis Affecting younger people than osteoarthritis and with a higher incidence among women than men, this disease results in a gradual deterioration in all joints, leading to permanent stiffness and debility. Some joints may be more seriously affected than others, and the back is usually one of the last regions to be affected.

Disorders and pain
Examples of disorders affecting the spine are scoliosis (**a**), where the spine is curved to one side or the other, and lordosis (**b**), an inward curvature of the spinal column in the lumbar region. Particular disorders produce pain in specific areas; illustrated here are the areas affected by cervical disk problems (**c**), lumbar disk problems (**d**), and sciatica (**e**).

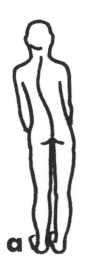
a

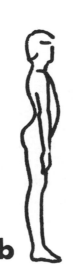
b

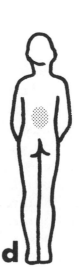
c

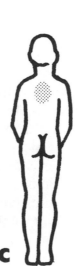
d

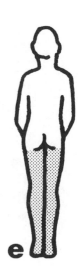
e

Coping with everyday life
You may find that following these hints helps to ease back pain.
1 A pillow under the shoulders will keep your spine curved when you are lying down relaxing.
2 When sitting in a chair, put a pillow behind your bottom and raise your feet on a stool to make yourself comfortable.
3 When sitting on the toilet, try to curve your spine and, if possible, raise your feet slightly.
4 Bending at the knees rather than the hips will take the strain off your back when you are lifting heavy objects.
5 If you have to carry a heavy load on one side, use the other arm to balance the weight.

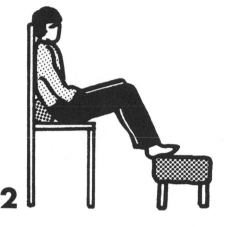

1

2

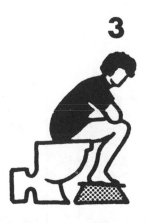

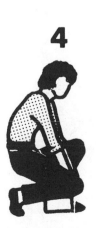

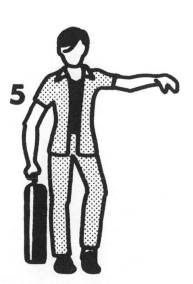

3

4

5

©DIAGRAM

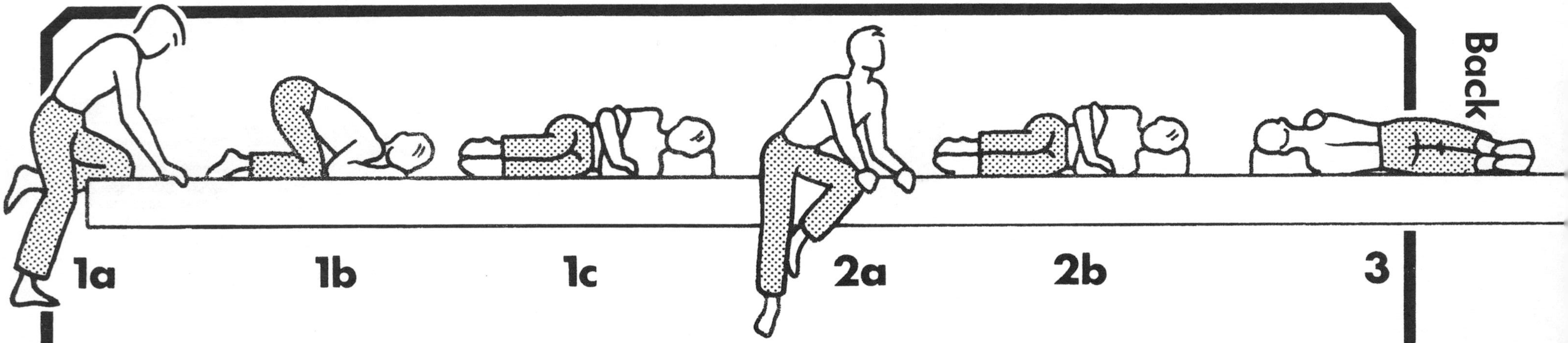

ADVICE

Back

Getting into bed

Sufferers from back pain know what agony the apparently simple action of getting into bed can bring; two comparatively painless methods are given here.

1a Face the bed. Lower your hands to support youself, at the same time lifting one knee onto the bed.

1b Bring the other knee up so you are kneeling on the bed.

1c Crawl forward and roll onto your favored side.

2a Sit gently on the bed, holding its side for support.

2b Bend your arms and then your knees to take the weight off your legs, and roll sideways onto the bed.

3 Recommended lying position
Always lie with your head sideways on the pillow, i.e. with your face pointing neither up nor down, and your head level with your spine.

Getting out of bed

With a bad back don't take chances with a sudden movement, particularly getting out of bed; two possible techniques are described below.

4a Slowly point your feet toward the end of the bed.

4b Gently ease one leg over the edge of the bed, knee first.

4c Lower the other leg to the floor.

4d Sit on the side of the bed and walk your hands up your thighs until you are standing.

5 Bring your knees to your chest, roll onto them, and then back off the bed one leg at a time. Straighten up slowly.

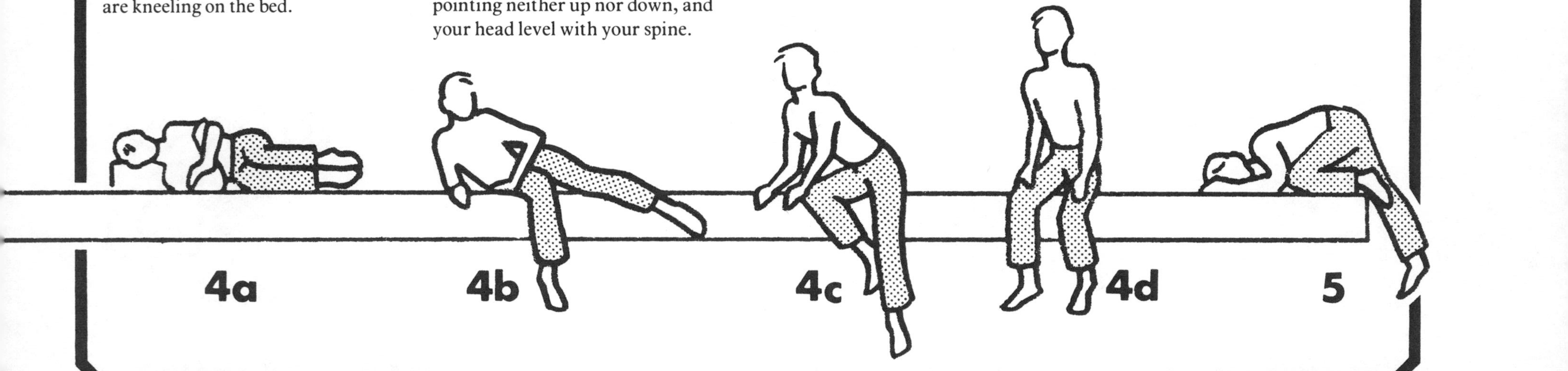

1a 1b 1c 2a 2b 3

4a 4b 4c 4d 5

ADVICE/EXERCISES

Lying comfortably

All back sufferers know the difficulty of getting comfortable in bed. Here are some suggestions for using pillows to make you more comfortable — keeping the head level with the spine, and the spine level with the bed.

1 Sleep on your side, using a pillow to keep your head level with your spine.

2 If you have thin legs and a wide pelvis you may find that pillows between your thighs and ankles are also helpful.

3 If you have wide shoulders and narrow hips, try pulling your shoulders forward or putting a thin pillow under your hips.

4 If you have narrow shoulders, a pillow under your shoulder and chest should help.

5 A pillow pulled in tightly against your stomach can ease back pains caused by sagging stomach muscles.

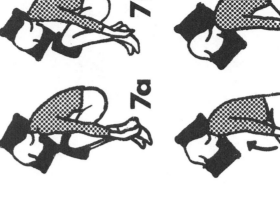

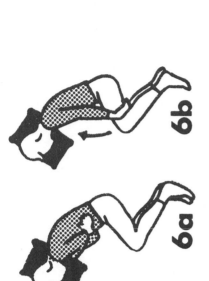

Simple back exercises

6a Lie in the fetal position, i.e. with your chin toward your chest, your knees bent slightly forward, and your arms folded over your chest.

6b With your hands under your knees, ease them gently toward your chest and hold them there.

7a From the fetal position, with your hands touching your feet, tuck your chin in gently toward your chest, inhaling as you do so.

7b Exhale as you relax.

8a From the fetal positon, tuck your chin in, as in 7a. With your hands behind your knees, ease them toward your chest, inhaling as you do so.

8b Exhale as you relax.

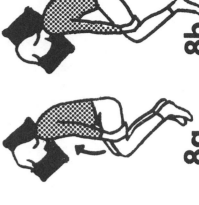

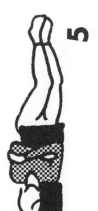

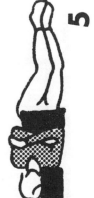

©DIAGRAM

Back pain

EXERCISES

Learning to tense your bottom
This will aid control over your posture in general.

1a Lie on your back with your knees slightly raised, your head and bottom supported by pillows. Inhale, and with pursed mouth exhale as you lower your back down onto the bed and tighten your stomach.

1b Inhale while relaxing and repeat several times.

2 Lie with only a shoulder pillow; turn your knees and feet outward and tighten your bottom muscles. Then tighten both stomach and bottom muscles and hold for as long as possible.

3a Start as in 2, with your toes facing forward. Keeping your hands on your thighs, tighten your bottom as much as possible.

3b Exhale, and your stomach muscles will also tighten; inhale as you relax, and repeat.

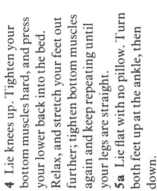

4 Lie knees up. Tighten your bottom muscles hard, and press your lower back into the bed. Relax, and stretch your feet out further; tighten bottom muscles again and keep repeating until your legs are straight.

5a Lie flat with no pillow. Turn both feet up at the ankle, then down.

5b Then turn one foot upward and one downward as if walking, and keep alternating.

6 Lie flat with your head on a pillow, your hands crossed on your stomach, and your knees bent. Roll your right knee out to the side as far as possible. Raise it, and repeat with alternate legs.

7 Lie on your back with your knees bent up to your chest. With your right hand, move your right knee in large circles, first clockwise and then counterclockwise. Repeat with the left hand and knee.

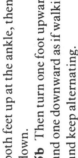
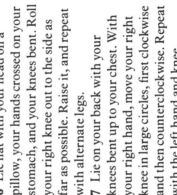
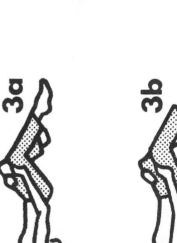
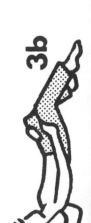
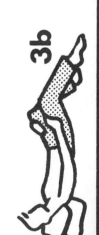

EXERCISES

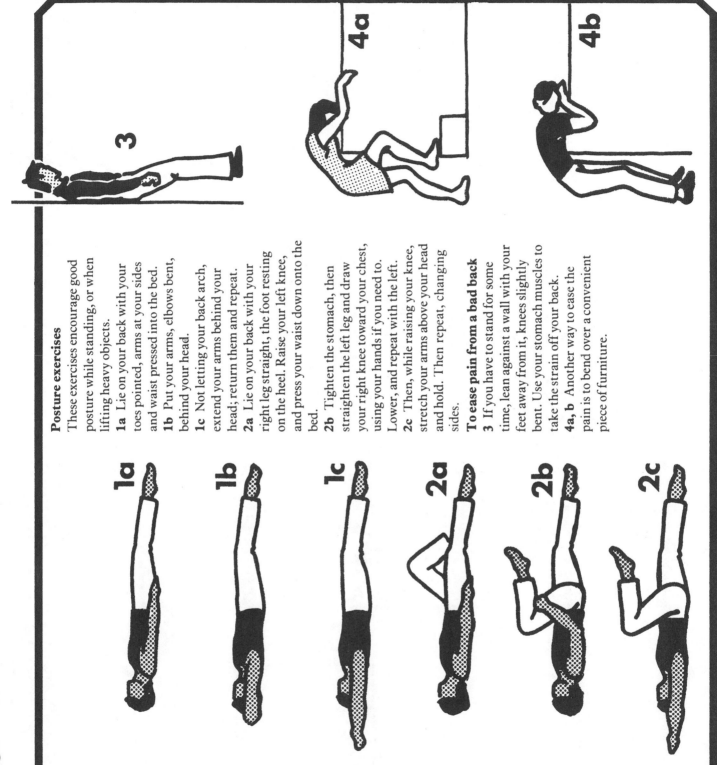

Posture exercises

These exercises encourage good posture while standing, or when lifting heavy objects.

1a Lie on your back with your toes pointed, arms at your sides and waist pressed into the bed.

1b Put your arms, elbows bent, behind your head.

1c Not letting your back arch, extend your arms behind your head; return them and repeat.

2a Lie on your back with your right leg straight, the foot resting on the heel. Raise your left knee, and press your waist down onto the bed.

2b Tighten the stomach, then straighten the left leg and draw your right knee toward your chest, using your hands if you need to. Lower, and repeat with the left.

2c Then, while raising your knee, stretch your arms above your head and hold. Then repeat, changing sides.

To ease pain from a bad back

3 If you have to stand for some time, lean against a wall with your feet away from it, knees slightly bent. Use your stomach muscles to take the strain off your back.

4a, b Another way to ease the pain is to bend over a convenient piece of furniture.

Back pain

EXERCISES

Stretching exercises

1 Rest your forearms on a heavy piece of furniture such as a bureau. Bend your knees and move your hips up and down, not from side to side. (Do this gently at first.)

2a This exercise is best done with that standard piece of home equipment — the kitchen sink. Stand facing the sink and grip the edge firmly. Lower your head and bend your knees slightly.

2b Push your bottom slowly backward and downward, breathing in as you do so. Then relax your back and return to your starting position, breathing out as you do so. Repeat 3–4 times.

3a Rest your hands on a piece of furniture and push your bottom out as in exercise 2.

3b Then, alternately straighten and hump your back, at the same time moving your hips up and down. Repeat as many times as you can.

4 This exercise requires an overhead bar, fixed so that you can grip it over your head, with your knees bent and your pelvis pushed back. Keeping your feet flat on the floor, slowly pull with your arms so that your weight hangs from your hands. This will gently ease the vertebrae apart. Repeat, this time pulling first one hip and then the other down and under. (Have a pillow on the floor beneath your knees in case your hands slip.)

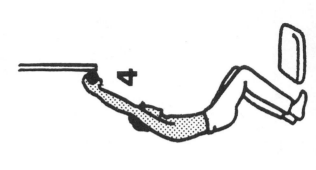

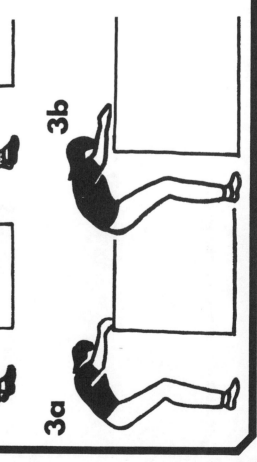

EXERCISES

Squatting exercises
Without easily working knees and strong thighs, back trouble is likely to occur. Squatting and related movements tone up and loosen the leg muscles.
1a Sit on a strong table with your legs hanging down, and allow them to swing freely from the knee, first one and then the other.
1b Lower the feet to the floor and repeat, swinging the legs from the knees.

2a Sit on a chair with your shoulder blades touching the back and your bottom well forward on the seat. Clasp both hands behind your right knee.
2b Draw your knee in as close to your chest as possible; repeat with the left. As your joints loosen, you will be able to draw your lower leg in toward your thigh.

3a Sit on pillows on a chair. Place one foot under the chair and one forward, with your legs slightly apart.
3b Without using your hands, slowly stand up, tightening your stomach muscles and pushing your bottom downward.

4 Hold onto a sink, with your knees and feet apart. Tighten your stomach muscles and push your bottom down and forward, bending the knees.

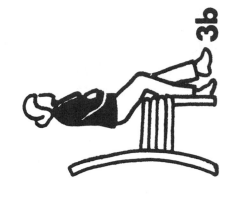
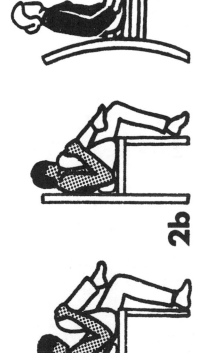
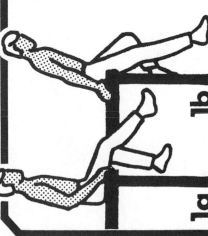
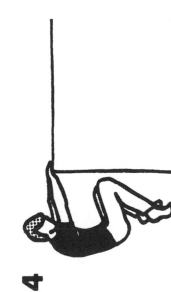

©DIAGRAM

Back pain

EXERCISES

5a Sit with your legs straight and your feet pressed against a wall.
5b Push forward repeatedly, trying to touch your toes.
6a Sit on the floor with your legs wide apart.
6b Bend forward with your arms outstretched, getting your body as close to the floor as possible.
7 Sitting with your legs wide apart, and your right arm behind your back, try to touch your right foot with your left hand. Repeat on the other side.

Exercises for scoliosis sufferers
The following exercises are intended for scoliosis sufferers. At first try the various exercises to each side, but then concentrate on strengthening the muscles on your weaker side, so helping to correct your spinal curve.
1a Kneel on the floor with your knees apart; bend from the hips, arms above your head, to rest your hands on the floor.
1b Press your chest as close to the floor as you can.
2 Start as in 1b, and then walk on your knees in a large circle, to the right and then to the left.
3a Kneel on the floor, and then bend forward to rest your head on folded arms on the floor.
3b Lift your left leg as high as possible. Repeat with the right.
4 Kneel with your thighs and arms at right angles to the floor. Simultaneously raise your left leg and right arm to form a straight line with your body. Hold, lower, and repeat with the right.

EXERCISES

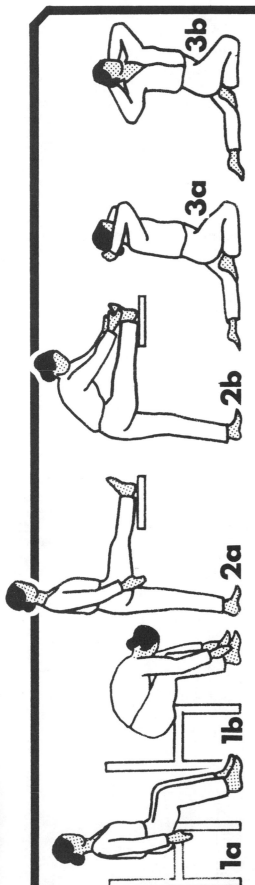

1a

1b

2a

2b

3a

3b

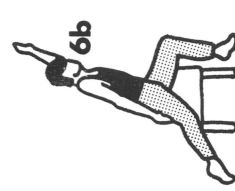

6b

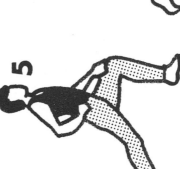

6a

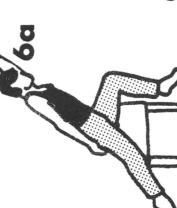

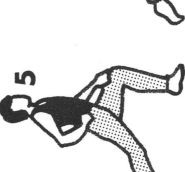

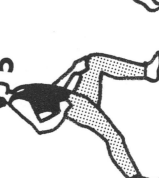

5

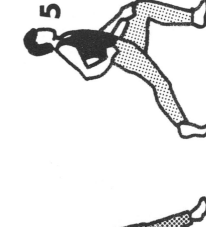

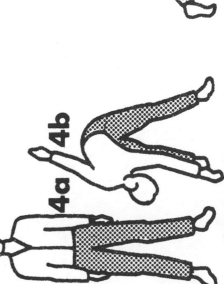

4a

4b

Exercises for scoliosis sufferers
1a Sit well forward on a chair, feet flat on the floor, knees slightly apart and arms hanging down.
1b Relax and let your head fall between your knees. Tighten your stomach muscles and sit up.
2a Stand with your right leg on a table, toes pointing upward.

2b Bounce your body forward to try and reach your toes with outstretched hands. Repeat with the left leg.
3a Kneel on your right knee with your left leg straight behind you; clasp your hands behind your head.
3b Turn your head and torso firmly to the right; hold for a count of 5. Repeat to the left.

4a Stand with your feet astride, legs straight.
4b Repeatedly reach for the right foot with the left hand, swinging the other arm back and up; straighten and repeat to the left.
5 Stretch your right leg behind you, bending the knee and turning the foot slightly inward. Place your right hand on your hip and your left hand on your left leg as shown. Then repeatedly rock your trunk back from the waist. Repeat, reversing legs and arms.

6a Sit astride a low stool, with your left leg bent and your right leg behind so that only the toes are resting on the floor. Hold your right arm by your side and the left straight up in line with your body.
6b Bend your body and straight arm backward several times. Repeat on the other side.

© DIAGRAM

RELAXATION

The stress factor

Inability to relax is commonly caused by stress, a consequence of the body's physiological reactions to external events. Stressful situations can be pleasant (supporting your team), unpleasant (an accident), physical (running), mental (worrying over past or future events), emotional (a bereavement), prolonged (business problems), or instantaneous (cutting a finger). Faced with these or similar situations the body tenses as part of the "fight or flight" response (see below). This response is essential to the

Fight or flight response
When your body prepares for action, these changes take place:
1 forebrain receives stimulus;
2a pituitary gland (see p.29) releases the alarm messenger hormone (ACTH);
2b lower brain alerts the nervous system;
3 ACTH causes the adrenal glands (see p.29) to release the hormones adrenaline (or epinephrine), noradrenaline (or norepinephrine) and cortisones. These cause:
4 heart rate to increase — blood is diverted to muscles and brain;
5 respiration rate to increase — nostrils and bronchi dilate;
6 liver to release sugar and fatty acids into the blood;
7 pupils to dilate;
8 sweating to increase;
9 blood clotting to speed up;
10 bowels and bladder to empty;
11 muscles to tense.

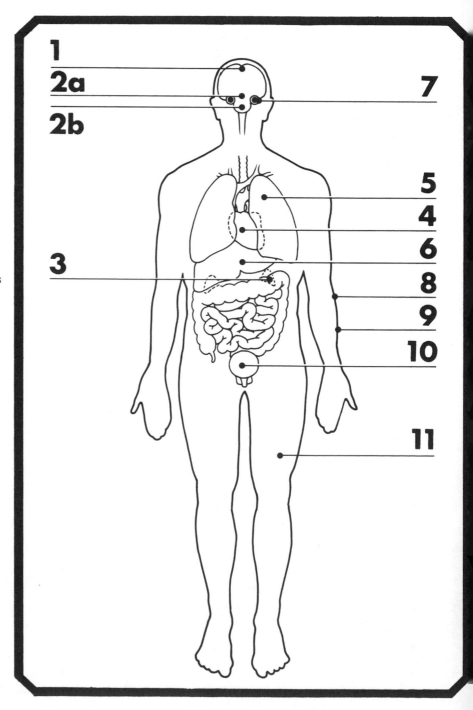

survival of animals in the wild. In the modern world, however, man no longer runs after his food, and faced with a dangerous situation cannot always run away. You cannot run in the driving seat of a car or in a overcrowded commuter train, nor can you flee financial trouble, divorce or city noise. Instead, stress is internalized. The unexpressed anger, irresolvable anxiety and frustration become trapped and cause depression, nervousness and irritability. These in turn cause more negative situations until they are expressed as physical, "psychosomatic," illnesses, e.g. hypertension, ulcers, muscular pain, aches, neuroses and breakdown. Prolonged stress simply runs the body down, in the same way as a machine wears out. The extra sugars and fatty acids released into the bloodstream, if not burned up with violent exercise, can be converted into cholesterol and give rise to atherosclerosis and other circulatory disorders. Environmental factors, especially noise, uncomfortable living or working conditions and crowding can cause stress. Misdirected energy (as in constant bad posture), colors (such as red), and working in opposition to your natural rhythms are also contributory factors to stress.

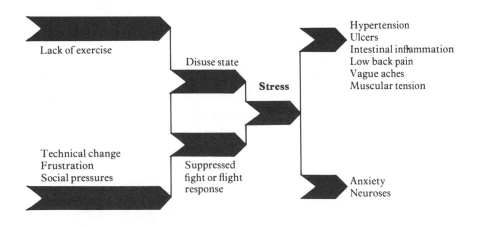

Causes and effects of stress
The diagram shows the major causes and effects of stress.

Signs of stress
The following is a list of the most common indications of stress. Check through the list. If you display seven or more of these reactions you are most probably suffering an undue amount of stress and would do well to follow a relaxation program.

1 Poor sleep
2 Waking up feeling unrested and dispirited
3 Jumping at unexpected noises
4 Impatience and irritability
5 Dissatisfaction with life in general, relationships or job
6 Any constant, pointless, repetitive action, e.g. teeth grinding or clenching, nail-biting, chainsmoking, tapping feet, fingers or pencils
7 Habits you know to be bad for you — overeating, smoking, drinking too much
8 Shallow breathing
9 Hunched, tense posture
10 Obsessions
11 Physical symptoms: migraine, skin complaints, indigestion, stuttering, flatulence, asthma, constipation, severe menstrual pain
12 Constantly being frustrated in your aims by others
13 Being late for buses, appointments, etc.
14 Use of sedatives
15 Pains in neck, shoulders, chest or back
16 Sweating for no apparent reason
17 Loneliness
18 Inability to show emotion
19 Inability to enjoy actions
20 A constant preoccupation with times and events other than now
21 A constant desire to change the unchangeable or to be or to do something else

Relaxation

Techniques of relaxation
Many systematic techniques of relaxation are now widely known; all combat stress by bringing the "fight or flight" response under control. There are two main groups: those that concentrate on the mind, and those that work on the body. Relax one, and you will relax the other.

Mental techniques These are forms of meditation, which combat stress by bringing the mind under conscious control. Different techniques derived originally from the esoteric elements of the major religions; all have the effect of increasing the powers of concentration. The mind is, in its usual state, a never-ending series of associations. Every impression that enters it sets off a chain of associations which, especially in stressful situations, rebound like a ricocheting bullet, setting up a wall of mental interference between the mind and outer reality. Meditation aims to bring this process under control, allowing you to concentrate on the moment, and not to worry about past or future possibilities. This increase in attention eventually leads to a new clear-sightedness; it helps you to see objects, people and situations as they are, not as you want them to be or as they appear to your subjective associations. This can lead to a new sense of peace with a new perception of your place in the world and your relation to external circumstances. It gives you a mental breathing space. This can help you to stop wasting energy in pointless anxiety and activity. By bringing the mind under control you also control your actions and undermine the "donkey and carrot" syndrome in which you do things automatically without knowing why, or even when or how. Meditation helps you to act, and not react automatically in fear, anger or greed.

Physiological effects of meditation
These are the opposite of those of the "fight or flight" response. The following conclusions emerge from the results of experiments designed to test scientifically the benefits of transcendental meditation (TM).

1 Sleep The reduction of oxygen — and so also of the metabolic rate — during meditation means a deeper level of rest. Meditation may also help insomniacs to get to sleep more easily.

2 Skin resistance to electricity decreases under stress and increases during meditation.

3 Cortisol level The amount of cortisol in the blood plasma increases under stress and decreases during meditation.

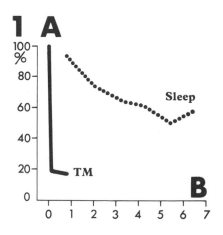

1 Sleep The first diagram compares the change in oxygen consumption during sleep and during TM. **A** shows the percent change in oxygen consumption. **B** shows the time in hours.
The second diagram compares the average time taken by an insomniac to fall asleep, for 30 days before starting TM, and for 30 days after starting TM.
C is the time in $\frac{1}{4}$ hour intervals.

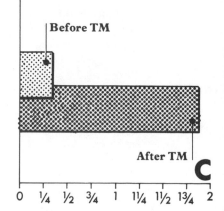

There are three methods of meditation. Most common is the use of physical or mental objects on which the meditator tries to focus his attention. Every time other thoughts, or even verbal definitions enter the mind they must be pushed off, and attention brought back to the object. Physical objects should be natural objects, such as stones or shells, or small personal objects like jewels or plain rings. Other objects include: the verbal or mental repetition of sounds (transcendental meditation's "mantras," "OM" or prayers); images with uplifting associations (the lotus flower, pictures of saints and gurus); and body rhythms, especially breathing. Bhakti, Sufi and transcendental meditations, Raja yoga and Kundalini yoga all use this method.

The second major method is to concentrate on yourself; to cultivate a constant awareness of your actions, thoughts and surroundings. This means that you begin to see how your mind works, to discover the automatic nature of your actions and to see the possibilities of the self or, in some philosophies, the essential nothingness, behind the transient automation. Krishnamurti's "self-knowledge" and Gurdjieff's "self-remembering" typify this method.

The third method combines aspects of the other two; the best known examples being Zen Buddhism's "zazen" meditation and use of the "koan s" (unsolvable problems), and Tibetan Buddism.

Despite their differences, all forms of meditation have the same basis — conscious control of attention. Choose the method suitable for your own personality and circumstances, and stress will be relieved. Remember, however, that because of its personal nature, meditation can only really be learned from a teacher on a one-to-one basis.

Conditions for meditation
Meditation by self-awareness and self-observation should be carried out in varying conditions so that you can see the many different aspects of your personality. Try to follow these simple guidelines.
1 Sit in a comfortable position (cross-legged or in a chair) with your back straight.
2 Choose a quiet time and place with no fear of interruption.
3 Let your thoughts and body settle for a few minutes before you begin.
4 Try to meditate for ½–1 hour, if possible at the same times each day.
5 As with all exercises, results are dependent upon the constancy and strength of your effort.

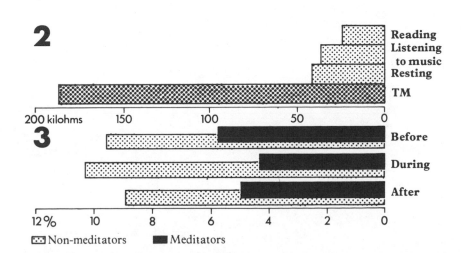

2 Skin resistance The diagram compares skin resistance during meditation and during various other activities. Resistance is measured in kilohms.
3 Cortisol level The diagram compares the percentage of cortisol in the blood plasma of non-meditators before, during and after relaxation, and of meditators before, during and after meditation.

©DIAGRAM

Relaxation

Physical relaxation techniques These aim to release the energy trapped or blocked in the body. By causing the body to relax, the mind itself will also relax. The direct relationship between mind and body is the essence of relaxation.

In the West, massage and the application of the Alexander principle (see page 96) are the main methods used. Western massage aims to stimulate the blood and lymph systems, to increase their flow and to work out knots of hard, tense tissue in the muscles. Techniques vary in intensity from steady stroking to Rolfing, in which each muscle is intensively worked.

Oriental techniques, such as acupuncture or shiatsu are complete methods of treatment for organic illness and are very effective in relieving stress, anxiety and depression. Their methods are based on a completely different philosophy from that embodied in Western physiology, and concern the flow of universal energy — Chi — along certain paths — "meridians" or "keiraku" — around the body. On each of these paths are 361 vital points or "tsubos." When the unity of the body is harmed by illness or injury, the harmony of the body processes is disrupted and the energy flow impaired. The afflicted part affects the tsubos on their corresponding meridian, usually causing them to hurt under pressure. By stimulating the tsubos on the correct meridian, the blockages to the energy are removed; the correct energy flow and, therefore, the harmony and health of the body are restored. Acupuncture works by stimulating the tsubos with needles; Shiatsu by the pressure of the thumbs, fingers, hands, knuckles and elbows; moxa uses heat; anma is a form of massage much like that of the West. Auricular therapy sees the ear to be shaped like the human embryo and to represent, therefore, a microcosm of the human body; stimulation of parts of the ear (usually with needles) affects corresponding parts of the body.

Massage strokes
Rubbing and stroking Here the palm, heel or four fingers of one or both hands stroke or rub the surface of the area. The movement should be toward the heart and can be superficial or deep.
Circular motion The palm or finger tips move in circular motions on the area.
Kneading massage The muscle or muscles are kneaded between the thumb and forefinger.
Pressure massage Pressure is applied to the tense or relevant area through the palm, thumbs or fingers. The pressure should be 6½–11lb (3–5kg) applied for 3–5 seconds. In certain areas, especially the shoulders, pressure should be applied through the thumbs, which are moved in a circular motion.

Use of thumbs and fingers in massage
When applying pressure, always use the balls not the points of your fingers and thumbs. **A** is the correct way to use fingers and thumbs. **B** is incorrect.

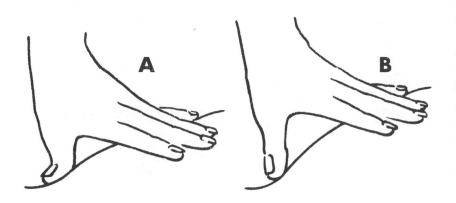

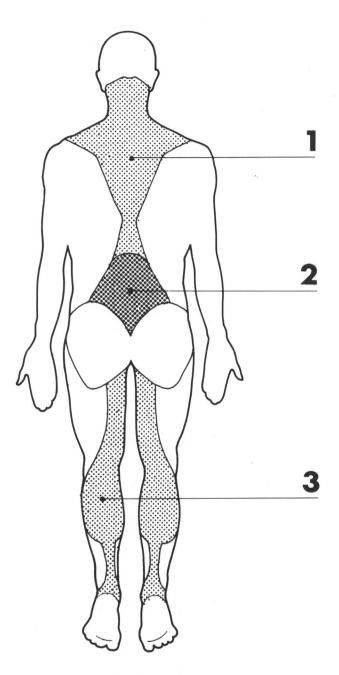

Main areas of tension
Tension in **1** usually results from anxiety and mental states; **2** is affected by overwork and strain in the lower back; **3** by strain in running and exercise.

Massage hints
When massaging use oil or talc to stop friction. Relax your hands and allow them to fit the contours of the body. Make sure each stroke has an evenness of speed and pressure. Begin lightly and increase the pressure and type of stroke as necessary. Use your weight, not your muscles, to apply pressure and let your movements flow. Do not break contact until you have finished the complete massage.

Environmental factors Relaxation can be increased by removing stress-creating factors from your environment. Try to organize activities beforehand so you know when you'll be doing things. Try to keep tidy so you do not lose things. Maintain good posture, and learn to enjoy physical exertion. Make sure you have complete breaks of attention during the day. Avoid being too hot or too cold, and keep noise to a minimum. Make time to be on your own, and give up any negative habits you know to be bad for you, like smoking or overeating.

©DIAGRAM

Relaxation

Sleep

This is the most important form of relaxation. About one third of our lives is spent in a state of near unconsciousness. There are two types of sleep.

Orthodox sleep forms about 75% of our sleep. The body is relaxed, and during the deepest periods of sleep the production of growth hormone and protein are at their highest while the body repairs itself with new cells.

Paradoxical, or REM, sleep accounts for the remaining 25%. This is the stage in which dreams occur. There is rapid eye movement (REM) behind the closed lids, the heartbeat and breathing become irregular, the brain receives more blood than when awake and its electrical activity is like that of the waking stage.

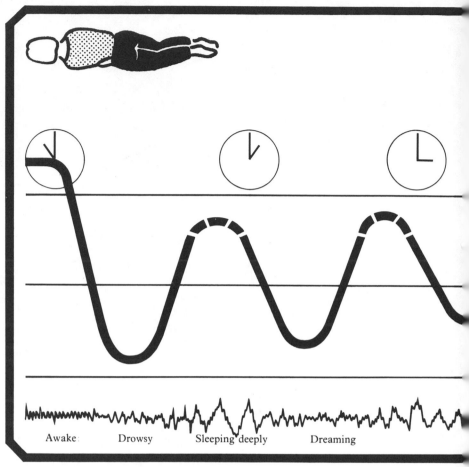

Awake   Drowsy   Sleeping deeply   Dreaming

Sleep

The amount of sleep a person needs gradually declines with age, but remains fairly constant from age 30. On average, a newborn baby sleeps for 16 hours a day, a 6-year-old for 10 hours, a 12-year-old for 9 hours, and an adult for 7 hours and 20 minutes. Although sleep needs are not dependent upon sex or intelligence, the amount needed is very personal; some adults need as much as 10 hours sleep daily while others need only 2 or 3 hours. We are so accustomed to thinking of 8 hours as being the necessary amount that many people use chemical means unnecessarily to prolong their sleep period.

Insomnia is habitual sleeplessness. It takes two major forms: in the first the person cannot get to sleep at all, and in the second the person wakes up after a few hours and cannot get to sleep again, or wakes and sleeps continuously through the night. People sometimes think they have not slept when, in fact, they have just woken at regular intervals and cannot remember sleeping! There are often easily rectifiable physical causes for sleeplessness, such as feeling cold or uncomfortable, or having bad eating habits. Make sure your room is warm but well aired and that the bed gives even and

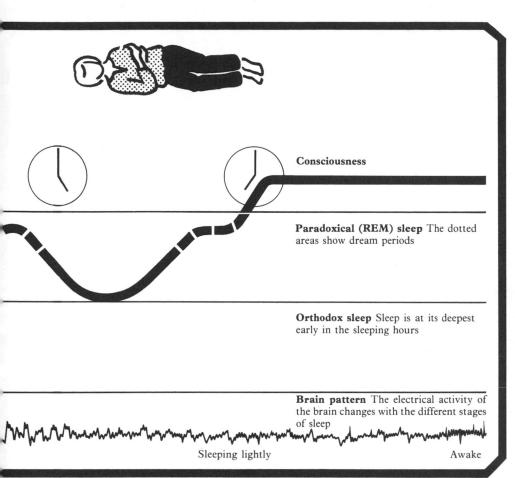

Consciousness

Paradoxical (REM) sleep The dotted areas show dream periods

Orthodox sleep Sleep is at its deepest early in the sleeping hours

Brain pattern The electrical activity of the brain changes with the different stages of sleep

Sleeping lightly   Awake

Why do we sleep?

Different theories suggest that sleep may be due to: a reduction in the brain's oxygen supply; a reduction in the number of impulses reaching the centers of consciousness; chemical processes; or conditioned responses.

Dreams

Everybody dreams whether they remember their dreams or not. A person who is deprived of paradoxical sleep — and hence of dreaming — will rapidly become insane and die.

The actual function of dreams is not known. Dreams have been used in prophecy for centuries. Freud saw them as indications of unconscious fears and desires. The computor analogy sees them as periods in which the brain sorts out the new data from the day and fashions revised programs.

firm support. Don't eat, and especially don't drink tea or coffee, late at night. Take exercise every day, to tire the body.

The most common causes of insomnia are psychological factors: worry, tension, depression or emotional upset. The main rule is not to worry over your lack of sleep — this only starts a vicious circle of tense worrying. If you really cannot get to sleep, don't lie there and worry about it, but get up and do something until tiredness overtakes you. Try and reeducate yourself into a positive frame of mind about sleep and have a gentle routine for preparation: a warm bath, a warm drink and quiet reading or talking to relieve tension. Whatever the psychological reason for insomnia, find a method for taking your mind off it; try concentrating on one part of the body or regularizing your breathing. The yoga "corpse" method of relaxing every part of the body in turn while breathing correctly is also helpful (see page 122). If you can, get a friend to massage your neck, shoulders, back and legs. Sleeping pills should only be used as a last resort; they do not give a satisfying sleep and should not be depended upon.

Relaxation

ADVICE

Standing

Incorrect posture is one of the main causes of physical tension and back trouble. If you stand correctly you can relax.

1a, b Good standing position

Place your feet straight so that your body weight is evenly distributed. Hold your head up and look straight ahead. Your neck should be straight, your shoulders down and held back. Breathe from your diaphragm, expanding your chest fully. Keep your stomach and your buttocks in, but do not hold your body stiffly. Practice standing in this way until it becomes quite natural and comfortable.

Sitting

Sitting badly is another common cause of back complaints.

2a, b Good sitting position

When choosing a chair ensure that it gives adequate support. Sit well back in the seat with your back straight and your head supported. Chair-arms should hold your elbows naturally, and your knee-joints should rest on the edge of the seat so that your feet reach the floor.

Lying

Lying comfortably is important for sleep and relaxation, and also for relieving back pain. A good, firm bed is essential. Additional pillows can be used to give extra support and to help keep your back straight (p. 107).

3a Good lying position

Lie on your right side (so that your heart is not constricted). Extend your right leg and bend your left knee up. Bend your left arm so that your hand is on a level with your face, and relax your right arm behind you, palm up. Close your eyes and relax.

3b Lying with your feet up

To rest and relieve aching or tired leg muscles and feet, lie for a few minutes with your feet on a pillow or book to raise them slightly above your head.

3c The corpse

This is a yoga position for deep relaxation. Lie flat on your back with your arms by your sides, palms up. Let your arms and legs go limp and allow your feet to fall gently apart. Raise your chin, close your eyes, and breathe deeply and regularly. Maintain this posture for several minutes. Get up slowly and gradually.

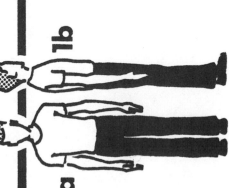

1a **1b**

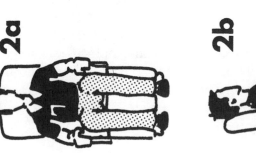

2a

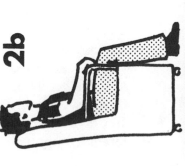

2b

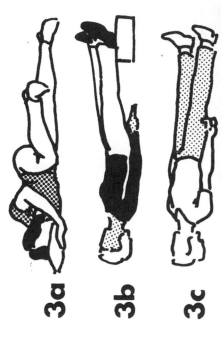

3a

3b

3c

EXERCISES

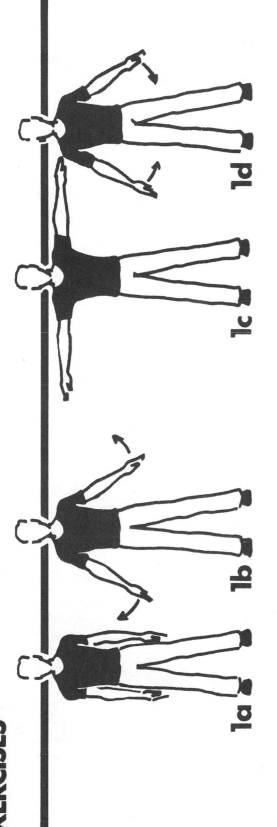

1a

1b

1c

1d

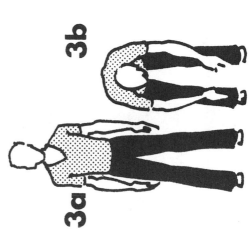

Relieving tension

1a Stand with your feet apart and your arms down by your sides.
1b Inhale deeply as you lift your arms to shoulder level.
1c Hold your breath for a moment as you stretch your arms and fingers out as far as you can.
1d Breathe out as you lower your arms back down to your sides.

2a Keeping your arm as relaxed as possible, start by shaking your right hand from the wrist. Next shake your elbow and then your shoulder. Finally shake your whole arm until it feels free from tension.
2b Repeat with your left arm.
2c With one leg and then the other, in turn shake your ankle, knee, thigh, and then your whole leg until every part is relaxed.

3a Stand with your feet apart and your arms hanging loosely by your sides.
3b Flop forward from the waist so that your head and arms hang loosely in front of you. After a few moments stand up straight again.

3b

3a

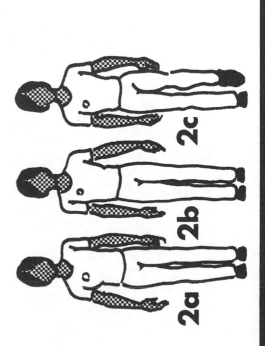

2c

2b

2a

©DIAGRAM

Relaxation

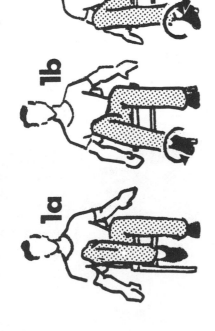

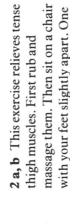

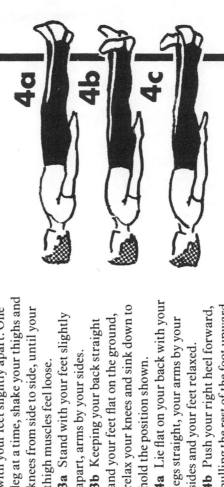

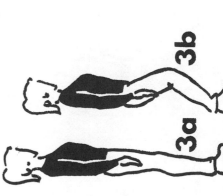

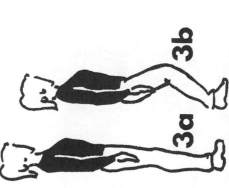

Relieving tension

1a Sit on a chair with your knees bent and both feet on the floor. Lift your right leg so that your foot can move freely.

1b Rotate your right foot, from the ankle, down and round to the right, moving it through as large a circle as possible.

1c Then rotate this foot in the opposite direction. Repeat exercise with your left leg.

2 a, b This exercise relieves tense thigh muscles. First rub and massage them. Then sit on a chair with your feet slightly apart. One leg at a time, shake your thighs and knees from side to side, until your thigh muscles feel loose.

3a Stand with your feet slightly apart, arms by your sides.

3b Keeping your back straight and your feet flat on the ground, relax your knees and sink down to hold the position shown.

4a Lie flat on your back with your legs straight, your arms by your sides and your feet relaxed.

4b Push your right heel forward, pulling the rest of the foot upward. You should feel this stretch in your calf, knee and thigh. Pull and relax repeatedly until your ankle joint is loose and your foot rises easily.

4c Let your right foot rest; repeat with the left leg.

EXERCISES

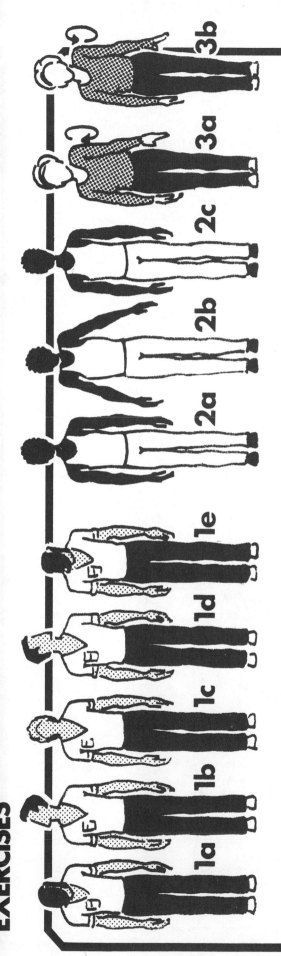

1a 1b 1c 1d 1e

2a 2b 2c 3a 3b

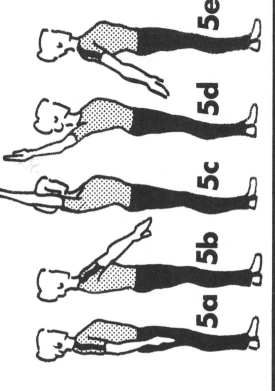

5a 5b 5c 5d 5e

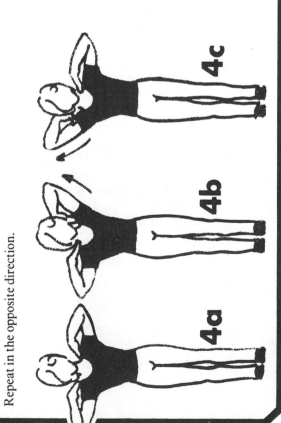

4a 4b 4c

Relieving tension
1a Stand with your arms hanging by your sides. Let your head hang forward and down.
1b Lift your head up to the right, keeping your shoulders straight.
1c Roll your head back and round.
1d Drop your head to the left.
1e Let it fall forward.
Repeat in the opposite direction.

2a Stand with your arms hanging by your sides.
2b Shrug both shoulders as high as you can.
2c Drop your shoulders. Repeat.
3a Lift your left shoulder as high as you can. Then swing it back and down. Roll it forward and up to complete a circle.

3b Still using your left shoulder repeat the circular movement forward.
Then roll your right shoulder.
4a Raise your arms to the side at shoulder level. Bend at your elbows to touch your shoulders.
4b, c Keeping your elbows bent, pull your left arm up. Lower it. Repeat with the right arm.
5a Stand with arms by sides.
5b Place the backs of your hands together down in front of you.
5c Keeping your arms straight, swing them forward and up.
5d, e Bring your arms down behind you in a circular action.

©DIAGRAM

PREGNANCY AND AFTER

During pregnancy a woman's body changes dramatically. Most noticeable is its increase in size and weight. As the breasts swell and the belly juts out farther and farther, many women become convinced that their bodies will never return to their normal shape, but the body need not alter permanently. Eating correctly ensures that a woman does not put on excess weight, and correct posture and gentle, controlled exercise ensure that, after the baby is born, the body returns easily and quickly to its former shape, if not an even better one.

Possible problems

The diagram shows possible problems occurring during pregnancy (**A**) and the postnatal period (**B**).

A1 Backache is caused by the extra abdominal weight throwing greater strain on the back.

A2 Hemorrhoids (piles) are stretched veins that occur around the back passage (anus). They can be aggravated by constipation.

A3 Varicose veins,

A4 cramp, and

A5 swollen ankles can all be caused by bad circulation and by standing for long periods.

B1 Sagging breasts may occur if a good supporting bra is not worn during pregnancy and after.

B2 Backache can result from failure to readjust posture after the baby's birth. (See p. 137.)

B3 Sagging stomach muscles can result from lack of exercise.

B4 Poor bladder control and prolapse of the womb may occur if the pelvic floor muscles are not strengthened by exercise.

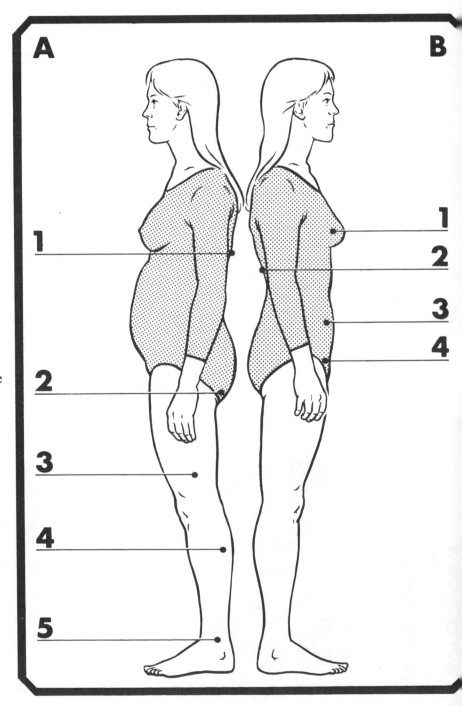

The following pages give advice on posture and relaxation and describe simple exercises for before and after the baby is born. Be sure to seek professional advice before any exercises are attempted.

Posture and daily activities This section begins with the right and wrong ways of doing such things as walking, sitting and lifting. Extra weight causes these actions to become difficult during pregnancy, and doing them incorrectly may throw extra strain on the abdomen and back. Good posture is important at any time; during pregnancy it becomes even more vital. The hollow, backward-leaning stance is one of the most common causes of backache among pregnant women.

Relaxation A pregnant woman tires easily and some rest every day is essential in the later stages of pregnancy. From 34 weeks onward, and before if possible, aim to lie down for 30 minutes to one hour, preferably after lunch. If you find it difficult to go to bed during the day, try lying on the floor with pillows for support.

Antenatal exercises Pregnancy places considerable strain on a woman's body, and labor itself is probably the most strenuous physical activity that any women undertakes. Provided that there are no complications, most women are encouraged to continue with their normal routine — although care should be taken to avoid becoming overtired. Walking is an excellent way of maintaining general fitness during pregnancy. Other exercises recommended in this book are specifically designed to improve posture and circulation, and to strengthen the muscles of the pelvic floor. These muscles support the abdominal organs and are slung like a hammock from the coccyx (tail bone) to the front of the pelvis; it is important to learn to contract them during pregnancy if their elasticity is to be retained.

Postnatal exercise Once the baby is born a woman wants to get her figure back as soon as possible; we have therefore included a selection of exercises for the postnatal period. As in the antenatal period, the emphasis is on the muscles of the pelvic floor, which must be strengthened in order to regain proper bladder control, for sexual intercourse and to help prevent prolapse of the uterus (womb) in middle age. Soon after the birth, exercising should be fairly gentle, but following the postnatal check-up six weeks after the birth it is usually safe for rather more strenuous exercises to be attempted.

Pregnancy and after

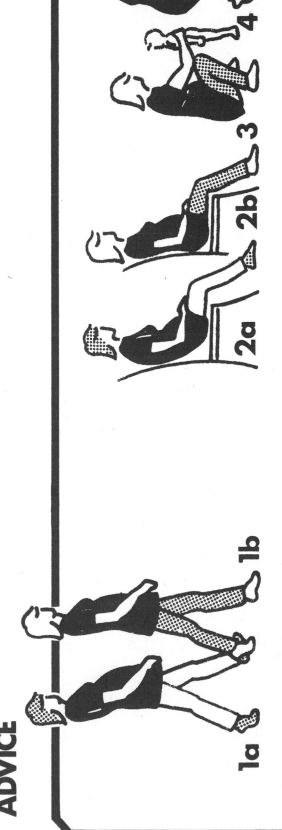

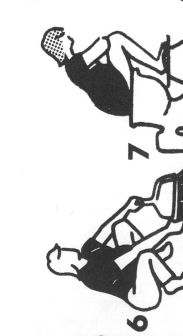

Posture and daily activities
Practicing good posture at all times
when you are pregnant will help to
avoid strain on your back and
stomach.
1a During pregnancy there is a
great temptation to walk badly,
with your pelvis tilted forward and
the hollow of your back increased
(also see p. 132).

1b The best walking posture is
upright; head erect, back straight,
abdomen and chest held well up.
The feet should be placed firmly on
the ground.

2a When you are tired it is easy to
slump into a chair, with your spine
rounded and inadequately
supported. The abdomen, breast
and ribs sag, causing backache.
2b Instead, sit well back into the
chair, with your back and thighs
supported and your feet resting on
the floor or on a pillow. Tuck your
pelvis under, and pull your
abdomen in. (In an easy chair use a
cushion to fill in and support the
hollow in your back.)
3 To lift a child easily, squat with
your knees bent and your feet
apart. Keeping your spine straight,
grasp the child close and straighten
up.

4 Avoid lifting heavy objects
during pregnancy. To lift an object
from the floor, bend and then
straighten your knees with your
feet in a walking position, keeping
your back straight throughout.
5 To put on your shoes, sit on a
bed or chair with your legs wide
apart, and put your foot across the
opposite knee.
6 When using a dustpan and
brush, bend down in a squat with
your knees apart and your back
straight.
7 When sitting on the toilet, place
your feet on a footstool and sit with
your knees comfortably apart,
leaning forward to prevent
straining.
8 Kneeling on all fours is ideal for
cutting fabric, etc.

ADVICE

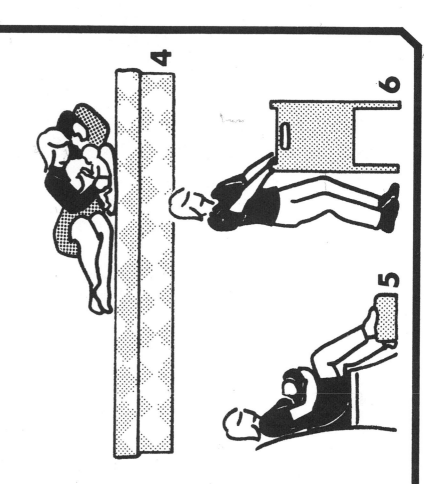

Posture and daily activities

1a Incorrect posture when ironing is a common cause of back strain; avoid bending your back and stooping over a low ironing board.

1b For maximum comfort when ironing, stand diagonally to the board with one foot in front of the other and your knees slightly bent.

2a Also avoid bending your back over a sink or worktop.

2b Instead, keep one leg in front of the other and bend them both slightly, keeping your back straight.

3 When sweeping with a broom, place one foot in front of the other and swing back and forward, keeping your back straight as you sweep.

Posture after the birth

Incorrect posture after your baby is born can all too easily result in troublesome aches and pains (also see p. 137).

4 When feeding your baby make sure that you are comfortable and that your back is supported. If feeding your baby in bed, prop yourself up with pillows while lying on one side with both knees bent up. Use another pillow to support the baby securely.

5 For another comfortable feeding position, sit in a chair with a pillow behind your back. Hold the baby on another pillow, helping to raise his head by placing one of your feet on a low stool as shown.

6 To lift your baby from his crib, stand with one side next to the crib and your feet in a walking position. Reach down by bending your knees while keeping your back erect.

©DIAGRAM

Pregnancy and after

Relaxing lying down

From 34 weeks onward, and before if possible, pregnant women should aim to spend 1 hour a day relaxing on a bed or lying on the floor with pillows. Any position that you find comfortable will be perfectly safe for the baby. The following suggestions may help women who have difficulty finding a comfortable position.

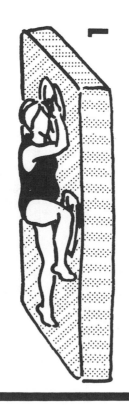

1

2

1 Try lying on one side with your head on a pillow, your lower arm down behind your back, your upper arm forward with the hand resting on your pillow, and your upper knee bent up to rest on a second pillow. Tense up completely and then relax, and then try to relax without tensing up first.

2 Some women prefer to bring both arms forward, or not to use a pillow under the knee.

Getting up

When rising from a lying position, pregnant women should not bend forward to sit up as this places too much strain on the abdominal muscles. The following is a recommended safe alternative procedure for getting out of bed. It can be easily modified for getting up from the floor.

3a If lying on your back, first bend your knees up.
3b Then roll over onto one side, bringing your top arm over.
3c Put your hands down on the bed and push yourself up into a sitting position.
3d Now swing your legs round and onto the floor.
3e Finally push yourself up into a standing position.

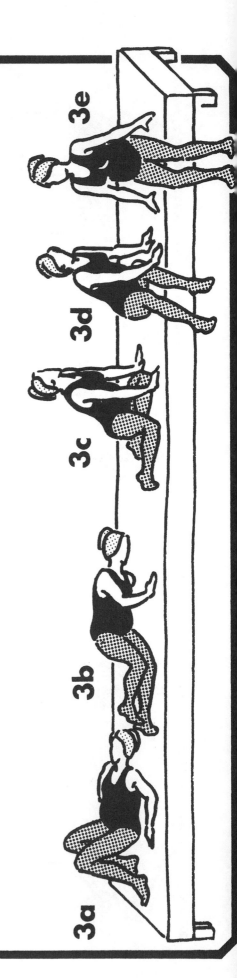

3a

3b

3c

3d

3e

ADVICE

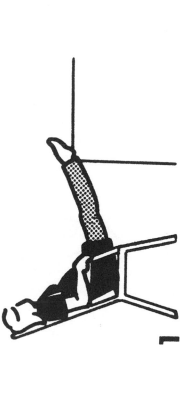

1

Putting your feet up
It is extremely good for women in the later stages of pregnancy to spend some time each day relaxing with their feet up. Raising the feet higher than the hips relieves pressure on the pelvic veins, aids circulation in the legs and helps to prevent varicose veins and swollen ankles.

1 Sit well back in a chair with a pillow in the hollow of your back and your feet raised on a table or stool.
2 Or lie on a sofa with a pillow to support your back and your feet raised on the sofa arm.
3 Alternatively lie on your back on the floor, with your head on a pillow and your feet resting on the edge of a low table or stool.

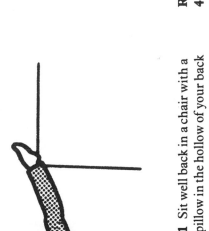

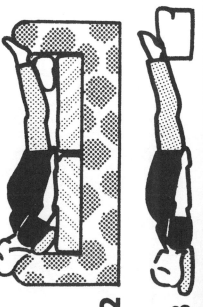

2

3

4

5

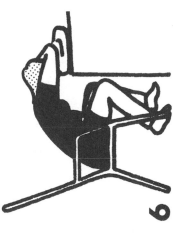

Recuperative positions
4 To relieve backache when sitting, sit well back in the chair with a pillow in the hollow of your back and one foot raised on a small stool or a pile of books 4–6in (10–15cm) high. About every $\frac{1}{2}$–1 hour get up and walk around.
5 Pain in the coccyx (tail bone) is quite common during pregnancy. Try placing a cushion under your thighs for relief when sitting.

6 To ease stiffness after working at a desk or table, lean forward and rest your head on your hands. Then try to relax your entire body.

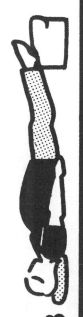

6

©DIAGRAM

Pregnancy and after

EXERCISES

0 — 16 — 28 — 36 — 40

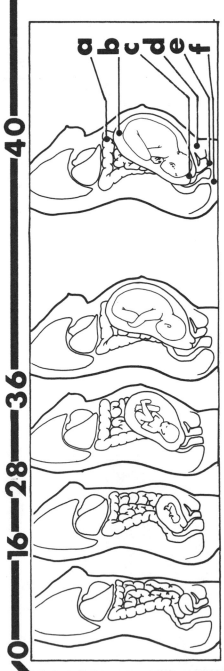

Identification of body parts

a Intestines
b Uterus (womb)
c Cervix (neck of the womb)
d Pelvic floor
e Vagina (birth canal)
f Anus (back passage)

Developments during pregnancy

Growth of the baby, in pregnancy causes the uterus (womb) to expand, so displacing some of the mother's internal organs. The diagrams above show the mother before pregnancy, and at weeks 16, 28, 36 and 40 (full term). Possible consequences in the later stages are shortness of breath, indigestion, frequent urination, and backache.

Posture during pregnancy

Standing badly will increase your tendency to backache.
1a This diagram shows incorrect posture during pregnancy. The natural hollow of the woman's back is increased and the uterus tips forward as illustrated.
1b For correct posture, try to hold your back straight so that the uterus is kept in a more upright position.

Posture exercise

This exercise will teach you how to control the tilt of your pelvis, improve your posture, and help to relieve backache.
2 Lie on your back with your knees bent up. Breathing normally, tighten your buttock muscles by squeezing the two sides of your bottom together and at the same time pull in your abdominal muscles to feel the hollow of your back press against the bed or floor. Hold for 5 seconds, then relax. Repeat 5 times slowly.
3 The same exercise can be done seated, feeling the hollow of your back press against the back of the chair.
4 Alternatively do it standing up, without bending your legs. Feel the hollow of your back flatten as you pull your muscles in and up.

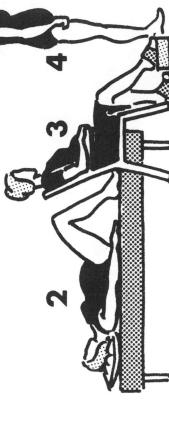

1a   1b

2   3   4

EXERCISES

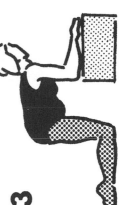

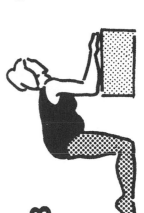

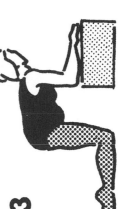

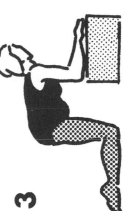

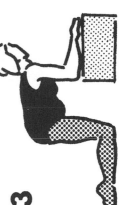

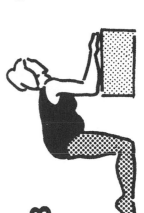

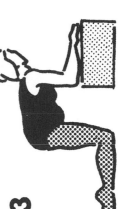

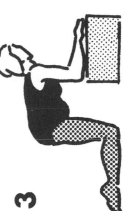

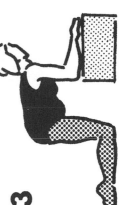

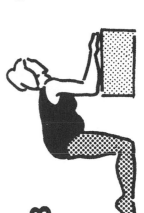

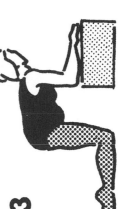

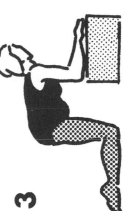

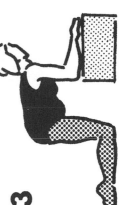

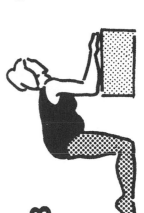

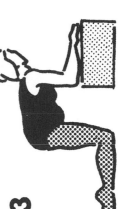

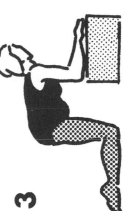

General exercises

Do each exercise 5–10 times at 3 daily sessions.

4a Lie on your back with your knees raised and your feet flat on the ground.

4b Straighten your left knee to extend your leg along the ground.

4c Repeat with your right leg.

5 Lie on your back with your knees raised and your feet flat on the ground. Tighten your buttock muscles, hold for a moment, and then relax.

2a Kneel on all fours with your knees directly below your hips and your hands directly below your shoulders.

2b Slowly arch your back and draw in your pelvis, tucking in your seat. Hold this arched position for 5 seconds and then relax. Repeat 6–8 times.

3 The same exercise can be done resting the forearms on a box or chair. Hump your back by tightening your abdominal and buttock muscles simultaneously.

Pelvic floor exercises

During pregnancy the muscles of the pelvic floor have to work harder than usual, supporting the weight of the developing baby. It is important to learn how to contract these muscles during pregnancy if their elasticity is to be retained after the birth.

1 When lying, standing or sitting and without holding your breath, first pull up the muscles of your anus as though preventing a bowel movement. Then continue the action forward to squeeze and lift the vagina as though preventing the flow of urine. Hold this position for a count of 5, and then relax. Repeat a few times at each session, up to a total of about 30 times a day.

Pregnancy and after

EXERCISES

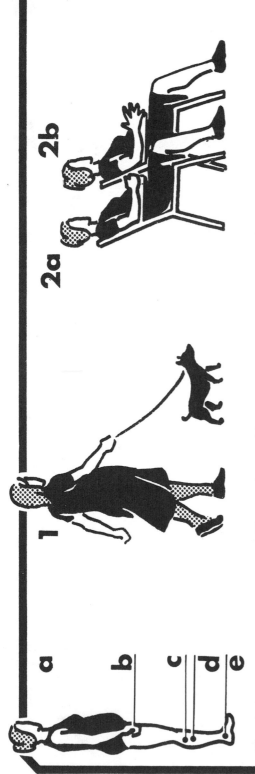

1

2a

2b

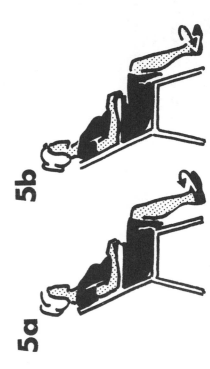

3a 3b

4a 4b

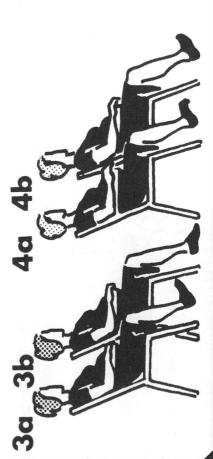

5a

5b

Circulation problems
During pregnancy, the weight of the fetus can press on the main leg veins in the groin and cause poor or sluggish circulation. Any of the following symptoms may occur:

a Fainting
b Swollen fingers
c Cramp
d Varicose veins
e Swollen ankles

The exercises on this page will alleviate the uncomfortable symptoms and improve general circulation. Exercises 2, 3, 4 and 5 can be done sitting comfortably, as shown, or lying down.

1 Walking is the best exercise of all for helping to prevent circulation problems; ideally you should take regular walks outdoors.

2a Clench your fists tightly.
2b Stretch all your fingers out very straight. Repeat this exercise frequently to alleviate swollen fingers; if your rings become tight or your fingers stiffen, tell your doctor.
3a With your heels resting on the floor, bend your feet upward from the ankle.
3b Bend your feet down again. Repeat often during the day.

4a With your heels resting on the floor, curl your toes under tightly.
4b Straighten your toes, and repeat
5a With your heels on the ground, move your feet round in small inward circles.
5b Then circle both feet outward several times.

EXERCISES

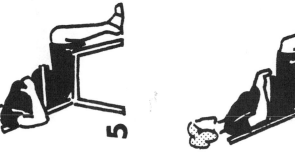

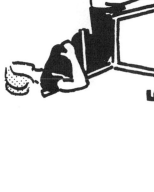

3

2

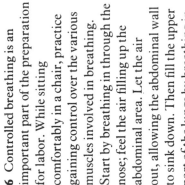

Circulation
Coping with cramp

Cramp is associated with poor circulation and often troubles pregnant women in the night or at other times when the body is inactive. The acute discomfort of cramp in the calves can be alleviated in the following ways.

1 If cramp occurs during the night, straighten the affected leg and bend the foot hard upward for 40–60 seconds. Then gently circle the foot or walk around the room. Pointing your toes will aggravate the cramp.

2 The same exercise can be done from a sitting position if cramp occurs during the day.

3 If possible ask someone to push your foot back into the cramp-relieving position; this can be very effective in reducing the discomfort.

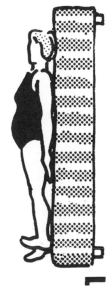

1

Fainting

4 If you tend to feel faint, get into the habit of pressing your knees back and tensing the muscles on the front of your thighs. This improves the circulation, reducing the feeling of faintness by sending more blood to the brain.

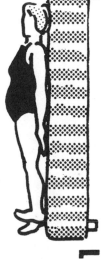

4

Breathing

5 You can improve your general circulation by learning to breathe efficiently. Sit on a chair, put your hands on your lower ribs, and feel the ribs expand as you breathe in deeply. Exhale, and repeat several times.

6 Controlled breathing is an important part of the preparation for labor. While sitting comfortably in a chair, practice gaining control over the various muscles involved in breathing. Start by breathing in through the nose; feel the air filling up the abdominal area. Let the air out, allowing the abdominal wall to sink down. Then fill the upper part of the lungs by breathing in through the nose, allowing the sternum, or breast bone, to lift up. Sigh the air out and feel the ribs and sternum sink down again.

5

6

©DIAGRAM

EXERCISES

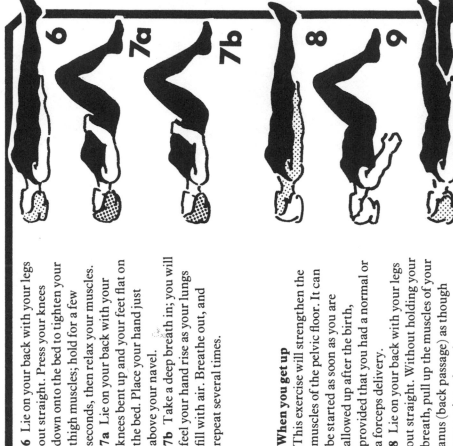

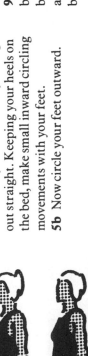

Postnatal relaxation

After the baby's birth you should rest for at least 1 hour every day. Relax completely in one of the following positions.

1 Lie flat on your stomach on the bed, with a pillow under your abdomen to prevent pressure on your breasts.

2 Lie on one side with your upper leg bent at the knee and your head on a pillow.

3 Lie flat on your back, with your legs out straight and your arms relaxed at your sides.

Postnatal exercises

Exercises 4–7 are designed to improve your circulation, and should be started as soon as possible after delivery. Do them lying down, as shown, or when sitting comfortably. They should be repeated at frequent intervals during the first 2 days after the birth, or for longer if you are kept in bed.

4a Lie on your back with your legs out straight. With your heels on the bed, bend your right foot up and your left foot down.

4b Push your left foot up and your right foot down; continue alternating the positions of your feet in this way several times.

5a Lie on your back with your legs out straight. Keeping your heels on the bed, make small inward circling movements with your feet.

5b Now circle your feet outward.

6 Lie on your back with your legs out straight. Press your knees down onto the bed to tighten your thigh muscles; hold for a few seconds, then relax your muscles.

7a Lie on your back with your knees bent up and your feet flat on the bed. Place your hand just above your navel.

7b Take a deep breath in; you will feel your hand rise as your lungs fill with air. Breathe out, and repeat several times.

When you get up

This exercise will strengthen the muscles of the pelvic floor. It can be started as soon as you are allowed up after the birth, provided that you had a normal or a forceps delivery.

8 Lie on your back with your legs out straight. Without holding your breath, pull up the muscles of your anus (back passage) as though preventing a bowel movement. Then continue the action forward to squeeze and lift the vagina as though preventing the flow of urine. Hold this muscle pull for a count of 5, and then relax. Repeat this exercise as often as possible, up to 50 times a day.

9, 10, 11 The same exercise can be done lying flat with the knees bent up, or with the legs straight and the ankles crossed; it can also be performed seated or standing.

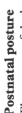

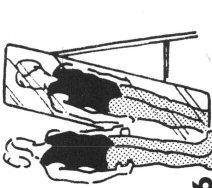

EXERCISES

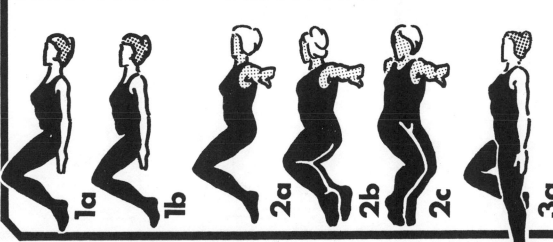

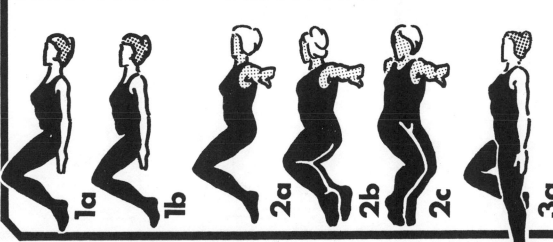

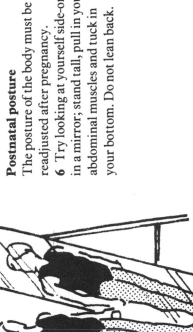

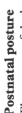

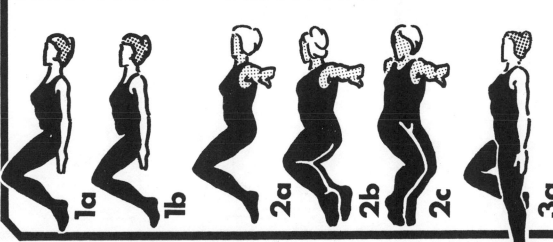

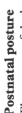

AFTER FORTY

Life, they say, begins at forty — but of course that is scarcely accurate. When you were in your middle or late twenties, aging had already begun; your nerve cells were starting to decay, and the faint beginnings of bodily deterioration had set in. Now, by the age of forty and after, you will be coming to admit that you are no longer as fit as you were.

At first you are conscious of a growing difficulty in performing physical tasks that were easy before; hills seem steeper and your breath shorter, and there is a feeling of a

Deterioration in bodily efficiency

In due course this affects general well-being and outward appearance in the following areas.

1 Deterioration in eyesight
2 Deterioration in hearing
3 Poor circulation and short breath as a result of hardened arteries and drooping chest
4 More skeletal frailty and stiffness, leading to aches, pains and bad posture
5 Sagging muscles
6 Fat deposits
7 Flat or aching feet, caused by bad posture and circulation

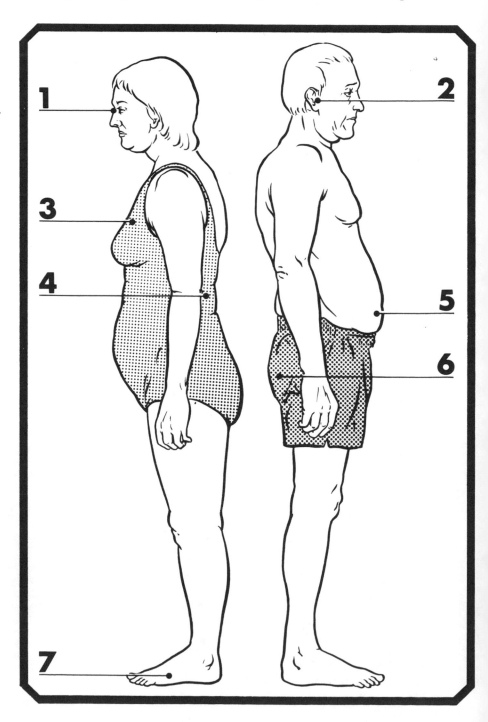

decrease in bodily efficiency. In women the menopause usually occurs in the late forties or early fifties, involving bodily changes and often emotional stress of which the victim alone is fully aware; but in due course these produce visible signs of aging. In both sexes, loss of muscle strength and redistribution of body fat cause the figure to change in the years after forty. Men tend to develop an abdominal bulge, and in women embarrassing new fat appears around the chin, waist, hips and bottom. In both sexes the skin becomes drier, leading to facial wrinkles, while atrophy (wasting) of the facial bones, deterioration of eyes and teeth, and graying or balding, all contribute to the outward evidence of aging. Arteries begin to harden, and joints to swell and work less easily. Some people find these changes difficult to accept, and become depressed by weight changes, sleep loss, poor appetite and a growing disgust with their bodies. This sad and usually unnecessary state can often be largely remedied by deliberate countermeasures such as regular repetition of the simple exercises described on the following pages. They won't halt the process of aging, of course, but they can slow it and almost certainly will diminish the feeling of aging by producing a greater sense of well-being and more confidence in your appearance. No elaborate apparatus is required and, although later you may go on to more complicated routines, you can choose those exercises that suit you best at different times. You don't need to do them all, and you don't need to do them in any particular order. If you have special problems — weight or posture, for instance — the table on page 141 will help you to find which exercises are best to remedy them, and if you would like to try some yoga you will also find a section on yoga for those over forty.

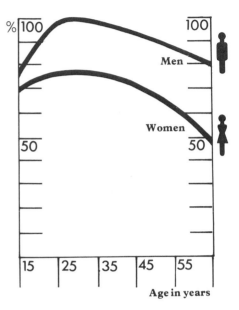

Muscle strength
Different aspects of fitness reach their peak at different times, and physical abilities such as strength, speed and endurance vary between individuals, and very noticeably between the sexes. Women have a longer life expectancy, but men are stronger and faster. The graph shows the average muscle strength of men and women at different ages.

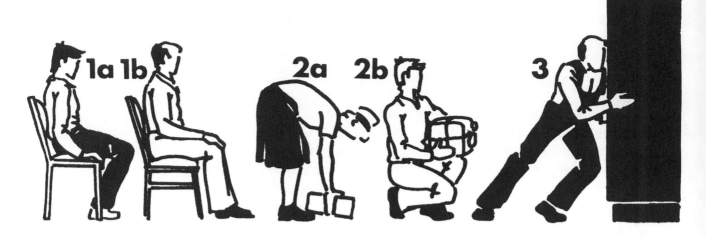

Posture

Good posture in everyday actions can do much to maintain health and retard deterioration.

1a Many people sit incorrectly, with their bottom forward in the seat and their back bent.

1b To avoid strain when seated, always sit with your back upright so that your spine and not your abdomen takes the weight of your chest and head.

2a Serious back injuries can result from this incorrect method of picking up a heavy object from the ground.

2b To avoid straining your back, try to keep your trunk vertical as you pick up a heavy object; place one foot in front of the other, bend your knees to crouch down, take hold of the object, then straighten your legs to raise it from the ground.

3 Pushing heavy objects can also result in injury unless you take care. In all forms of pushing, using the back, arms or shoulders, bend and then straighten the legs to exert pressure.

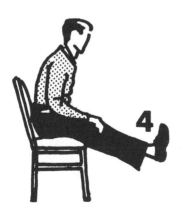

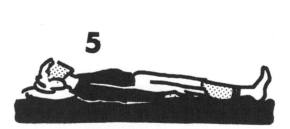

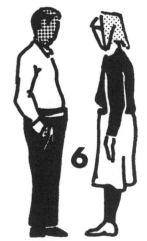

Exercising in the home

The advantage of exercising in the home is that you can do it to suit your own convenience and your own routine. Elaborate keep-fit apparatus is not essential.

4 For example, you can exercise effectively by stretching out your legs straight in front of you while sitting in a chair.

5 Some exercises can be done in bed, and most can be done at any time — but not within an hour after a large meal. An important home exercise is relaxation, which should form a regular part of your routine; a ½ hour flat on your back after lunch works wonders.

6 The home exercises you choose will, of course, relate to the degree of physical activity in your life as a whole, but in the pages that follow you will find exercises designed for such specific problems as overweight, sagging breasts, fat legs, etc.

Exercise chart
All exercises have a purpose other than just moving your limbs about. Some can induce general relaxation; some improve circulation or develop particular muscles. Use this chart to choose those that suit your own particular needs and problems; you will soon discover those that most increase your feeling of well-being.

Bold type indicates the page number
Lighter type indicates the exercise number

General conditions

Posture	**140** 1, **140** 2, **140** 3
Respiration	**142** 3, **151** 16
Circulation	**142** 3, **148** 5, **152** 5, **152** 6, **152** 7, **154** 4
Relaxation	**146** 1, **153** 1, **153** 2, **153** 3
Overweight	**144** 1, **144** 5, **146** 5, **149** 1, **149** 2, **149** 3, **149** 4, **149** 5, **149** 6, **149** 7, **149** 8, **149** 9, **149** 10, **149** 11, **150** 1, **150** 3, **150** 4, **150** 5, **150** 6, **150** 7, **150** 8, **150** 9

Specific areas

Neck	**143** 7, **145** 4, **145** 5, **146** 1, **151** 4, **151** 5, **151** 6, **151** 14, **152** 6, **152** 7, **152** 8, **154** 3, **154** 4
Shoulders	**142** 1, **142** 3, **145** 6, **145** 7, **145** 8, **146** 3, **146** 4, **147** 7, **148** 7, **151** 1, **151** 2, **151** 13, **151** 15, **154** 2, **155** 5
Arms	**142** 1, **142** 3, **144** 4, **146** 2, **146** 3, **146** 4, **146** 6, **147** 5, **151** 1, **151** 2, **151** 3, **151** 7, **151** 15
Chest and bust	**145** 8, **146** 2, **147** 6, **151** 2, **151** 3, **155** 5
Back	**142** 2, **144** 2, **144** 4, **145** 4, **145** 6, **145** 7, **145** 8, **146** 4, **146** 5, **146** 6, **147** 6, **148** 4, **148** 5, **148** 7, **152** 5, **152** 6, **152** 7, **152** 8, **154** 1, **154** 2, **154** 3, **154** 4, **155** 1, **155** 2, **155** 3, **155** 6, **155** 7
Waist	**144** 1, **144** 3, **144** 4, **144** 5, **145** 3, **146** 6, **147** 4, **151** 10, **151** 11, **155** 1, **155** 2
Abdomen	**142** 2, **144** 1, **144** 2, **144** 3, **144** 4, **144** 5, **145** 1, **145** 2, **145** 3, **145** 4, **145** 6, **145** 7, **145** 8, **146** 5, **146** 6, **147** 5, **148** 1, **148** 2, **148** 3, **148** 4, **148** 5, **151** 11, **151** 13, **151** 15, **152** 8, **153** 5
Hips	**142** 2, **143** 1, **143** 2, **144** 1, **144** 3, **144** 4, **144** 5, **146** 5, **146** 6, **148** 6, **155** 1
Buttocks	**148** 8, **153** 6, **154** 2
Thighs	**143** 1, **143** 2, **143** 3, **143** 5, **144** 2, **146** 3, **146** 4, **147** 1, **147** 2, **147** 3, **147** 5, **147** 6, **148** 1, **148** 2, **148** 3, **148** 6, **148** 8, **151** 11, **151** 13, **155** 3, **155** 5, **155** 6, **155** 7
Calves	**142** 3, **143** 3, **143** 4, **143** 5, **146** 3, **147** 3, **151** 12
Feet and ankles	**142** 3, **143** 5, **146** 3, **147** 2, **147** 3

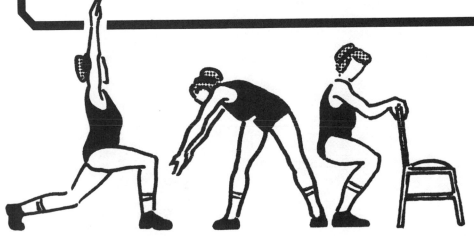

Variety
Although exercises should be performed regularly, preferably at about the same time each day, don't become a creature of habit. Not only will a mixture benefit different parts of your body, it will prevent you from becoming bored.

©DIAGRAM

EXERCISES

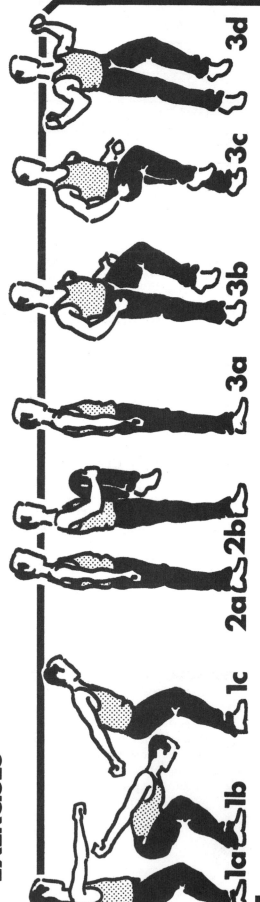

1a 1b **1c** **2a 2b** **3a** **3b** **3c** **3d**

Warming-up exercises for men

These require no apparatus, and each exercise can be performed on its own or as a sequence with any of the others. Before you start, decide on the best time of day for you to exercise, and stick to this as closely as possible. Avoid the time before breakfast if you have no opportunity to relax and cool off afterward. Build up slowly to about 20 repetitions of each exercise.

1a Stand with your feet about 6in (15cm) apart, knees slightly bent and arms stretched forward.
1b Swing your arms backward, bending your knees more and leaning forward as though skiing.
1c Straighten up as your arms swing forward.

2a Stand erect.
2b Raise one leg, bending your knee and hugging it as close to your body as possible, keeping your back straight. Repeat with your other leg.
3a For this exercise, hold your hands as though you had a rope in them for jumping.
3b, c, d Raise the feet as though jumping the rope, and at the same time move the hands as though turning it. Keep the rhythm as smooth as possible.

More examples

Other simple warming up exercises can be used. For instance, stand erect with your feet flat on the floor and your arms hanging down. Keeping your arms and feet in the same position, bend your knees to a squatting position and repeat rhythmically several times.
Or, start with your feet astride and your arms stretched forward. Keeping your feet in the same position and your body erect, twist your body from one side to the other, allowing the arms to swing round and turning the head as far as you can.

Deep breathing

A steady blood flow depends on a good supply of oxygen, and that depends on good deep breathing. While doing any of these exercises you should breathe deeply and exhale as hard as you can. Also you can use specialized breathing exercises. For example, stand with your toes and heels together and stretch your arms above your head, inhaling as you do so and raising your chest as high as possible. Exhale as you lower your arms.

EXERCISES

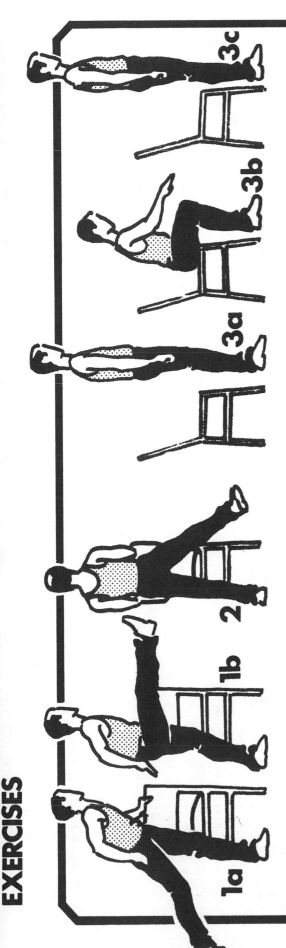

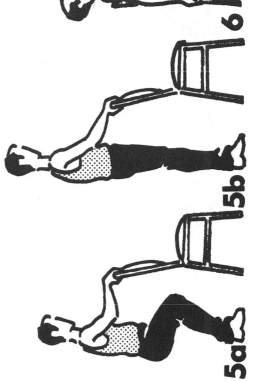

Men's exercises with a chair
These are good for loosening up.

1a, b With your left side facing the back of a chair, hold its back in your left hand. Keeping your left leg straight, swing your right leg (also straight) backward and forward several times, bending your body slightly forward as you swing. Change sides and repeat.

2 Hold the back of the chair with both hands. Swing your right then your left leg sideways, several times each.

3a Stand in front of the chair, then bend your knees as though to sit down but don't sit.
3b Just allow your buttocks to touch the chair.
3c Stand again, and repeat.
4a Stand facing the chair, then swiftly step onto it.
4b Stand up straight on it.
4c Step backward off the chair. Repeat the exercise.

5a Stand holding the back of the chair; bend your knees, which should be pointed straight ahead.
5b Stand straight, and repeat.
6 Sit with your back firmly against the back of the chair, holding its back legs with your hands. Stretch your neck backward as far as it will go, then return; inhale as your neck goes back, exhale as it goes forward.

After forty

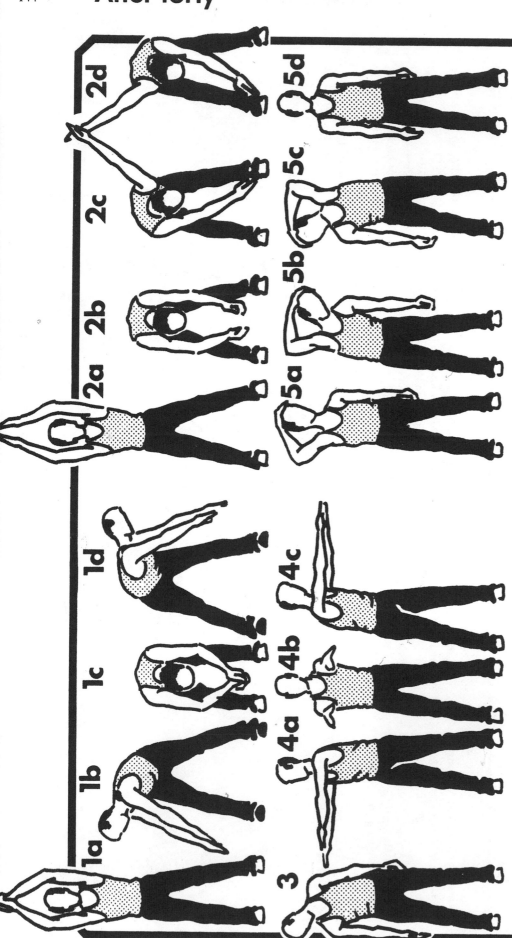

Men's trunk exercises

These exercises will loosen and relax stiff joints.

1a Stand with your feet apart, your arms raised and your hands loosely gripped overhead.

1b, c, d Bending from your hips, swing your trunk and arms in a graceful circle to return to the starting position. Repeat in the opposite direction.

2a Stand with your feet astride.

2b Bend forward.

2c Swing your right arm to touch your left toe.

2d Repeat to the other side.

3 With your arms at your sides, stand with your feet astride. Keeping your trunk facing forward, bend from side to side, allowing your head to move freely.

4a With your arms forward at shoulder height, stand astride and then twist your trunk to the right, allowing your arms to swing round the body and your head to turn as far as possible.

4b, c Swing your arms round the front to the other side.

5a Stand with your feet astride, your left arm hanging down and your right arm bent over your head.

5b Bend your trunk to the left several times.

5c Reverse your arm positions and repeat to the right.

5d Straighten up and relax.

EXERCISES

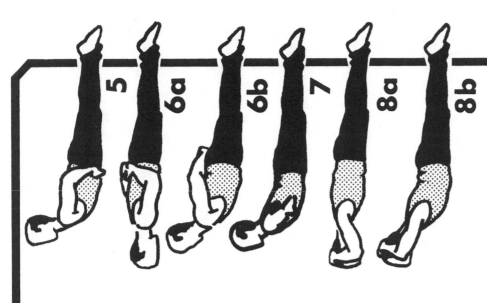

Men's exercises on the floor
Lie on a blanket or carpet, and move all furniture away.

1a Lie flat on your back, arms by your sides and feet slightly apart.
1b Raise your head and shoulders until you can see your ankles; lower them, and repeat.

2a Start as in 1a.
2b Raising your head and shoulders, without sitting up, move your body forward and touch your knees.

3a This exercise should only be done by very fit people, preferably under supervision. Lie on your back with your knees raised and your feet flat on the floor, arms stretched above your head.

3b Raise your trunk, stretching out your legs and swinging your arms over your head to touch your feet.

4a This exercise is also only for very fit people, preferably under supervision. Lie flat on your back with your arms stretched above your head.

4b Keeping your shoulders and arms pressed down, raise your legs and body so that your feet touch your hands.

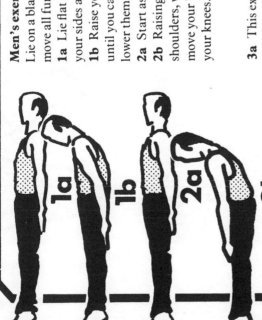

5 With your head turned to one side lie facedown, feet together and hands on your hips. Raise your head and shoulders, turning your head to the front and inhaling. Exhale as you relax.

6a Lie facedown and, keeping your arms straight, clasp your hands behind your back.
6b Raise your head and shoulders and try to make your shoulder blades meet. Relax and repeat.

7 Lie facedown with your arms stretched out sideways, palms down. Raise your head and shoulders as high as possible, bringing your arms back in line with your shoulders. Relax and repeat.

8a Lie facedown with your hands behind your head, palms down.
8b Lift your shoulders and head from the floor, bringing your shoulder blades together. Relax and repeat.

©DIAGRAM

After forty

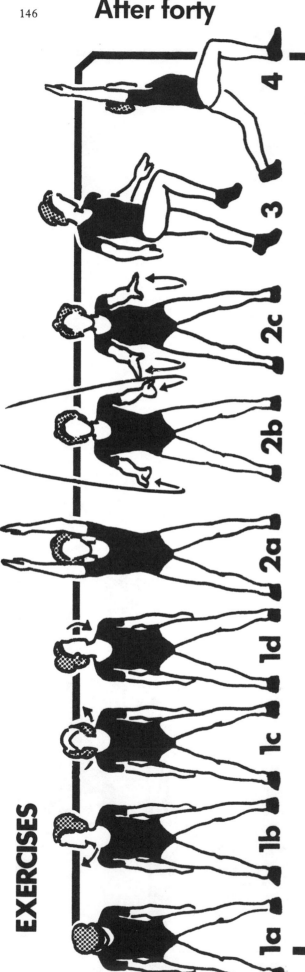

1a **1b** **1c** **1d** **2a** **2b** **2c** **3** **4**

Women's warming-up exercises
1a Stand erect, feet astride, and drop your head to rest your chin on your chest.
1b, c, d Swing your head slowly across your right shoulder, back and round to your left shoulder, then down again. Repeat in the opposite direction.

2a Stand with your feet astride and your arms above your head.
2b, c Keeping your head erect, swing your arms back and round in large circles. Repeat making forward circles.
3 Move your arms and feet vigorously as though jumping an imaginary rope.

4 With your arms above your head and your trunk kept upright, lunge forward first with your right leg and then with your left.
5a Stand with your feet astride, hands clasped slightly forward above your head.
5b, c, d Bending at the waist, lower your head, trunk and arms and swing them rhythmically in a complete circle. Repeat in the opposite direction.

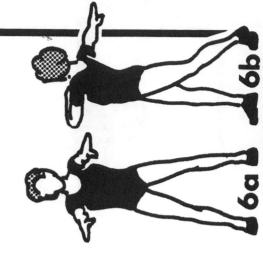

6a Stand with your feet astride, arms outstretched in front.
6b Twisting at the waist, swing your arms so that your right arm is extended behind you and your left arm is across your chest. Repeat with your left arm behind.

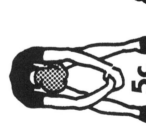 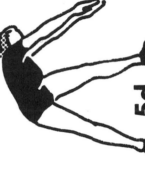

5a **5b** **5c** **5d**

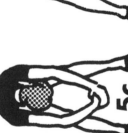 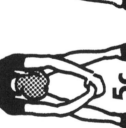 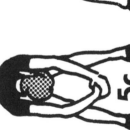 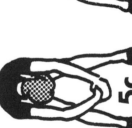

6a **6b**

EXERCISES

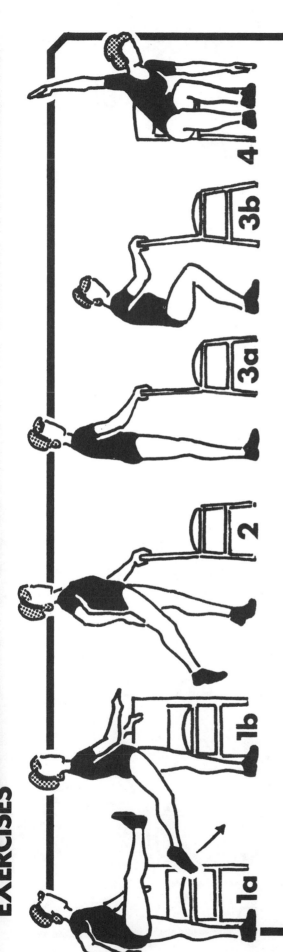

1 **3b** **3a** **2** **1b** **1a** **4**

Women's leg and waist exercises

1a, b Holding the back of a chair with your left hand, swing your right leg forward and backward several times to make full semicircles. Change hands and repeat with the other leg.

2 Holding the back of a chair, stand on tiptoe on your left foot while you kick your right leg back. Then slowly lower your foot and your leg. Repeat, changing legs.

3a Stand behind a chair, holding its back with both hands.
3b Breathing out, bend your knees until you are squatting. Then stand up straight again, breathing out.

4 Sit firmly on a chair with your arms out to the sides, then bend to the left and touch the floor, balancing carefully. Repeat to the right.

5a Raise your bottom from the floor to balance on your hands and feet, with your knees bent and your back held straight and parallel to the floor.
5b Then kick each leg in turn as high as you can, pointing your toes as you do so.

6a Stand straight with your arms behind your head.
6b Keeping your trunk upright, lunge forward onto each leg in turn.

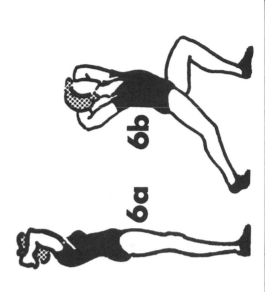

6a **6b**

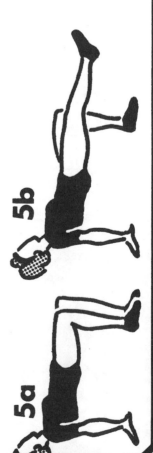

5a **5b**

© DIAGRAM

EXERCISES

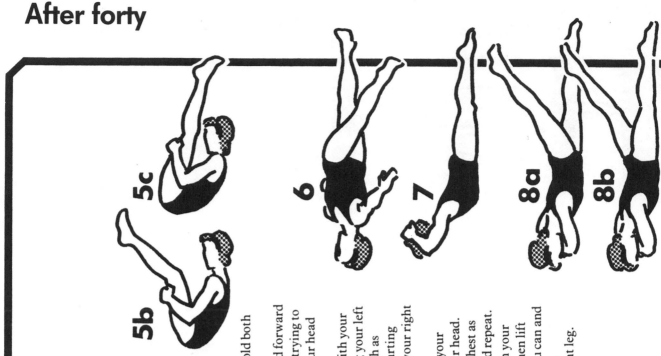

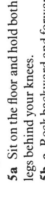

Women's exercises on the floor

1a Lie on your back with your knees bent up.

1b Clasp your hands below your left knee and draw it up to your chest. Repeat with your right leg.

2 Lie on your back with your knees bent up. Raise your left leg in the air, toes pointed, and rotate your foot several times. Repeat with your right leg.

3 Lie on your back with your arms, palms down, at your sides. Raise your left leg vertically, then lower it slowly. Repeat with your right leg.

4a, b Lie on your back with your arms at your sides and your knees raised. Starting with your head and shoulders, bend forward and touch your knees with your hands. Lower and repeat.

5a Sit on the floor and hold both legs behind your knees.

5b, c Rock backward and forward a little farther each time, trying to touch the floor behind your head with your toes.

6 Lie flat on your back with your arms outstretched. Swing your left leg over your right, as high as possible. Return to the starting position and repeat with your right leg over your left.

7 Lie on your front with your hands clasped behind your head. Lift your head and your chest as high as you can; lower and repeat.

8a Lie on your front with your hands under your chin, then lift your left leg as high as you can and swing it to make 6 circles.

8b Repeat with your right leg.

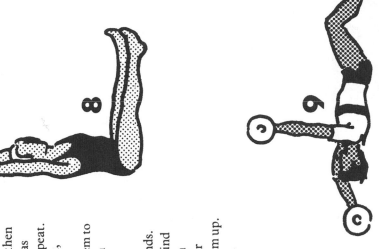

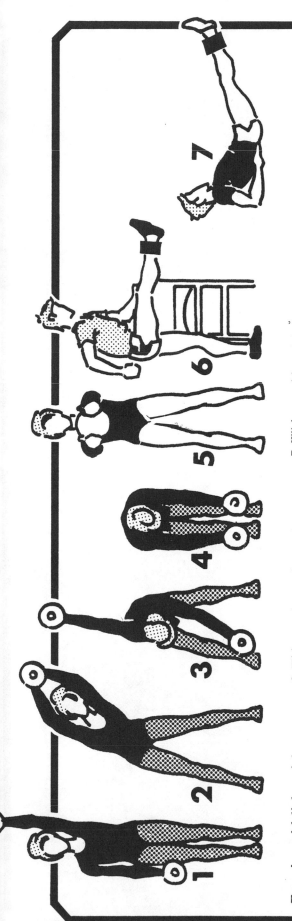

Exercises with light weights
These can be done by men and women. If you haven't any dumb-bells, use a couple of heavy magazines, tightly rolled. Start with only a few exercises at a time.
1 Stand straight with your feet together and your arms hanging so that the dumb-bells are at your thighs. Swing your left arm up and over your head, inhaling as you do so. Then exhale as you return to the starting position. Repeat with the right arm.
2 Stand with your feet astride, holding a light weight in both hands over your head. Bend your body from the waist rhythmically from side to side.

3 This exercise needs practice. Stand straight with your feet astride and the dumb-bells hanging in front of your thighs. Keeping your arms and legs straight, swing the left dumb-bell toward your right foot and the right one above your head. Repeat to the other side.
4 Stand with the dumb-bells hanging in front of your thighs. Keeping your legs straight, bend over and touch your toes. Rise again and repeat.
5 Stand with your feet astride and hold in both hands in front of you a medicine ball or some other soft object. Press hard with both hands.
6 Around your right ankle wear a strap with a light weight attached. Stand sideways with your left hand holding the back of a chair, and swing your right leg backward and forward several times. Reverse and repeat.

7 With an ankle weight on each leg, lie on your back. Raise your head and shoulders until you are supported by your forearms, then lift your straight legs as high as possible. Lower slowly and repeat.
8 Sit with your back straight, dumb-bells raised above your head. Rhythmically lower them to the floor and raise them again several times.
9 Lie on the floor, holding a dumb-bell in each of your hands. Stretch your left arm out behind your head and your right arm straight up. Then stretch your right arm out and your left arm up. Change arm positions several times.

After forty

EXERCISES

Exercising together
These exercises are specially designed for two people. Partners should be of roughly similar height and weight.

1 Stand back to back, then bend down to pass a ball between your legs.

2 Stand back to back and pass a ball over your heads.

3 Stand back to back and pass a ball round to the sides and across your fronts.

4 Stand facing each other, holding the ends of two sticks. Then pull and push each arm in turn.

5 Lie on your back with your partner holding down your feet. Then lift your head and shoulders off the ground.

6 Lie on your front and lift your head and shoulders off the ground while your partner holds down your feet.

7 Sit back to back on the floor. Holding hands above your heads, alternately push and pull your partner.

8 Sit facing each other on the floor. Hold hands and pull each other backward and forward.

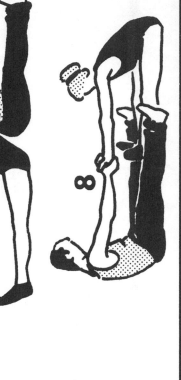

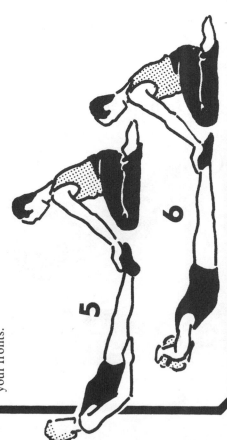

EXERCISES

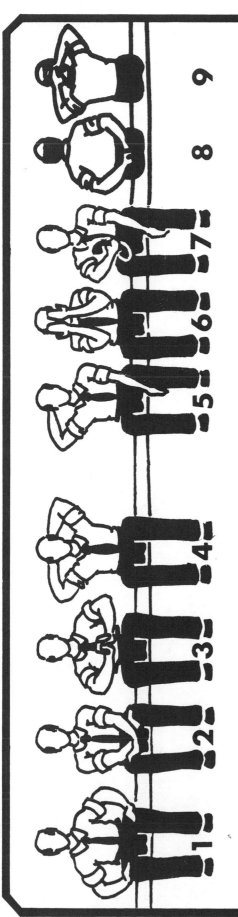

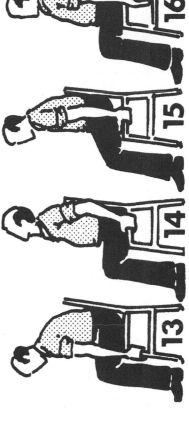

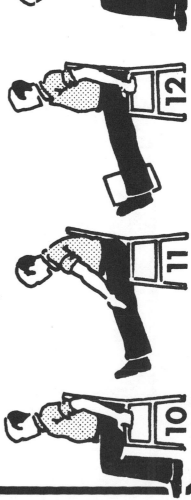

Quick exercises sitting down
Isometric exercises

These exercises take very little time, but are dangerous for anyone with heart trouble or high blood pressure. Seek medical advice before attempting them. No position should be held for longer than 6 seconds and no exercise done more than once a day. (Also see p. 226.)

1 With your hands on your knees, resist with your legs as you try to push them apart.

2 With your hands on opposite knees and your legs apart, try to push your legs together.

3 Put your palms together and push them hard.

4 Clasp your hands firmly behind your head. Resist with your hands as you push your head back.

5 Do the same with one hand.

6 Press your palms on your cheeks and try to push your head forward against them.

7 Grip a telephone receiver as tightly as you can.

8 Clasp your hands behind your back and push them together.

9 Do the same behind your neck.

10 Try to lean to one side as you resist this movement by gripping your chair seat.

11 Stretch out your legs and rest your hands on them below your knees; push up with your legs and down with your hands.

12 Stretch out your legs with a waste basket between your ankles; try to push your feet together.

13 Grip the front of your chair to provide resistance as you try to lean back.

Non-isometric exercises

14 Roll your head slowly round and round.

15 Grip the sides of your chair seat and use your arms to raise your body.

16 Sit with your arms at your sides and expand your chest to breathe really deeply.

©DIAGRAM

After forty

POSES

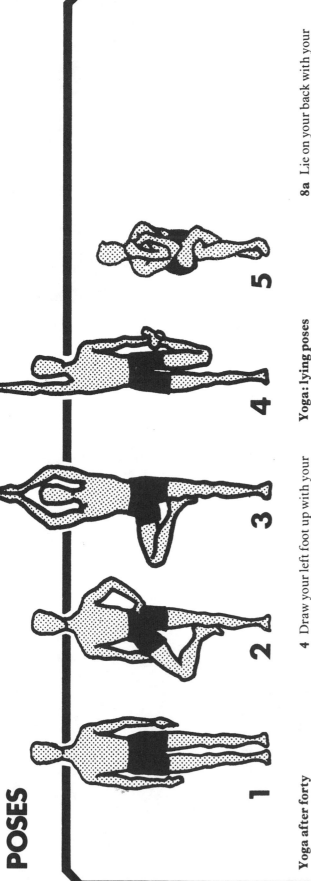

1   **2**   **3**   **4**   **5**

Yoga after forty

You don't need to be young to practice yoga — in fact, it has many advantages for people over forty as a way of toning sagging flesh and muscles and improving poor circulation. (See p. 256 for general introduction to yoga.)

Yoga: standing poses

1   Start in a relaxed stance.

2   Place the flat of your right foot against your left knee, your right hand on your thigh, and your left hand on your hip.

3   Place your right foot flat against your left inner thigh; put your hands, palms together over your head.

4   Draw your left foot up with your left hand, and hold your right hand open above your head.

5   Cross your knees in a crouching position, with your right foot tucked behind your left calf, and your right elbow resting on your upper knee. Rest your left elbow in the crook of your right arm, then cross your right arm behind the left and place your palms together, supporting your chin with both hands.

Yoga: lying poses

6a   Lie flat on your back with your hands on your hips.

6b   Roll back to rest on your head, shoulders and upper arms, with your hands supporting your hips as shown. Hold this pose as long as you can.

7   From a lying position, roll back as in 6a but this time straightening your body at the waist to bring your feet in line with your head. Shut your eyes, press your chin against your chest, and breathe deeply.

8a   Lie on your back with your arms straight on the ground behind your head.

8b   Keeping your bottom on the ground, swing your straight legs up over your body, aiming to form an angle of 45° between your body and your legs.

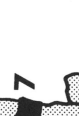
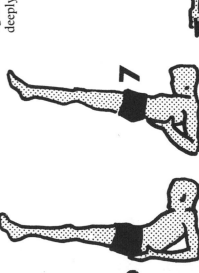

6a   **6b**   **7**

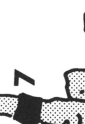
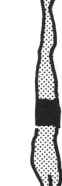

8a   **8b**

POSES

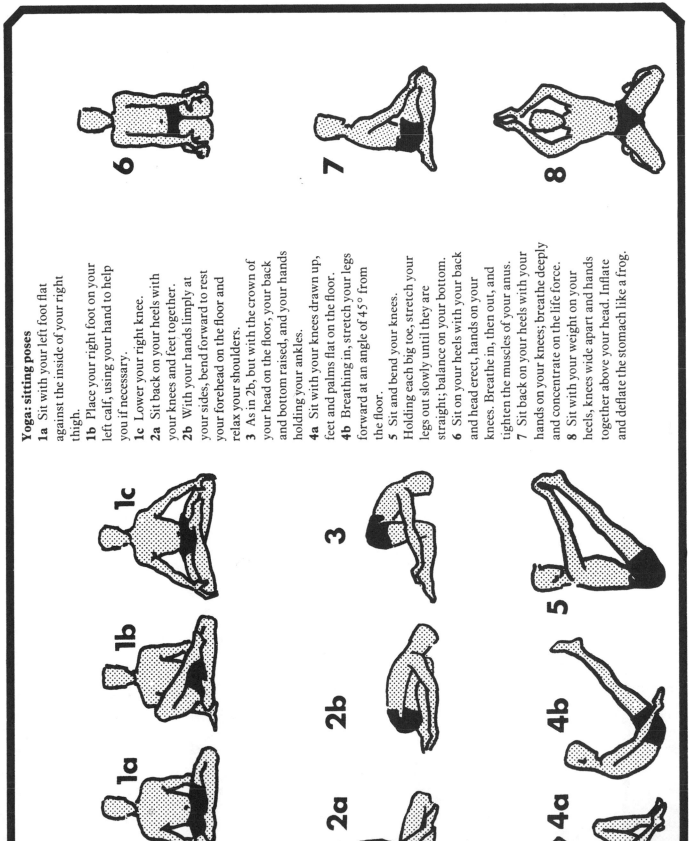

Yoga: sitting poses

1a Sit with your left foot flat against the inside of your right thigh.

1b Place your right foot on your left calf, using your hand to help you if necessary.

1c Lower your right knee.

2a Sit back on your heels with your knees and feet together.

2b With your hands limply at your sides, bend forward to rest your forehead on the floor and relax your shoulders.

3 As in 2b, but with the crown of your head on the floor, your back and bottom raised, and your hands holding your ankles.

4a Sit with your knees drawn up, feet and palms flat on the floor.

4b Breathing in, stretch your legs forward at an angle of 45° from the floor.

5 Sit and bend your knees. Holding each big toe, stretch your legs out slowly until they are straight; balance on your bottom.

6 Sit on your heels with your back and head erect, hands on your knees. Breathe in, then out, and tighten the muscles of your anus.

7 Sit back on your heels with your hands on your knees; breathe deeply and concentrate on the life force.

8 Sit with your weight on your heels, knees wide apart and hands together above your head. Inflate and deflate the stomach like a frog.

After forty

POSES

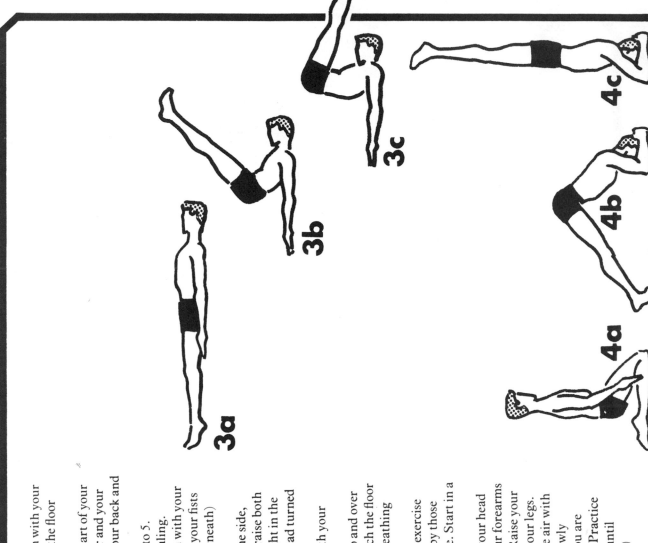

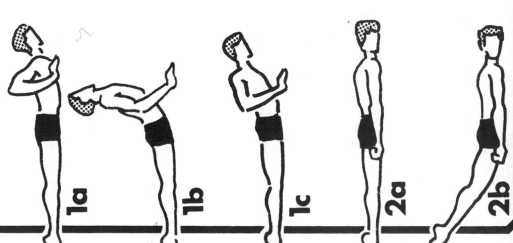

Yoga: stretching

1a Lie on your stomach with your hands, palms down, on the floor level with your chest.

1b Keeping the lower part of your body pressed to the floor and your shoulders down, arch your back and look upward.

1c Breathing in, count to 5. Return to the floor, exhaling.

2a Lie on your stomach with your arms straight down and your fists clenched (thumbs underneath) under your thighs.

2b Turn your face to one side, breathe in, and quickly raise both your legs together straight in the air. Repeat with your head turned to the other side.

3a Lie on your back with your arms at your sides.

3b, c Raise your legs up and over your head, trying to touch the floor with your toes. Hold, breathing rhythmically.

4a This is an advanced exercise and should not be done by those with high blood pressure. Start in a kneeling position.

4b Lean over and rest your head on the floor between your forearms and interlaced fingers. Raise your bottom and straighten your legs.

4c Raise your feet in the air with your knees bent, and slowly straighten out so that you are standing on your head. (Practice this pose against a wall until your balance is reliable.)

POSES

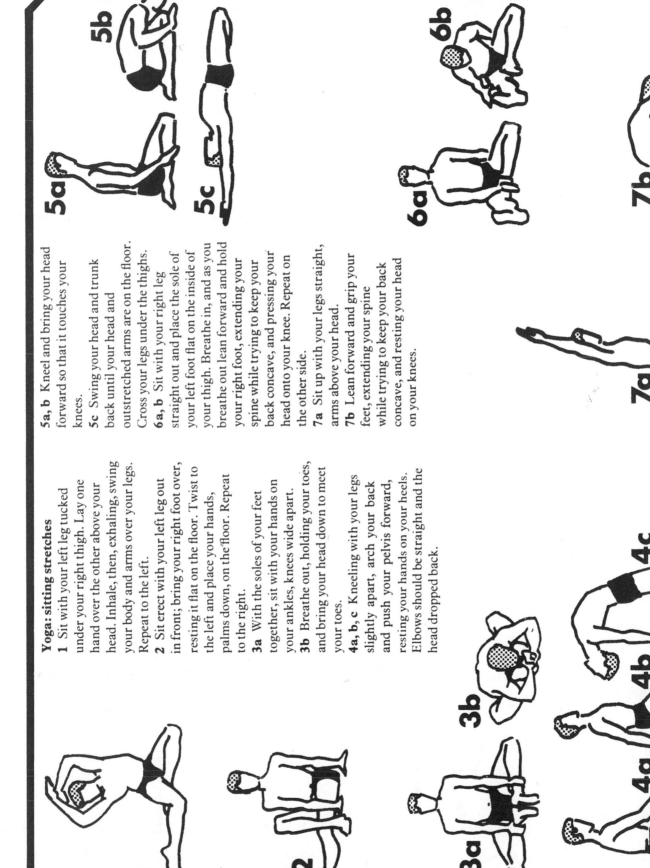

Yoga: sitting stretches

1 Sit with your left leg tucked under your right thigh. Lay one hand over the other above your head. Inhale, then, exhaling, swing your body and arms over your legs. Repeat to the left.

2 Sit erect with your left leg out in front; bring your right foot over, resting it flat on the floor. Twist to the left and place your hands, palms down, on the floor. Repeat to the right.

3a With the soles of your feet together, sit with your hands on your ankles, knees wide apart.

3b Breathe out, holding your toes, and bring your head down to meet your toes.

4a, b, c Kneeling with your legs slightly apart, arch your back and push your pelvis forward, resting your hands on your heels. Elbows should be straight and the head dropped back.

5a, b Kneel and bring your head forward so that it touches your knees.

5c Swing your head and trunk back until your head and outstretched arms are on the floor. Cross your legs under the thighs.

6a, b Sit with your right leg straight out and place the sole of your left foot flat on the inside of your thigh. Breathe in, and as you breathe out lean forward and hold your right foot, extending your spine while trying to keep your back concave, and pressing your head onto your knee. Repeat on the other side.

7a Sit up with your legs straight, arms above your head.

7b Lean forward and grip your feet, extending your spine while trying to keep your back concave, and resting your head on your knees.

AFTER SIXTY

Most of the exercises included for the over-forties can be done to the age of sixty, but increased bodily deterioration or illness will make a gentler regime advisable after sixty. Physical deterioration will now be openly perceptible: the facial bones have atrophied (wasted), teeth are missing or have been replaced by dentures, the skin of the face is wrinkled, and the hair graying or balding. Muscles have lost shape, size and strength, bones are more brittle, joints worn and stiff. Lung capacity is lowered, arteries have hardened and narrowed, and the blood pressure has probably

Bodily deterioration
The general deterioration of the body becomes outwardly evident in the over-sixties.
1 Graying or balding
2 Deterioration in eyesight
3 Atrophy of the facial bones
4 Deterioration in hearing
5 Wrinkles
6 Loss of teeth
7 Loss of upright posture
8 Sagging muscles
9 Fat deposits
10 Decrease in sexual interest
11 Stiffness and weakness in joints.
12 Unsteadiness in walking or standing.

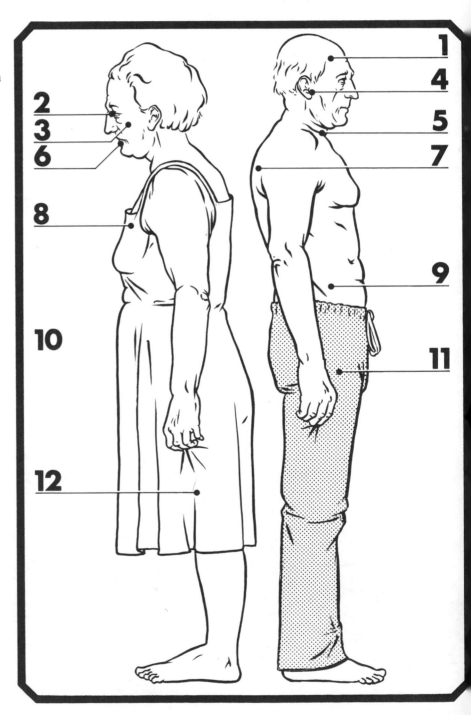

increased. The brain has lost weight while the body has gained it.

People over sixty need not feel that they are rushing into rapid decay, but they will become aware that they are slowing down generally. It takes longer to recover from even minor illnesses or wounds, and they have difficulty in remembering things. They may feel the cold more, and may lose interest in sexual activity. The process is a gradual one, however, and it has been going on for the entire adult life, so it can be accepted without the panic that the list of signs of aging might engender; also, the onset of aging can be resisted by physical and mental activity. This depends on the personality of the individual, and often the physically active over-sixties are also the mentally active. The pages that follow describe some ways in which both men and women can moderate the effects of aging by an improved appearance and a greater sense of well-being.

To derive maximum benefit from the exercises, keep to a regular program, doing your exercises at about the same time each day. Try to do them as rhythmically as possible; you will probably find that exercising to music will help with this as well as making exercise sessions more enjoyable. Stop as soon as you feel tired. Before meals is the best time to exercise; certainly not less than an hour after a meal. Make yourself comfortable by removing shoes and jacket, even pants or skirt. If you have been ill, check with your doctor before starting a course of exercises so that he can give his approval.

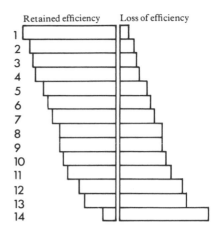

Decline in efficiency
The extent of the decline in efficiency of various parts of the body by age 75 is shown in the diagram. The different bars represent the following:
1 Body weight
2 Basal metabolic rate
3 Body water content
4 Blood flow to brain
5 Cardiac output at rest
6 Filtration rate of kidneys
7 Number of functioning nerve fibers
8 Brain weight
9 Number of functioning kidney glomeruli
10 Maximum ventilation volume
11 Kidney plasma flow
12 Maximum oxygen uptake
13 Number of taste buds
14 Return of blood acidity to equilibrium

Age	60	65	70	75	80
	28.0%	35.3%	42.8%	50.5%	58.3%

Slowing down
Everyone suffers a general slowdown as they grow older. In your mid-twenties your body is, generally, at its peak of ability. The percentages shown here demonstrate the decline in speed of a middle-distance runner. Other fitness activities decline in a similar fashion.

After sixty

EXERCISES

1a 1b 1c 1d 2a 2b 3a 3b 4a 4b 4c 5

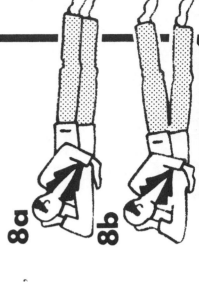

8a

8b

Exercises for feet and legs
These exercises will aid mobility and posture. Gradually increase the number each day.

1a Stand straight but relaxed.
1b Raise your heels so that you stand on your toes.
1c Rock back gently so that you stand on your heels.
1d Continue rocking to and fro.
2a Stand upright with your feet flat on the floor, then turn your toes in and heels out, raising your heels.

2b Turn your toes out and your heels in, raising your toes.
3a Stand upright, then rise up on your toes.
3b Bend your knees outward, lowering your body as if sitting; rise slowly.
4a Stand upright with your arms by your sides.
4b Bend your knees, then straighten up.
4c Raise first one knee then the other as high as possible, keeping your back straight.

5 Placing each foot flat on the ground, run slowly on the spot.
6 Sit on a chair with your right leg extended in front of you, your foot slightly off the ground. Wriggle the toes of your right foot. Repeat, changing legs.
7 Sit with one foot raised as for exercise 6. Turn your raised foot from the ankle to the right and to the left. Repeat with the other foot.
8a Lie on your right side with your head on your right hand and your left hand flat on the bed.
8b Raise your left leg a few inches, keeping it straight. Lower it.

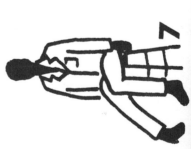

7

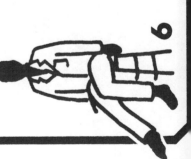

6

EXERCISES

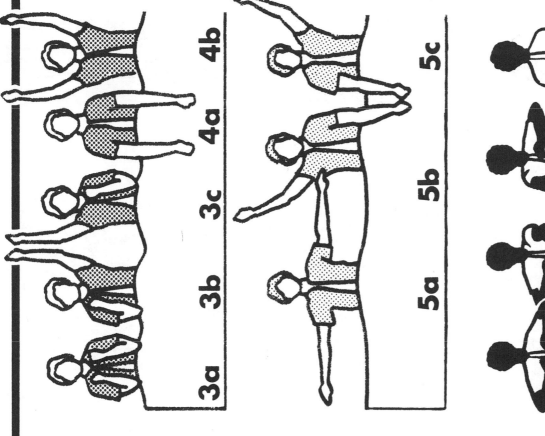

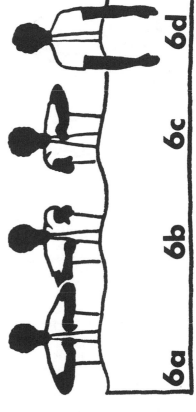

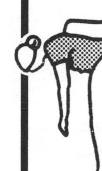

Exercises for hands and wrists

These exercises are invaluable for the bedridden, but they can be done by anyone, anywhere.

1a Stretch your arms out in front with your hands open and your palms down. (Or keep your elbows bent if you find it difficult to hold your arms straight out.)

1b Close your hands.

1c Open them with your fingers extended. Repeat several times.

2a Start as for exercise 1.

2b, c Raise your hands alternately up and down, several times.

3a Sit up straight; close your fists up against your shoulders, elbows well in.

3b Reach up with one arm, keeping the fist closed.

3c Repeat with the other arm.

4a Start with both arms resting on your thighs.

4b Reach up with both arms at the same time.

5a Sit with your arms stretched out as far as possible.

5b, c Raise one arm while lowering the other, then alternate.

6a Clench your hands and bring them up to your chest, raising your elbows to the sides.

6b Push your left arm straight out in front.

6c Repeat with your right arm.

6d Raise, and then lower both arms.

©DIAGRAM

After sixty

EXERCISES

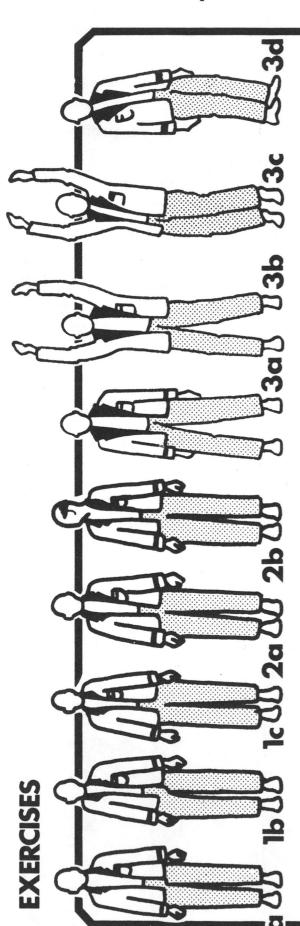

1a **1b** **1c** **2a** **2b** **3a** **3b** **3c** **3d**

Exercises for shoulders, neck and trunk

1a Stand straight with your feet together, shoulders well back and fists clenched at your sides.

1b, c Raise and lower your right shoulder, then your left.

2a Stand relaxed.

2b Turn your head to the right, then to the left. Next let it fall forward and back.

3a Stand with your feet apart, arms at your sides.

3b Raise your arms over your head.

3c Sway your hips backward and forward, keeping your knees straight as you sway.

3d When your arms get tired, put them by your sides and continue swaying your hips.

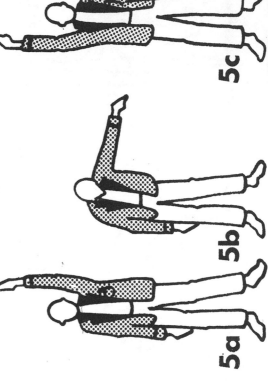

4a Stand with your legs astride, arms by your sides.

4b Bend to touch your left foot with your right hand.

4c Straighten up again.

4d Repeat, touching your right foot with your left hand.

5a Stand with your feet apart, arms at your sides. Raise your left arm above your head.

5b With straight legs bend from the waist, letting your right hand slide down the thigh.

5c Straighten up and repeat with the other arm.

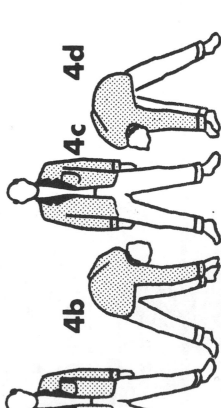

4a **4b** **4c** **4d** **5a** **5b** **5c**

EXERCISES

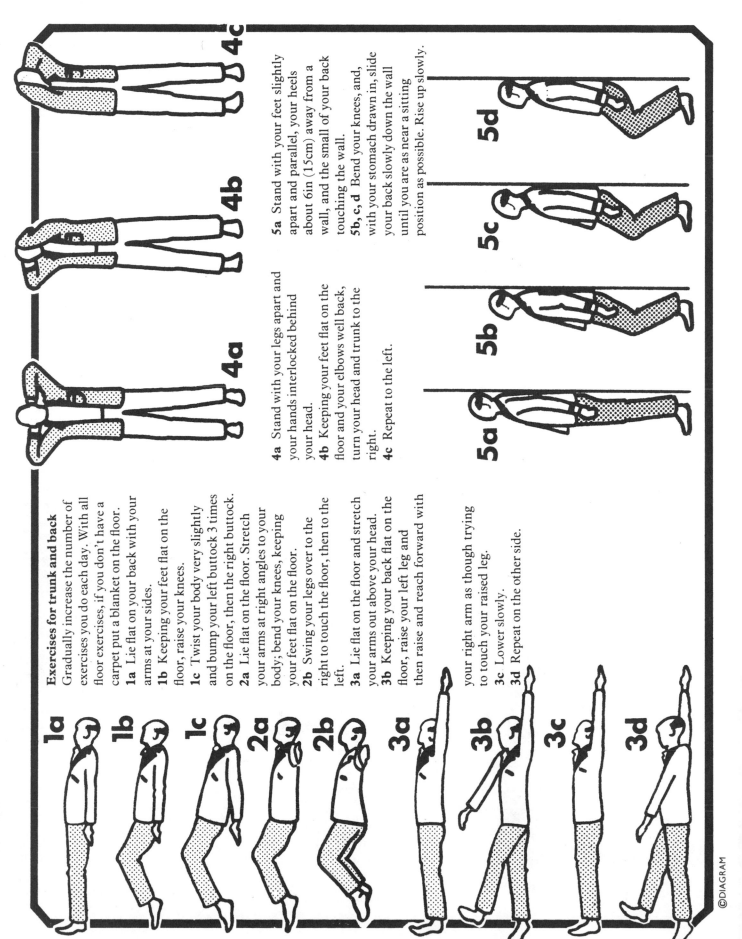

Exercises for trunk and back

Gradually increase the number of exercises you do each day. With all floor exercises, if you don't have a carpet put a blanket on the floor.

1a Lie flat on your back with your arms at your sides.

1b Keeping your feet flat on the floor, raise your knees.

1c Twist your body very slightly and bump your left buttock 3 times on the floor, then the right buttock.

2a Lie flat on the floor. Stretch your arms at right angles to your body; bend your knees, keeping your feet flat on the floor.

2b Swing your legs over to the right to touch the floor, then to the left.

3a Lie flat on the floor and stretch your arms out above your head.

3b Keeping your back flat on the floor, raise your left leg and then raise and reach forward with your right arm as though trying to touch your raised leg.

3c Lower slowly.

3d Repeat on the other side.

4a Stand with your legs apart and your hands interlocked behind your head.

4b Keeping your feet flat on the floor and your elbows well back, turn your head and trunk to the right.

4c Repeat to the left.

5a Stand with your feet slightly apart and parallel, your heels about 6in (15cm) away from a wall, and the small of your back touching the wall.

5b, c, d Bend your knees, and, with your stomach drawn in, slide your back slowly down the wall until you are as near a sitting position as possible. Rise up slowly.

©DIAGRAM

Chapter 5 PARTNERS AND EQUIPMENT

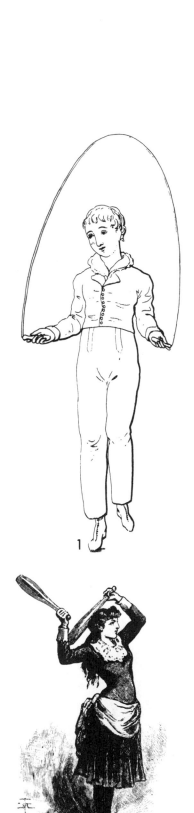

1

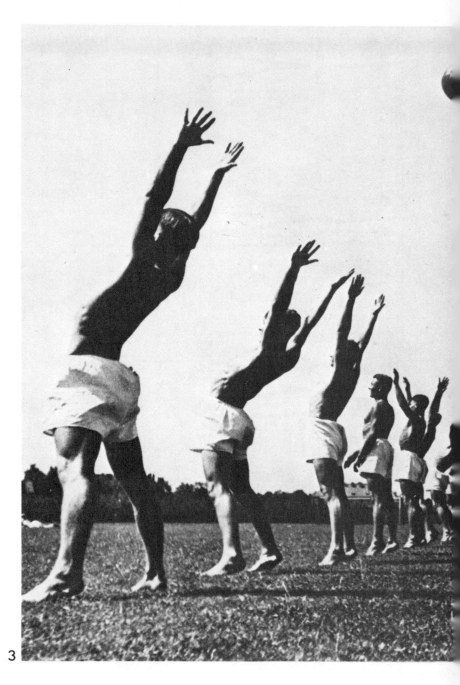

3

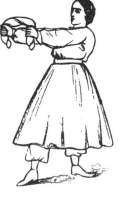

2

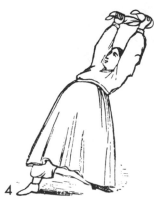

4

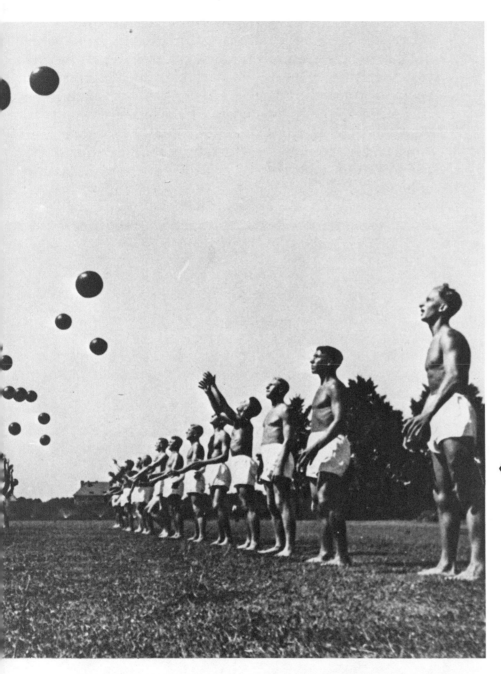

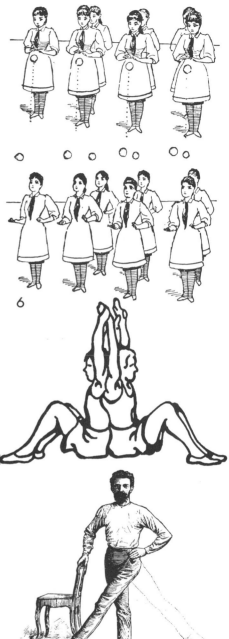

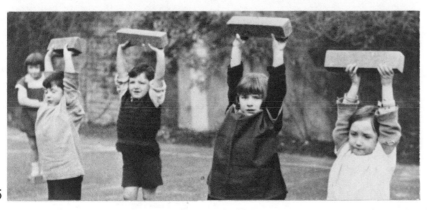

1 *Gymnastic Exercises* Capt. P. H. Clias (London 1825)
2 *The Family Magazine* (London 1890)
3 German soldiers at morning training, 1930s (The Mansell Collection)
4 *The New Gymnastics* by Dio Lewis (London 1866)
5 Schoolyard exercises (Radio Times Hulton Picture Library)
6 *Healthful Exercises for Girls* by A. Alexander (London 1902)
7 *Home Gymnastics for the Well and the Sick* by E. Angerstein (USA 1889)

EXERCISING TOGETHER

Exercising with other people has numerous advantages. Some people are temperamentally unsuited to an individual exercise program; exercising alone can easily result for them in feelings of loneliness, boredom and lack of progress. Even people who generally enjoy exercising alone are likely to benefit from varying their routine to include exercising with others. Some people find that the best answer for them is to join a regular keep-fit class; for others, the ideal solution is to find a partner and embark on a joint program of exercises at home.

Exercises for two
In the exercise illustrated here both partners are benefiting, but in different ways. One partner is developing his strength and balance by taking the other on his back. The other is exercising her stomach muscles with a variation of the basic leg-lift exercise.

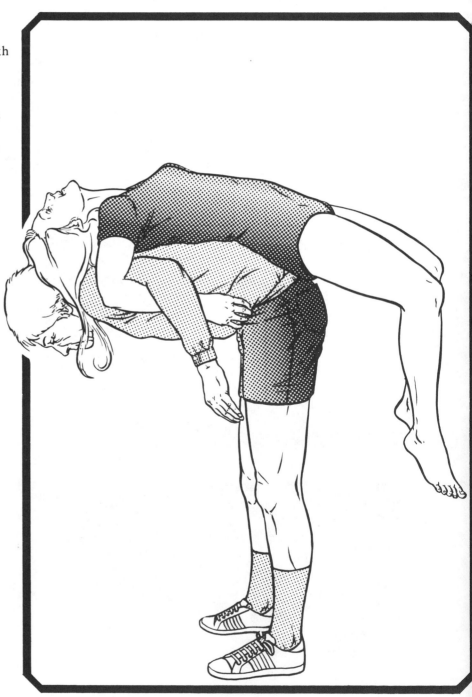

By sharing in an exercise program, you and your partner can benefit in many ways. Both of you can increase your fitness while enjoying the pleasures of physical and mental togetherness. Exercising with a partner can be tremendous fun, but try not to laugh too much and ruin your concentration! If you are enjoying your exercise program, and if you make a joint commitment to set aside certain times for exercising together, you are more likely to succeed in your fitness aims. An exercise partner can provide valuable encouragement, and help you by suggesting ways in which you can improve your performance. Many people also find that an element of competition helps spur them on to make an extra effort; but be careful not to overdo things in trying to compete with a partner who is fitter than you are. Some people find that exercising with a friend helps them overcome inhibitions and embarrassment about their body; this may be particularly helpful to the figure-conscious.

When exercising with a partner you can do many of the individual exercises included elsewhere in this book. Try facing each other and synchronizing your movements as though you were looking in a mirror. Included in the next few pages, however, is a selection of exercises designed specifically for two people. They are arranged according to position — standing, sitting, and lying down — but you can combine them in any way you like to make up your own joint program.

In some exercises for two, one of the partners acts almost like a piece of equipment, supporting his partner or holding one part of his partner's body while the partner exercises some other part. In other exercises, both partners benefit equally through performing similar actions together. In yet others, the partners perform different actions but each one benefits in a different way; this is true of many of the isometric exercises in which one partner provides resistance to a force exerted by the other.

Whenever you and your partner have a different role to play in a particular exercise you should always repeat the exercise and reverse roles so that you both obtain maximum benefit. Obviously you will have to take into consideration any great differences in physical capabilities between you and your partner, but learning to adapt the exercises or to control your own actions to suit the capabilities of your partner can increase your rewards by helping you find a new physical and mental harmony that will enrich your whole relationship.

©DIAGRAM

Exercising together

EXERCISES

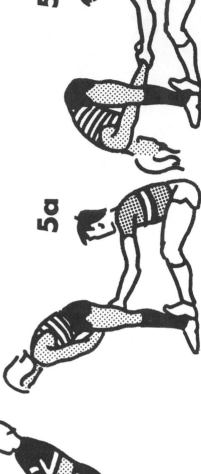

Standing exercises
Repeat each of these exercises, reversing your roles.

1a Stand facing your partner, about 15in (40cm) apart. Raise your arms out to the sides, and get your partner to place his hands behind your upper arms. Then pull your arms back against his hands as he resists.

1b Get your partner to push against the front of your arms while you try to move them forward against his pressure.

2 Stand side by side, facing forward, with your feet apart. Clasp hands as shown. Bend your right knee and lean to the right. Your partner must keep both feet on the ground as you pull him with you, stretching his left side. Repeat the exercise with your partner pulling you to the left.

3 Face your partner and hold his hands. Adopt a crouching position while your partner remains standing. Stretch your arms and keep your backs straight as each of you leans slightly backward to balance the other.

4a Face your partner, hold his hands, and stand with your feet placed between his. Keeping your backs straight, both of you should then lean backward until your arms are fully extended.

4b Continuing to balance each other and, keeping your backs straight, sink to a squatting position while your partner remains standing. Then slowly stand up again.

5a Ask your partner to sit behind you, holding hands between your legs as shown.

5b Keep your legs straight, and bend at the waist as he slowly pulls your hands back.

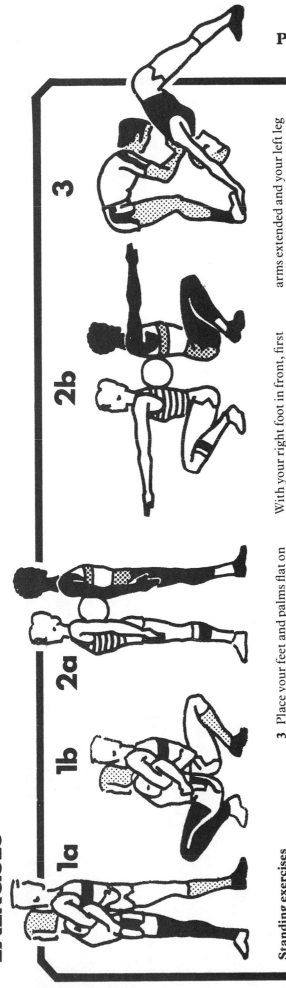

3

2b

2a

1b

1a

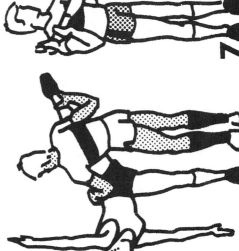

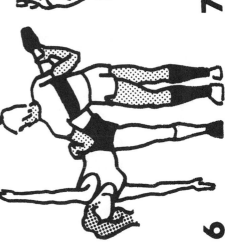

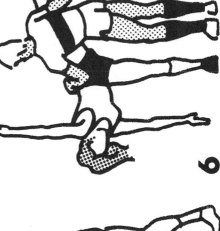

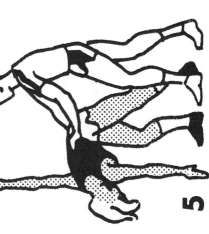

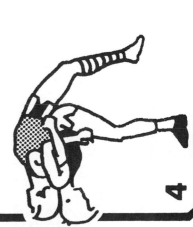

Standing exercises
Reverse roles where appropriate.
1a Stand with your backs together and your elbows linked.
1b Pressing back against each other, both sink slowly into a squatting position and then stand up again.
2a Stand back to back, holding a large ball between you as shown.
2b Both stretch your arms forward and, without letting the ball fall, sink to a squatting position and then stand up again.

3 Place your feet and palms flat on the floor and bend into an inverted V-shape. Your partner should then tread lightly on your fingers and slowly lean his weight against your back.
4 Stand back to back with your elbows linked. Lean forward to lift your partner off the ground.
5 Get your partner to support you by holding your hips from behind.

With your right foot in front, first lean over until your body is parallel with the ground. Then touch the ground with your left hand, stretch your right arm up, and twist your body to look at your right hand. Get your partner to help by pushing your left hip and pulling your right hip. Repeat to the other side.
6 Lean to the right, with your arms extended and your left leg raised. Get your partner to lean gently on your hip with one hand and to raise your left leg higher with the other. Repeat to the other side.
7 Stand about 1ft (30cm) from a wall, with your forearms against it. Raise your left leg and get your partner to pull it still higher. Repeat with your other leg.

7

6

5

4

©DIAGRAM

Exercising together

EXERCISES

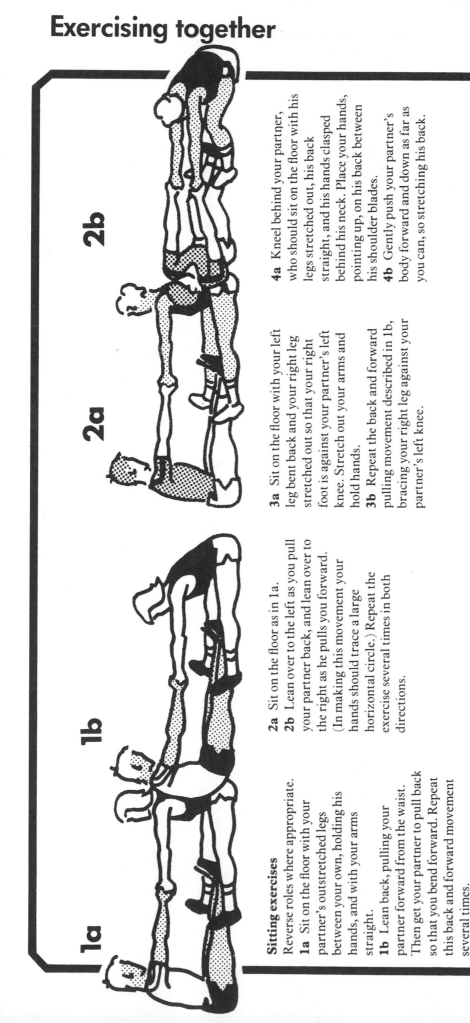

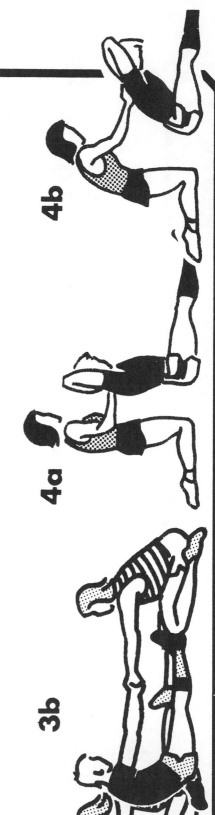

Sitting exercises

Reverse roles where appropriate.

1a Sit on the floor with your partner's outstretched legs between your own, holding his hands, and with your arms straight.

1b Lean back, pulling your partner forward from the waist. Then get your partner to pull back so that you bend forward. Repeat this back and forward movement several times.

2a Sit on the floor as in 1a.

2b Lean over to the left as you pull your partner back, and lean over to the right as he pulls you forward. (In making this movement your hands should trace a large horizontal circle.) Repeat the exercise several times in both directions.

3a Sit on the floor with your left leg bent back and your right leg stretched out so that your right foot is against your partner's left knee. Stretch out your arms and hold hands.

3b Repeat the back and forward pulling movement described in 1b, bracing your right leg against your partner's left knee.

4a Kneel behind your partner, who should sit on the floor with his legs stretched out, his back straight, and his hands clasped behind his neck. Place your hands, pointing up, on his back between his shoulder blades.

4b Gently push your partner's body forward and down as far as you can, so stretching his back.

EXERCISES

Crouching/sitting exercises
Reverse roles where appropriate.
1 Crouch down facing your partner. Grasp his arms at the elbows and get him to grasp yours. Then both lean back, with your feet flat on the ground and your bottoms kept off the ground.

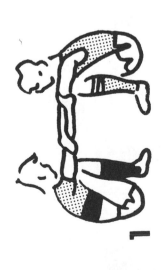

2 Get your partner to kneel down and bend forward until his forehead touches the floor, and then to raise his arms behind him. Straddle his body and sit on it gently, as far back as you can. Take hold of his wrists and slowly and gently lift his arms and push them forward.

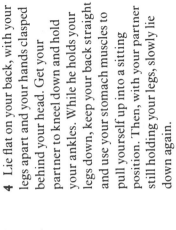

3a Lie on your back with your knees raised, your feet flat on the ground and your hands clasped behind your head. Get your partner to sit gently on your feet, taking some of his weight on his hands, and to lean back slightly against your legs.
3b Your partner should stay in this position while you use your stomach muscles to pull yourself up into a sitting position. Then bend farther forward until your elbows touch your knees.

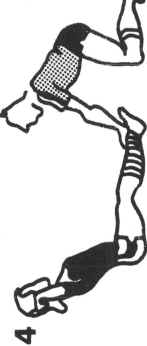

4 Lie flat on your back, with your legs apart and your hands clasped behind your head. Get your partner to kneel down and hold your ankles. While he holds your legs down, keep your back straight and use your stomach muscles to pull yourself up into a sitting position. Then, with your partner still holding your legs, slowly lie down again.

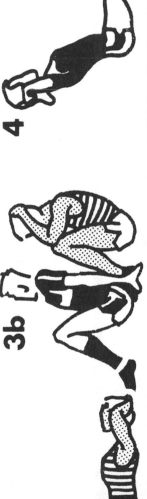

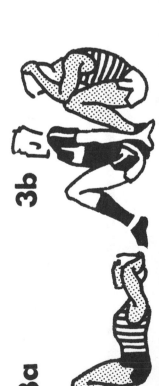

©DIAGRAM

Exercising together

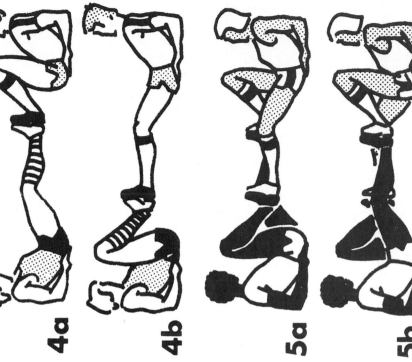

4a From a sitting position lean back onto your elbows. Get your partner to face you in the same position. Raise your feet and place your soles against those of your partner. Now extend your legs to push back your partner's legs as he gently resists you.

4b Your partner should then extend his legs to push back your legs as you resist him. Repeat this back and forward movement.

5a, b This exercise is similar to exercise 4 but this time move your right and left legs independently. Extend one leg to push back your partner's leg, while he extends his other leg to push back yours. Alternate your leg positions back and forward for perhaps 1 minute or more.

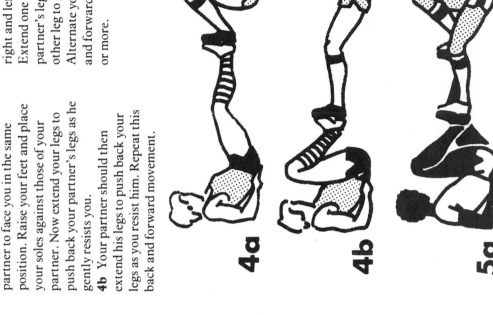

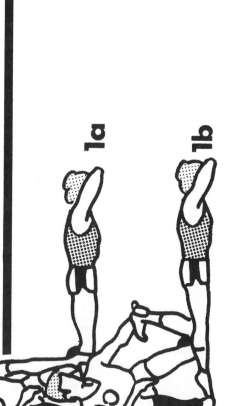

Lying down exercises
Reverse roles in exercises 1–3.
1a Lie on your front with your head on your hands. Get your partner to hold the heel of your left foot in one hand.

1b Your partner should then push against your heel as you bend your knee and raise your foot against his pressure. Then repeat with your other foot.

2 Lie on your back with your arms stretched out to the sides. Keeping your legs straight, raise your feet off the ground. Then get your partner to pull your feet toward him as you try to raise your feet still higher.

3 Lie on your back with your arms stretched behind your head. Get your partner to stand astride you and push down on your upper arms as you try to raise them.

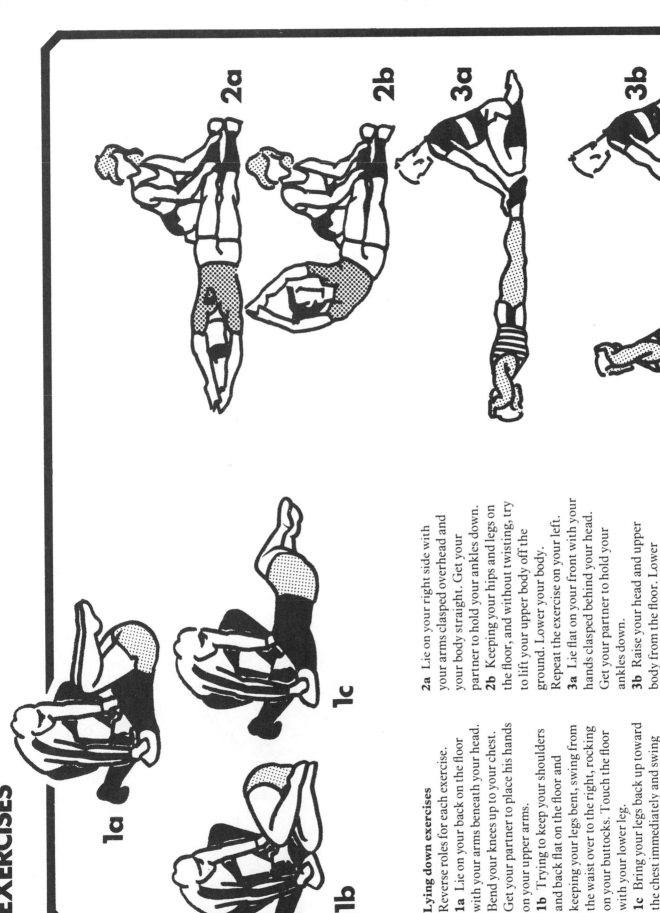

EXERCISES

Lying down exercises
Reverse roles for each exercise.
1a Lie on your back on the floor with your arms beneath your head. Bend your knees up to your chest. Get your partner to place his hands on your upper arms.
1b Trying to keep your shoulders and back flat on the floor and keeping your legs bent, swing from the waist over to the right, rocking on your buttocks. Touch the floor with your lower leg.
1c Bring your legs back up toward the chest immediately and swing them over to touch the floor on the left.
Repeat the rocking movement.

2a Lie on your right side with your arms clasped overhead and your body straight. Get your partner to hold your ankles down.
2b Keeping your hips and legs on the floor, and without twisting, try to lift your upper body off the ground. Lower your body.
Repeat the exercise on your left.
3a Lie flat on your front with your hands clasped behind your head. Get your partner to hold your ankles down.
3b Raise your head and upper body from the floor. Lower yourself slowly.
Repeat the exercise.

©DIAGRAM

SIMPLE EQUIPMENT

The use of equipment when exercising has two important advantages: it adds variety to an exercise program, and it makes particular exercises more efficient. A wide range of fitness machines is available in gyms or for home use (see page 197) but many exercises do not require expensive and complicated equipment. The following pages demonstrate how you can build up a complete exercise program at home or at work, using simple domestic equipment and other commonly available items.

Equipment is useful for exercising because it increases the

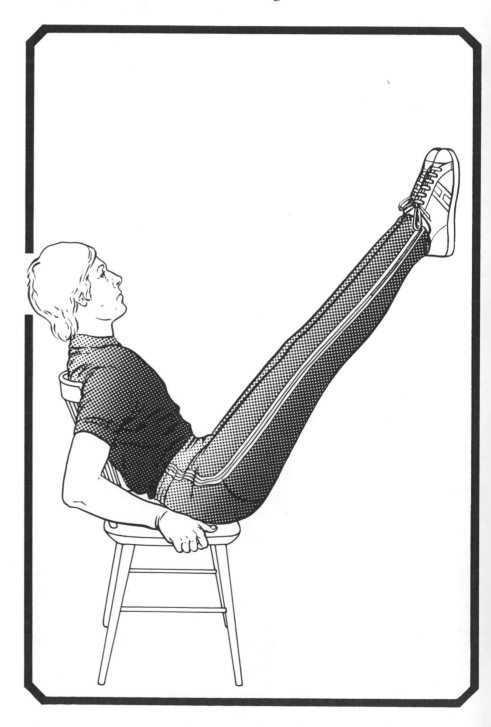

work done by your muscles, by offering resistance or opposition against which they can pull or brace themselves. Among the common household things you can use in this way are walls, stairs, chairs, tables, bureaus and even broom-handles! You can also use simple games equipment like beach balls, hula-hoops or skipping ropes. Exercises run in fashions; in the mid-nineteenth century Indian clubs were very popular, in the 1920s boxing gloves were widely used, and the hula-hoop was all the rage in the 1950s.

The main advantages of the equipment described here are that it is easily available and can be used whenever it is most convenient; at home, in the open air, or at work. It is ideal for the businessman or the busy housewife.

If you can, set aside a specific time for your exercises, and do them regularly, allowing a few minutes to relax afterward; wear simple, loose-fitting clothing, or a leotard or swimming-trunks. If this is not possible, just a few minutes exercising in the office, or even in your car, can help to keep you fit. Try to make exercise enjoyable; some of our examples are ideal for the beach — why not get your friends to join in too!

Remember that some of the equipment included here is not specifically designed for exercising, so you must always pay particular attention to safety. Give yourself a clear space and plenty of room. Make sure that the objects you use have no sharp edges or protruding corners and that they are strong and secure, unlikely to fall over or collapse. See that the floor is not slippery or uneven. Remember your aim is to be fit — so look after yourself!

EXERCISES

Exercises on a mat
These exercises can all be done on a mat, or just on the floor. Make sure you allow yourself plenty of room.

1a Lie on your back and point your toes, keeping your arms by your sides, palms up.

1b Bend your left knee as high as possible to your chest, keeping your right leg flat. Then repeat the exercise, bending the right leg. This exercise can be varied by raising both legs together and lowering them as slowly as possible.

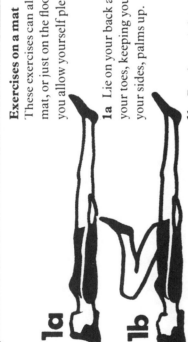

2a Lie on your right side, supporting your head on your right hand, with the other palm placed on the floor in front of you. Keep your legs together.

2b Keeping your body still, raise your left leg as high as you can. Make sure that you do not lean forward or back. Then repeat the exercise 10 times for each leg.

3a Lie flat on your back with your arms by your sides.

3b Keeping your body flat on the floor, raise your left leg and stretch it across to the right as far as possible. Then repeat this with the right leg.

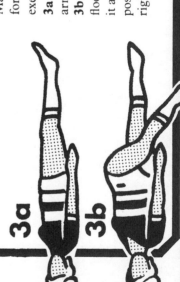

4a Lie flat on your back with your feet together, and extend your arms behind your head.

4b Keeping your legs straight and your heels on the mat, sit up and stretch forward until you can touch your toes.

5a Lie flat on your back with your arms extended behind your head.

5b Swing your legs upward and lean forward into a "jack-knife" position, reaching for your ankles and balancing on your hips.

6a The basic push-up. Lie flat on the floor with your face down, keeping your body straight. Place both hands on the floor at shoulder level, palms down with your elbows bent.

6b Breathing in as you push up, straighten both arms and raise your body, keeping it rigid. Lower your body, breathing out as you go down. Repeat up to 20 times.

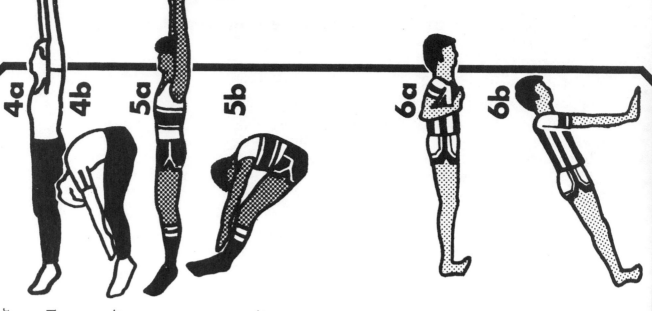

EXERCISES

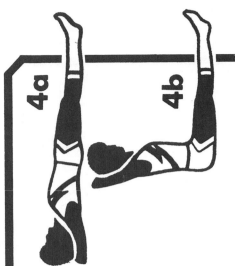

4a

4b

5

6b

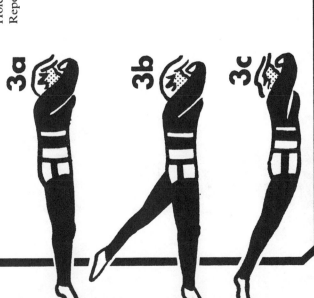

6a

Exercises on a mat

1 Lie on your back and swing your legs into the air, keeping your bottom on the ground. Then make large cycling movements with your legs.

2 For a more advanced cycling exercise, raise your bottom off the ground to support yourself as shown, with your hands under your hips.

3a Lie on your front with your legs together and your forehead resting on the backs of your hands.

3b Slowly raise your left leg as far as possible and then lower it again. Repeat with your right leg.

3c Finally raise both legs together and at the same time lift your head, keeping your hands on your forehead and your elbows well up. Hold this position for a count of 4. Repeat the exercise 5–10 times.

4 Lie flat on your back with your feet together and both hands behind your neck. Then raise your body to a sitting position.

5 Sit on the floor with your knees bent and your hands behind your neck. Then twist your body to touch your right knee with your left elbow. Then touch your left knee with your right elbow.

6a Sit on the floor with your legs apart and your arms outstretched to each side.

6b Twist and bend your body to touch your left foot with your right hand.

1

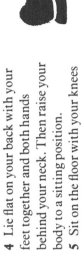

2

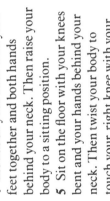

3a

3b

3c

Simple equipment

EXERCISES

Chair exercises

Choose a stout chair with no rough edges. Make sure it stands firmly and that the floor is not slippery. Exercises 1–4 are particularly good for older and overweight people. They can easily be done in a confined space.

1 Sit down, and then bring your head down and forward. Bending one knee for support, bring the other up to touch your forehead. Repeat 10 times. (This exercise mobilizes the spine and hip joints.)

2 Sit with your legs wide apart and your hands on your hips. Bend your head at a right angle to your body and move it alternately to the right and left. Repeat 10 times.

3 Sit as in exercise 2. Bending from the waist, slide your hands down one leg as far as the ankle. Repeat 10 times for each leg.

4a This exercise is also good for younger women. Sitting well back on a straight chair, raise your right buttock. Hold for a count of 4 and then lower it.

4b Repeat with the left buttock, and then raise alternate buttocks.

5a Stand with your back to the chair.

5b Sit down lightly. Repeat rapidly 30–40 times.

6a Mounting a chair often forms part of fitness tests. Stand about 1ft (30cm) in front of the chair and step up onto it.

6b Dismount backward. Repeat 15 times with each foot.

7a Stand 18in (45cm) behind a chair and rest your hands on the back.

7b Bend to a squatting position, then rise onto your toes. (This is like the bar exercises used by ballet dancers.)

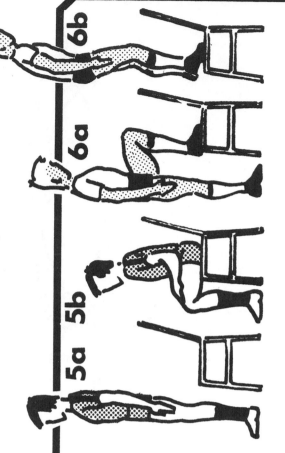

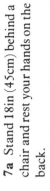

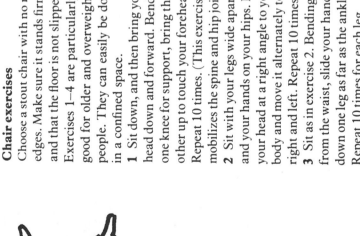

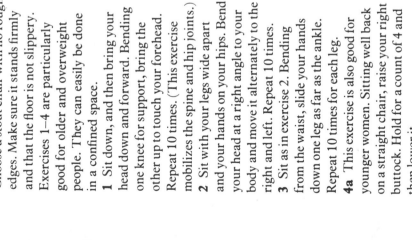

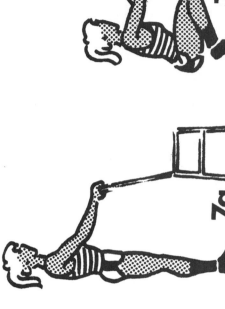

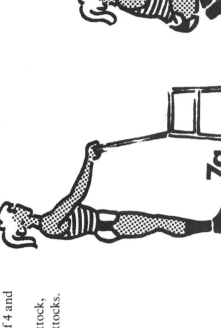

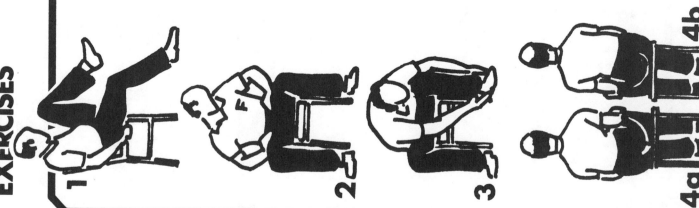

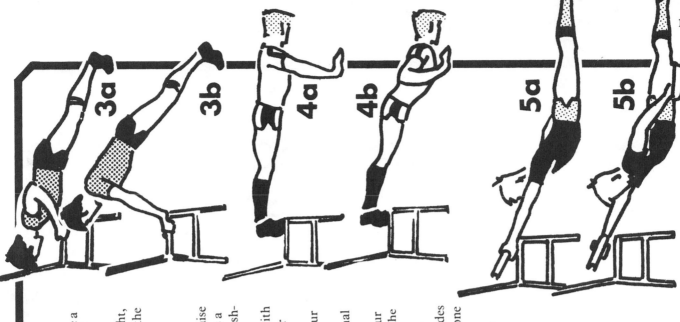

3a **3b** **4a** **4b** **5a** **5b**

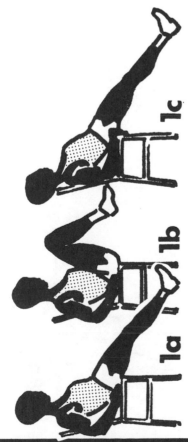

1a **1b** **1c**

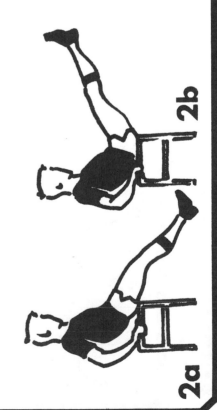

2a **2b**

Chair exercises

1a Sit at the front of the chair. Gripping the sides firmly, lean back with your legs out.

1b Bending your knees, bring your thighs up to your body. Hold this position. (Try gripping a cushion between your thighs and stomach.)

1c Stretch out to full length.

2a Sit as in 5a.

2b Keeping your legs straight, raise them above waist level, breathing in. Then lower them slowly and breathe out. Repeat the exercise.

More strenuous exercises

These exercises are designed for more athletic people. Always use a strong, steady chair.

3a Face the chair and grip the edges. Keeping your body straight, move your feet back away from the chair. Breathing out, bend your arms and lower your body until your chest touches the chair.

3b Straighten your arms and raise your body, breathing in. (This is a variation of the conventional push-up.)

4a Adopt the position shown, with your hands on the floor and your feet on a chair.

4b Bend your arms, keeping your body straight. Then straighten your arms to return to the original position. Repeat 3–5 times.
As an alternative, "walk" on your hands as far as you can around the chair in each direction.

5a Lie facedown in front of the chair, with your arms by your sides and a book in each hand. Place one book on the chair, remove it.

5b Repeat with the other book. Do the exercise 30 times, using alternate arms.

©DIAGRAM

Simple equipment

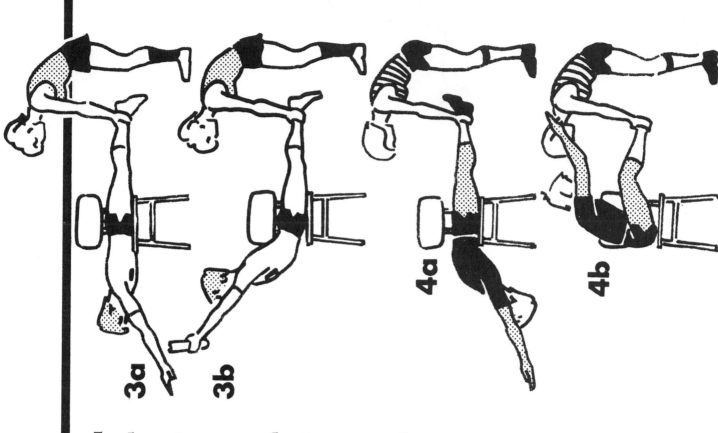

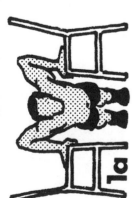

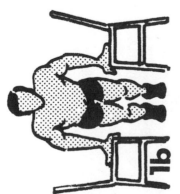

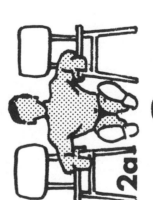

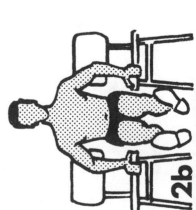

More complex chair exercises
For some of these exercises you will need two chairs. Ensure that they are strong and standing firmly on a non-slippery surface.

1a For this exercise you need two chairs facing each other. Place one hand on the seat of each chair and support yourself on your hands and toes. Move your feet back and straighten your body, then bend your arms to lower your body.

1b Straighten your arms and push up, raising your body.

2a Brace two chairs against a wall and sit between them, with your forearms and hands on the seats.

2b Push up with your arms, straightening your body and bringing your hips forward.

3a You will need a partner for this exercise. Lie on your stomach over a chair and get your partner to hold your legs. Then lean forward to grasp a book at arm's length on the floor.

3b Lift the book, raising your body as far as you can.

4a Lie backward over a chair. With your partner holding your legs stretch your arms back.

4b Sit up and lean forward until your head touches your knees (or stretch as far as you can).

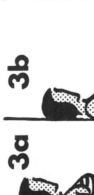

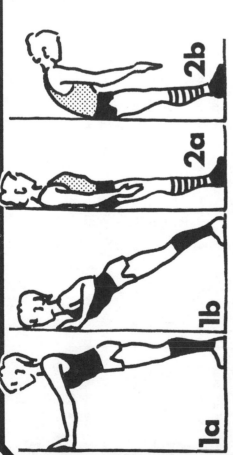

4a Tuck both feet under a bureau and lie back, stretching your arms above your head.

4b Pulling with your stomach muscles, swing your body up and breathe in. Touch your ankles with both hands and then lie back slowly, breathing out.

5a Rest your heels on the edge of a drawer or low table and lie back with your arms stretched above your head.

5b Pull up and lean forward from the waist until you touch your ankles with both hands.

6 Rest your hands about 1ft (30cm) apart on a firm table. Move your feet back and lean forward, keeping your body straight. Then bend your arms and lower your body, breathing out as you go down. Straighten your arms and push up, breathing in as you rise.

Exercises with a bureau or table
Make sure that any item of furniture is strong and securely fixed. Also see that the floor is not slippery.

Exercises using a wall
Again make sure that you do not slip on the floor.

1a This wall pushing exercise is designed to strengthen the arms and shoulders. Stand facing the wall about 3ft (90cm) away. Stretch out your arms at shoulder height, palms toward the wall. Keeping your body straight, fall forward to touch the wall with your hands.

1b Bend your arms until your head touches the wall. Then straighten them and push away from the wall to stand upright. Repeat 10–20 times.

2a Stand with your back to the wall and your feet about 6in (15cm) away from it.

2b Breathing out, flop forward from the hips, letting your head and arms hang freely. Then, breathing in, straighten up slowly and press your spine against the wall.

3a Brace your back against the wall. Keeping your feet flat on the ground, slide your back down the wall until your thighs are parallel to the ground.

3b Without shifting your body position, raise your heels as high as you can and stay on your toes for 6 seconds.

Simple equipment

EXERCISES

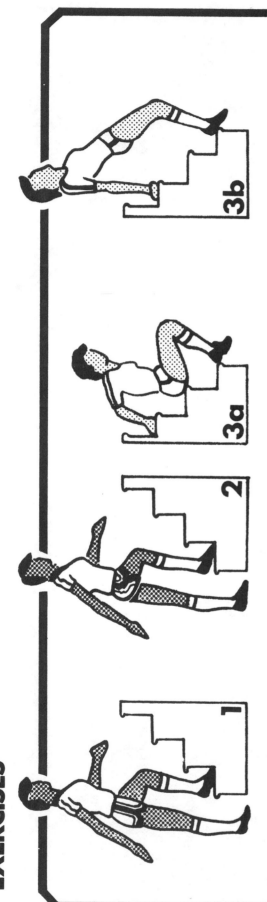

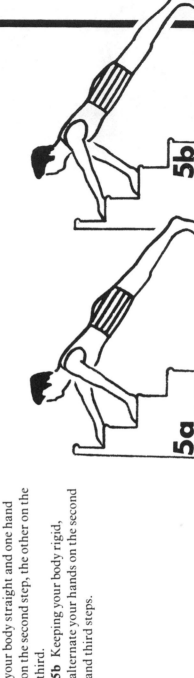

Exercises on the stairs

Climbing the stairs is a good indication of general fitness; the effect of this activity is also very useful to physicians making heart tests. The exercises included here are to be done on an ordinary straight flight of stairs. If there is a carpet make sure that it is securely fixed. Take care that you do not slip when coming down. Remember, you are aiming for fitness not a broken ankle!

1 Run up and down the stairs as many times as you can.

As a variation you can run up leaving out every other step, but use them all to come down.

2 Stand with one foot on the ground and the other on the bottom step. Jump up slightly and quickly exchange the positions of your feet. Repeat up to 20 times.

3a Sit on one step with your feet on the step below and your hands on the step above you.

3b Push your hips forward and straighten your arms so that your body forms a straight line from the knees.

4a Sit on one step with your feet on the step below and your arms straight in front of you.

4b Straighten your legs, and then bend them again without touching the step.

5a Adopt the position shown, with your body straight and one hand on the second step, the other on the third.

5b Keeping your body rigid, alternate your hands on the second and third steps.

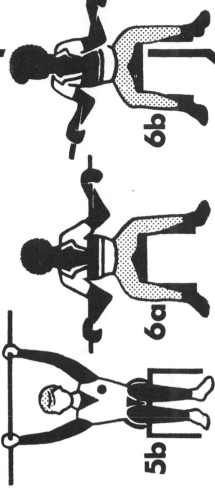

1a **1b** **1c**

2a **2b**

3a **3b**

Exercises with a stick

For these exercises you need a strong, light stick about 4ft (1.2m) long. A household broom-handle is ideal.

1a Grip the stick with both hands at arm's length above your head. Then bring it forward and down to rest across your thighs.

1b Swing it up above your head.

1c Bring the stick down across your buttocks.

2a Stand erect, holding the stick so that it passes along your shoulders, behind the neck.

2b Raise your left leg as high as you can, keeping it straight as shown. Repeat 8 times for each leg.

3a Stand as in exercise 2a.

3b Keeping your back and legs straight and your feet flat on the floor, slowly bend forward and exhale. Then straighten up and inhale.

4a Stand erect, holding the stick behind your thighs.

4b Bend your legs to squat on your toes, keeping your back straight and exhaling as you sink down. Inhale as you rise.

5a Sit on a low stool or bench, with the stick across your back.

5b Keeping your body straight, raise your arms behind your head. Then lower them again.

6a Sit firmly astride a stool. Place the stick behind your shoulder blades, resting in your elbow crooks.

6b Keeping your hips still, twist your trunk from the waist up to the right and to the left. Repeat 12 times.

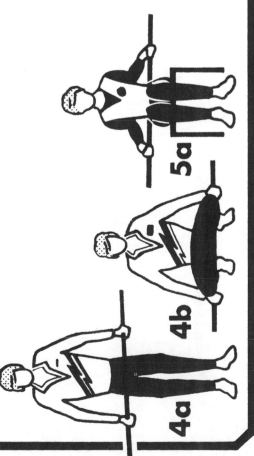

4a **4b**

5a **5b**

6a **6b**

©DIAGRAM

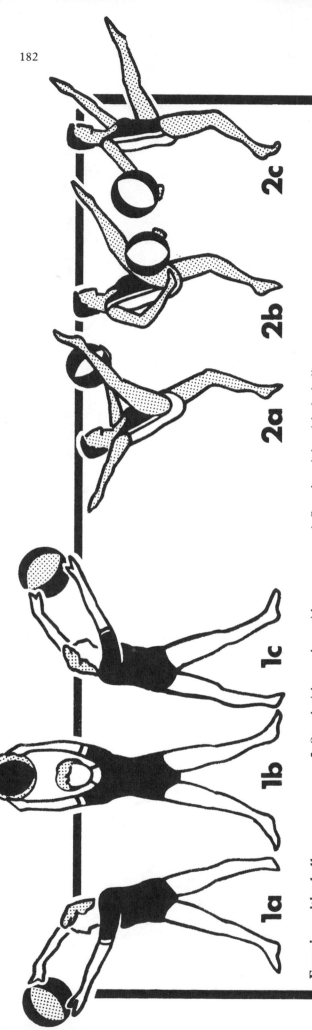

2c

2b

2a

1c

1b

1a

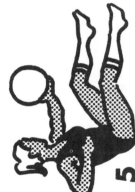

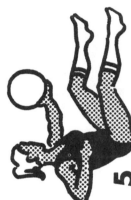

6

5

4

3

Exercises with a ball

For these exercises you need a large ball such as a beach ball.

1a Stand with your feet apart, grasping the ball with both hands. Stretch your arms out to one side.

1b, c Swing your body in large circles, bending from the waist. Change direction so that you do not become dizzy.

2a Holding the ball, swing your right leg high.

2b, c Quickly pass the ball from one hand to the other beneath your leg. Repeat, swinging the other leg up.

3 Stand with your legs wide apart, holding the ball with your arms outstretched. Bend back as far as you can and inhale. Then swing forward as far as possible, breathing out.

4 Stand upright with the ball on the ground in front of you. Raising your left leg behind you bend forward to support yourself with your right hand on the ball. Repeat with the other leg and hand.

5 Sit on the ground with your legs apart and slightly raised. Pass the ball from one hand to the other, passing it under one leg and over the other.

6 Throw the ball high and leap after it, stretching the whole of your body. Catch the ball and exhale as you lean slightly forward.

182

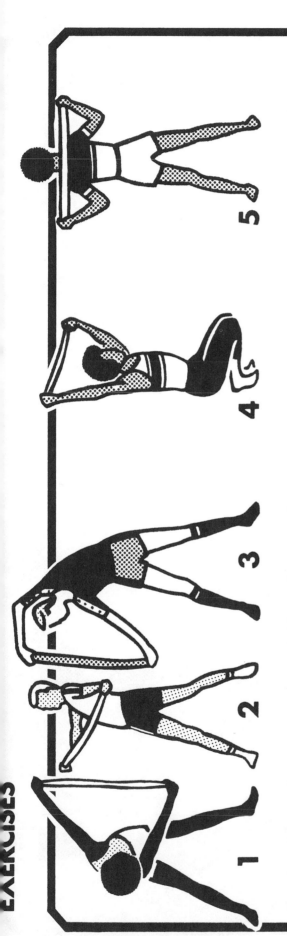

5

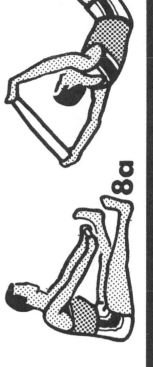

4

3

2

1

Exercises with a towel

Designed to improve posture, these exercises can be done in the bathroom or on the beach. Hold the towel tightly stretched, with one hand near each end.

1 Feet apart, let your body hang forward and then swing to one side, stretching as far as you can. Hold a moment, and then swing to the other side.

2 Stand with your feet apart and the towel in front of you. Turning from the waist, pull the towel back to the right and then to the left. Repeat.

3 Feet apart, hold the towel above your head. Without leaning forward, pull the towel from side to side.

4 Breathing in, crouch down with your arms above your head. Breathing out, drop your arms and rise to a standing position.

5 Hold the towel behind your shoulders and inhale. Then stretch your arms up, bend forward and exhale.

6 Kneel, with your body erect and the towel in front of you. Twist to the right and with your right hand touch the floor behind your feet. Exhale. Return to the starting position. Inhale. Repeat from side to side.

7 Lie flat on your front, with your arms stretched before your head. Then, as shown, raise your arms above your head and your feet from the floor, taking care not to bend your knees.

8a Sit with your feet stretched in front of you. Lean forward as far as you can, exhaling as you do so.

8b Raise the towel above your head and lean back, raising your legs from the ground without bending your knees, and inhaling as you do so. Repeat.

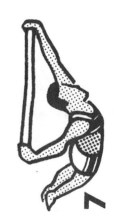

8b

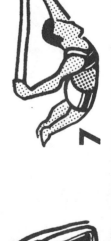

8a

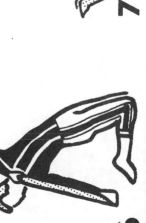

7

6

© DIAGRAM

EXERCISES

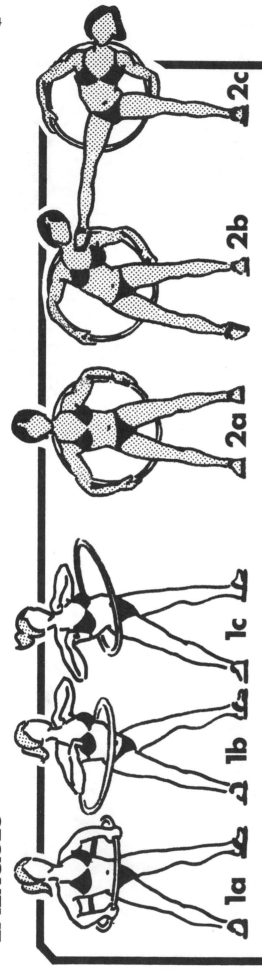

1a **1b** **1c** **2a** **2b** **2c**

Exercises with a hula-hoop
Once a popular child's toy, this makes a useful exercise aid.
1a Stand with your feet apart, one slightly in front of the other, holding the hoop around your waist.
1b Swing the hoop strongly forward to the left and let go. At the same time bring your hips forward and swing them back quickly.

1c Repeat this rocking and swinging movement as fast as you can, shifting your weight from front foot to back, and using your hips, so that the hoop is always moving and stays in the air. Try rotating the hoop on your neck, legs or arms.
2a Stand straight with your feet apart. Hold the hoop close behind you, with your arms wrapped round the outside.

2b Bend to the left from the waist, tipping the hoop.
2c Then lift your right leg high until it is parallel with the floor. Return to your starting position and continue the movement from side to side.
3a Sit within the hoop with your knees bent, and grasp the rim.
3b Shoot your arms up to hold the hoop overhead, stretching your legs out at the same time.

4a Sit on the floor with your legs stretched wide apart, holding the hoop upright in front of you with its rim on the floor.
4b Roll the hoop over toward your right toe and stretch as far as you can.
4c Roll it back and then to the left. Repeat from side to side.

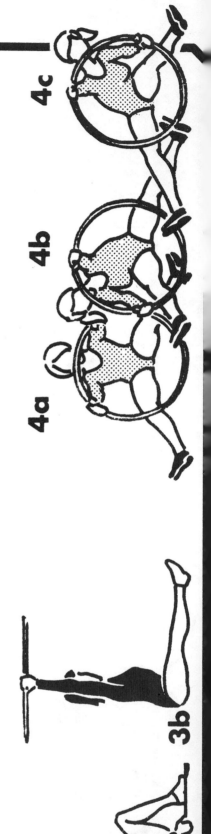

3a **3b** **4a** **4b** **4c**

Exercises with Indian clubs

Indian clubs first became popular for exercise purposes in the mid-nineteenth century. Interest in this activity has recently revived, with colored pennants and lights sometimes added to the clubs for greater effect. Exercise with clubs is designed to develop general fitness and coordination, and to increase shoulder agility and muscle power. The weight of the clubs increases the effectiveness of the large, medium, and small swinging movements typical of exercises using this equipment.

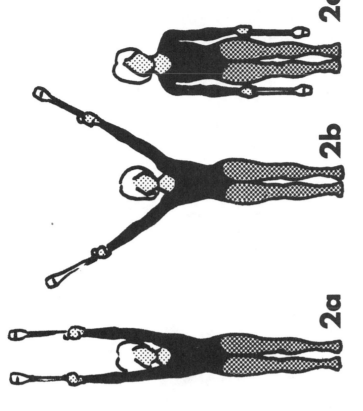

1a **1b** **1c**

2a **2b** **2c**

Large swings and circles

1a Stand in the starting position, feet together and arms down by your sides, with the clubs pointing up.
1b Stretch your arms out to each side level with your shoulders, holding the clubs in a straight line.
1c Swing your arms forward until they are parallel in front of you. Next swing them back to the side as in 1b, and then forward again. Repeat this swinging movement several times.

2a From the starting position shown in 1a, first raise your arms above your head.
2b, c Then swing your arms out to the side and down to your thighs, keeping the clubs in a straight line with your arms and letting the weight of the clubs pull your arms down. Your shoulder joints should move freely and form the axis for the swing. Next swing your arms back up to position 2a to repeat the swing down. As a variation, keep one arm raised as you swing the other one down and up again.

©DIAGRAM

EXERCISES

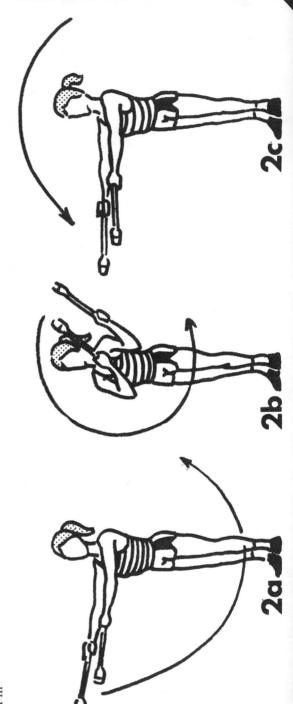

1a **1b** **1c** **1d**

2a **2b** **2c**

Exercises with Indian clubs
Medium swings and circles

1a Holding one club in your right hand, extend your right arm to the side so that the club is at shoulder level. Then swing the club down and across in front of your body.

1b, c Bending your elbow to act as the axis, circle the club in the air in front of you.

1d Follow through to finish the movement with your arm extended at shoulder level to the left. Repeat the exercise with your left arm.

2a With a club in each hand, extend your arms to the same side so that the clubs are held parallel at shoulder level.

2b With your elbows as the axis, swing the clubs in a circle in front of you, keeping the clubs parallel.

2c Swing the clubs over and round to finish in the starting position as at 2a. Repeat to the other side.

EXERCISES

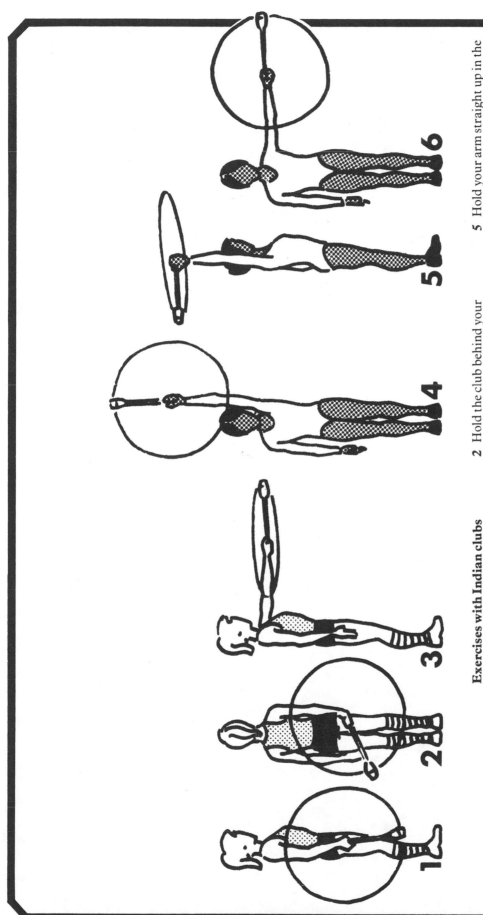

Exercises with Indian clubs
Small swings and circles
For these exercises all movement should be from your wrists, with your arms kept outstretched and immobile. Each exercise should be repeated to use both arms.

1 Hold the club down by your side and then turn it in a vertical circle parallel to your side.

2 Hold the club behind your buttocks and swing it in a vertical circle.

3 Stretch your arm out in front of you and rotate the club horizontally, parallel to your arm.

4 Hold your arm straight up in the air and then rotate the club vertically.

5 Hold your arm straight up in the air and then rotate the club horizontally over your head.

6 Extend your arm to the side, holding the club out straight, and then rotate the club vertically from the wrist.

©DIAGRAM

EXERCISES

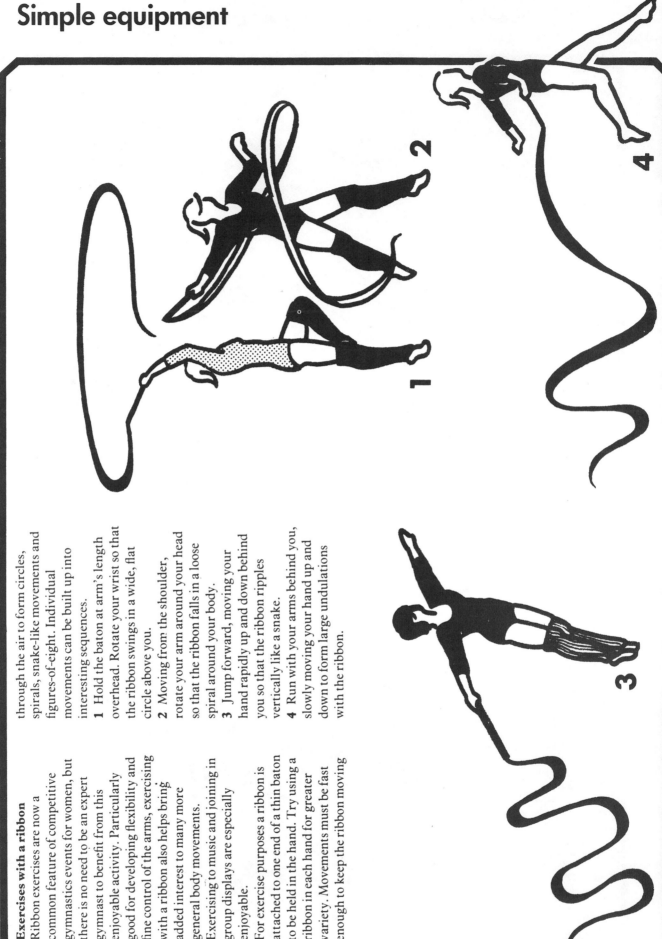

Exercises with a ribbon
Ribbon exercises are now a common feature of competitive gymnastics events for women, but there is no need to be an expert gymnast to benefit from this enjoyable activity. Particularly good for developing flexibility and fine control of the arms, exercising with a ribbon also helps bring added interest to many more general body movements.
Exercising to music and joining in group displays are especially enjoyable.
For exercise purposes a ribbon is attached to one end of a thin baton to be held in the hand. Try using a ribbon in each hand for greater variety. Movements must be fast enough to keep the ribbon moving through the air to form circles, spirals, snake-like movements and figures-of-eight. Individual movements can be built up into interesting sequences.

1 Hold the baton at arm's length overhead. Rotate your wrist so that the ribbon swings in a wide, flat circle above you.
2 Moving from the shoulder, rotate your arm around your head so that the ribbon falls in a loose spiral around your body.
3 Jump forward, moving your hand rapidly up and down behind you so that the ribbon ripples vertically like a snake.
4 Run with your arms behind you, slowly moving your hand up and down to form large undulations with the ribbon.

EXERCISES

Exercises with a ribbon

1 Swing your arm in front of you to make a large vertical circle with the ribbon.

2 Jump forward, swinging your arms up and back so that the ribbon curves with your body.

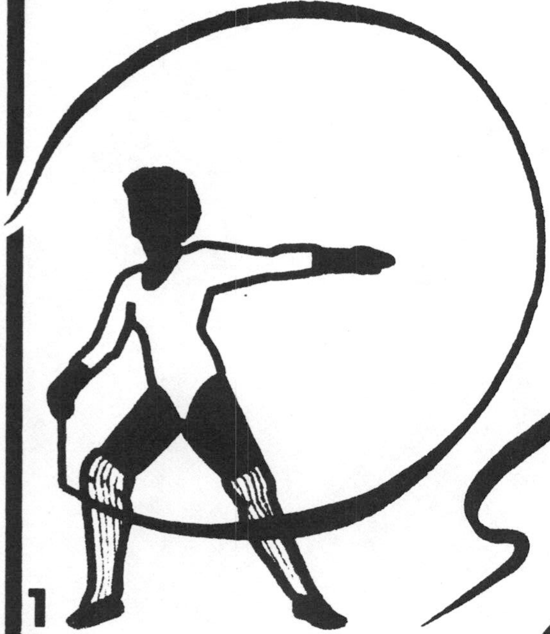

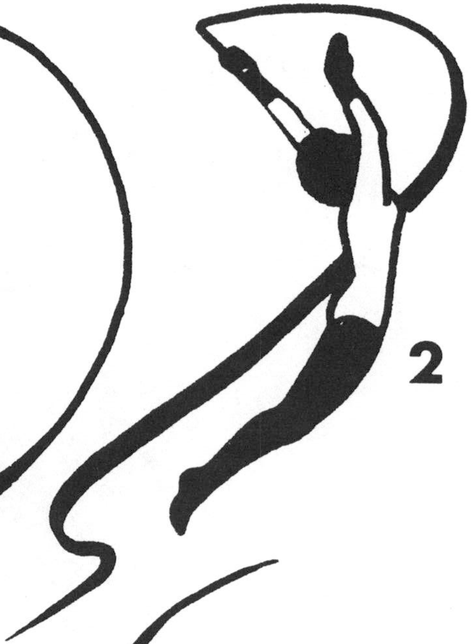

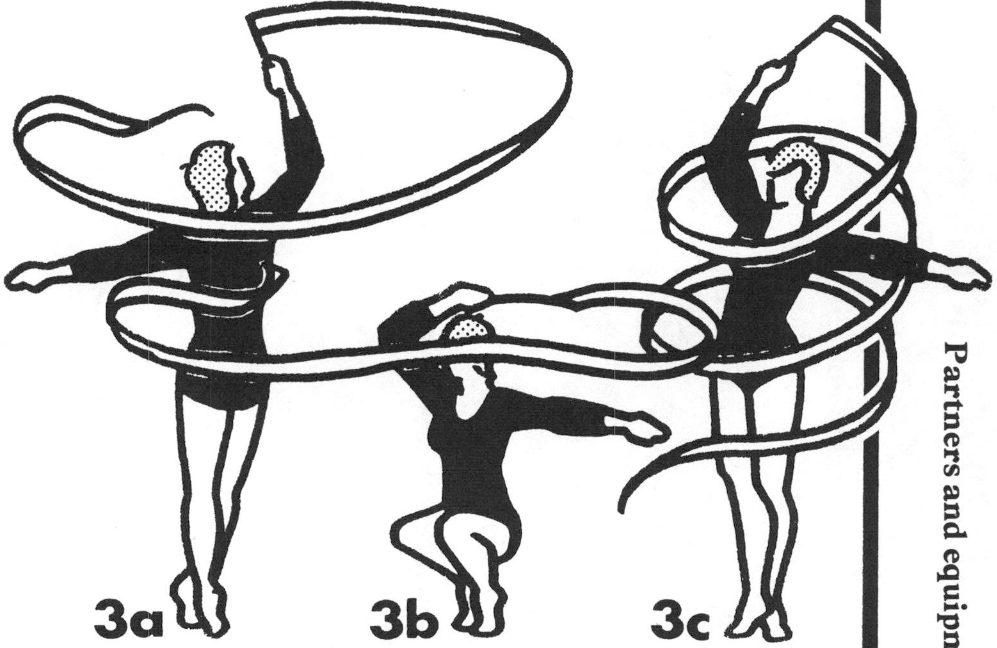

3a Stretch up on your toes and swing the ribbon in a circle overhead.

3b Bend your knees to squat, continuing to rotate the ribbon above your head.

3c Stand up quickly, reducing the width of the circle and allowing the ribbon to fall into a spiral around your body.

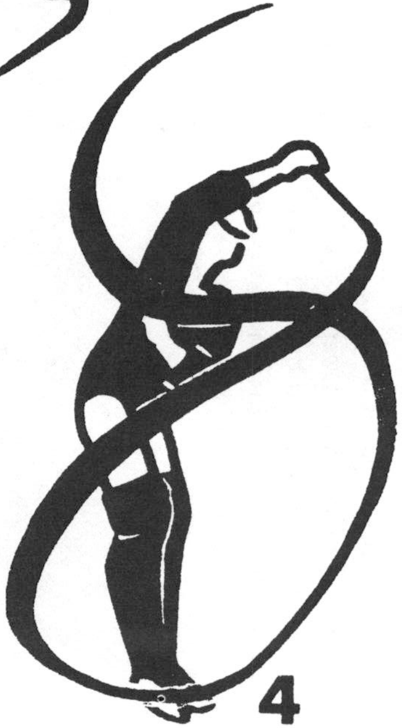

4 Twirl the ribbon in front of you to make a large, vertical figure-of-eight.

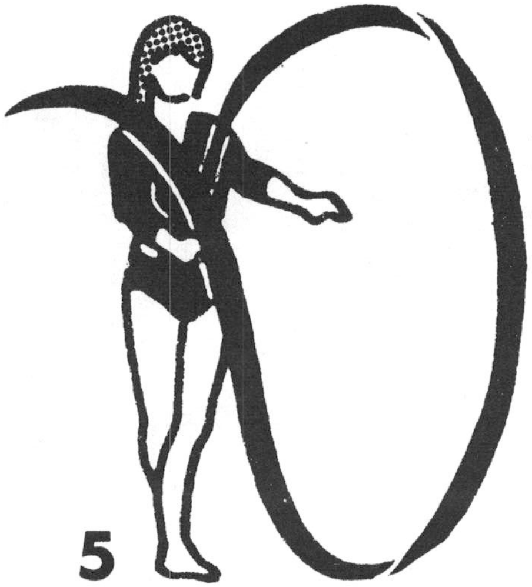

5 Twirl the ribbon to make a large figure-of-eight lying on its side.

©DIAGRAM

JUMPING/SKIPPING

Jumping or skipping with a rope is an excellent form of exercise. Jump ropes have been favorite children's toys for centuries; now they are gaining popularity with adults for use in keep-fit routines and reducing programs. Rope exercises are a good way of warming up before other exercise activities, and are ideal training for sports requiring stamina, coordination and rhythm. Jumping with a rope strengthens and tones the muscles, and is excellent exercise for the heart and lungs. In fact, this enjoyable way of keeping fit is really almost child's play!

Jumping benefits
In addition to general fitness benefits, exercise with a jump or skipping rope has effects that are of particular interest to specific groups of people.

As every boxer knows, exercise with a rope is good for bodybuilding. Arm and leg muscles are developed and strengthened while neck, shoulders and chest are firmed and filled out.

Women are likely to be more interested in the improvements skipping can make to the figure. It tightens flabby muscles and loose flesh on the arms, thighs and buttocks, makes thighs and calves more shapely and, especially if the rope is turned backward for jumping, helps to firm the bust and improve overall posture.

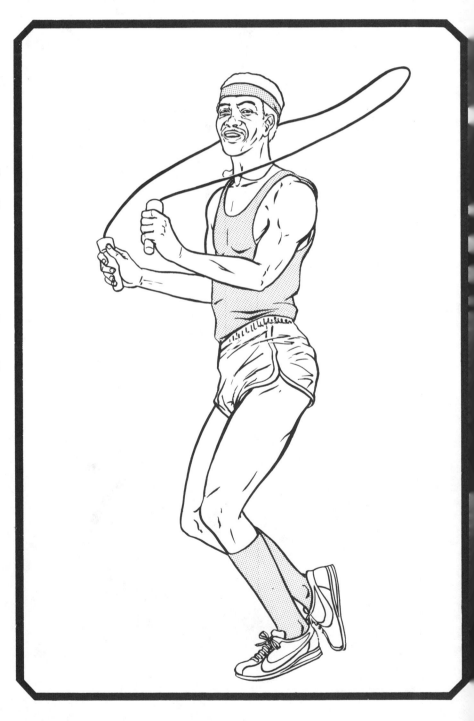

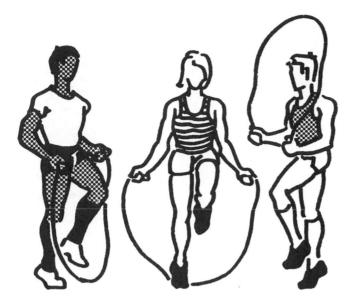

Health warning

Almost everyone will benefit from jumping, but if you are over 35 and unused to exercise, or if you have a history of back pain or arthritis, you are advised to consult your doctor before starting a jumping program. Aching muscles are quite common when people start jumping; treat with heat or analgesic rubs.

Jumping hints

It is a good idea to jump in front of a mirror to watch your technique. Keep your head facing forward and your back straight. Try to breathe through your nose, not through your mouth.

Turn the rope as smoothly as possible, using your wrists and forearms.

Push off with your toes. Flex your knees and, except when making fancy jumps, lift your feet only high enough just to clear the rope. Landings should be as light as possible, and always on the balls of the feet.

Time your jumping sessions, perhaps by listening to music. Between exercises, or when you are tired, try a few stretching exercises to ease your muscles and to help you relax.

Equipment and clothing

Of course you can use a simple length of rope for jumping, but specially made jump ropes are better. Good ones are made of leather or heavy fiber, about $9\frac{1}{2}$ft (2.9m) long, with strong handles fitted with ball bearings to help the rope turn.

Wear loose, light clothing, socks, and a pair of good running shoes with padded insoles.

Where to jump

You can jump indoors or out, where there is enough space to swing your rope. A wood floor is ideal for jumping on, preferably with a mat to cushion your landing and to help you jump lightly.

When to jump

Try to jump regularly at the same time each day. Choose whatever time suits you best, but do not jump for at least $1\frac{1}{2}$ hours after a meal.

Using a jump rope for 5–15 minutes daily should get you into shape. Then maintain your new level of fitness with 15–30 minutes jumping 3 times a week.

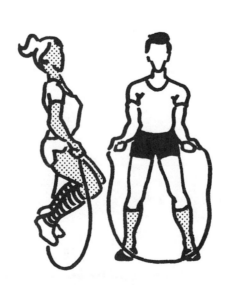

EXERCISES

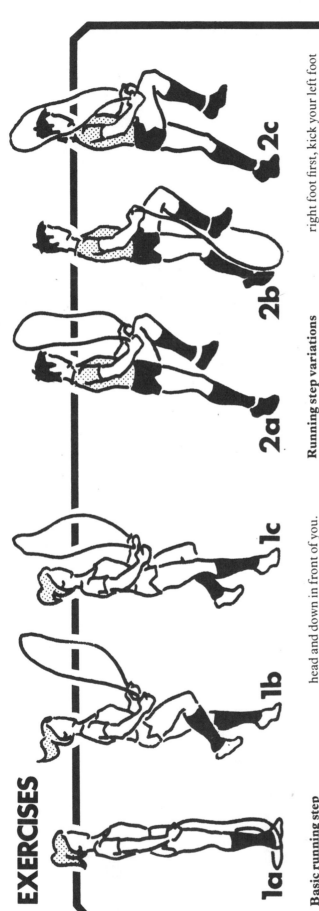

2c

2b

2a

1c

1b

1a

Basic running step

1a For all steps start with your feet together, back straight, head held up, arms down by your sides, holding the rope with the slack behind your feet.

1b Swing the rope up over your head and down in front of you. With the right foot leading, jump over the rope. Land only on the ball of the right foot, with the left foot raised behind you.

1c Swing the rope over again, this time jumping it to land on the left foot. Continue jumping the rope with alternate feet, staying on the spot.

Running step variations

2a, b, c Jump from foot to foot as in the basic running step, but for this variation raise your knees as high as you can while jumping the rope.

3a, b, c As for the basic running step, but after jumping the rope

right foot first, kick your left foot back to touch your left buttock. Alternate legs.

4a, b, c As for the basic running step, but after jumping the rope right foot first, bounce once on that foot before jumping the rope left foot first. Alternate legs.

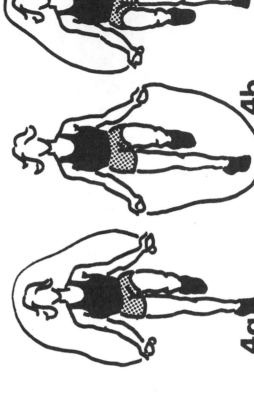

4c

4b

4a

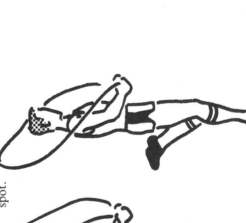

3c

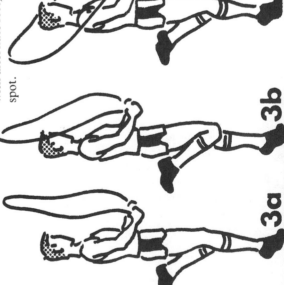

3b

3a

EXERCISES

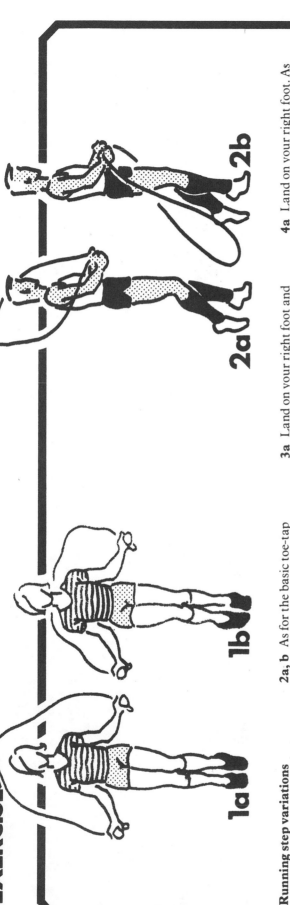

1a

1b

2a

2b

Running step variations
1a After landing on your right foot, quickly tap the ground beside it with your left toe. Then bring the rope over to jump it left foot first.
1b Land on your left foot and tap with your right. Continue with alternate feet.

2a, b As for the basic toe-tap exercise (1a, b) but this time quickly tap the ground just behind your landing foot.

3a Land on your right foot and quickly tap your left heel on the floor just in front of you.
3b Land on your left foot and tap with your right heel. Continue, alternating feet.

4a Land on your right foot. As you swing the rope overhead, bend your left knee and kick your left leg against the back of your right leg.
4b, c Land on your left foot and kick the back of your left leg with your right leg. Continue, alternating legs.

3a

3b

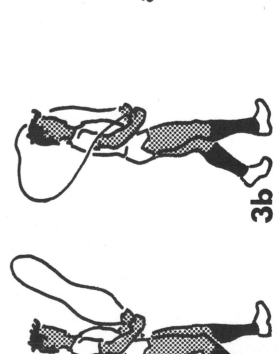

4a

4b

4c

©DIAGRAM

Jumping/skipping

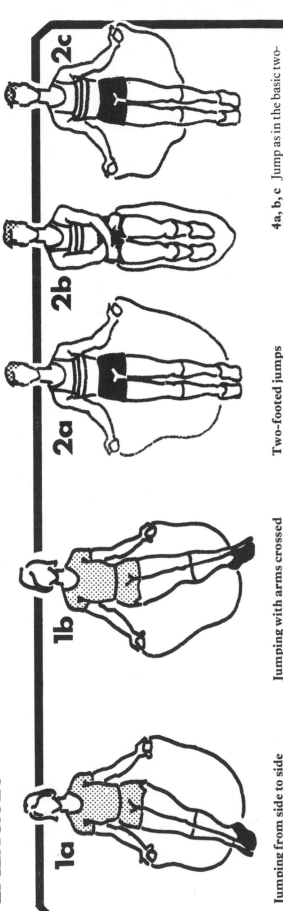

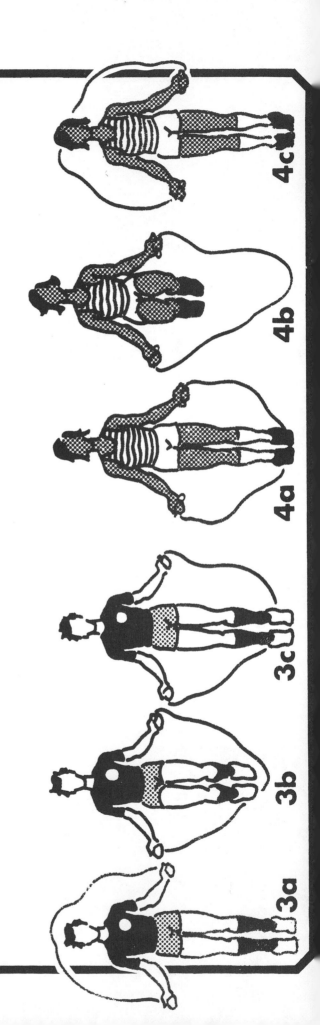

Jumping from side to side
1a Jump to the right, leading with your right foot and landing with your two feet close together.
1b Repeat to the left, with your left foot leading. Then continue from side to side.

Jumping with arms crossed
2a Hold the rope normally for your first jump.
2b Next time you bring the rope forward cross your arms.
2c Continue alternating regular and cross-arm jumps.

Two-footed jumps
3a Start with your feet together and the rope held behind you.
3b Bring the rope over and jump it, pushing off with your toes and keeping your feet together.
3c Land on the balls of your feet.

4a, b, c Jump as in the basic two-footed jump (3a, b, c) but after a few jumps turn the rope very quickly and jump higher than usual so that you can fit in 2 or even 3 turns of the rope before you land.

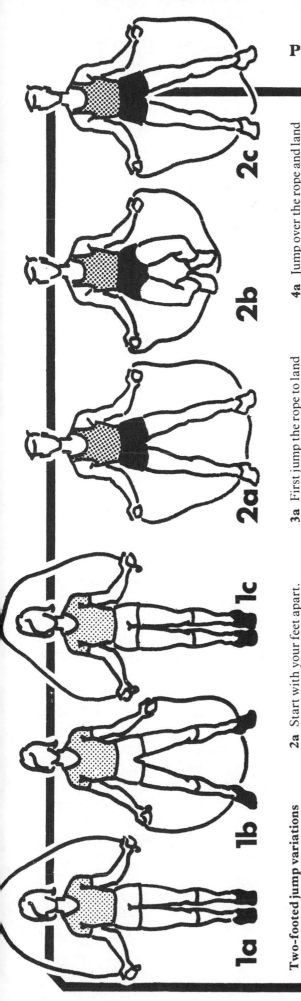

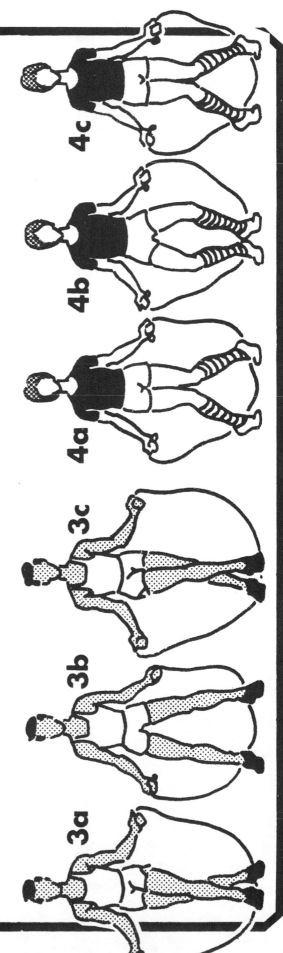

2c

2b

2a

1c

1b

1a

Two-footed jump variations

1a First jump the rope with your feet together.

1b Next time land with your feet apart as shown.

1c Alternate jumps with the feet together and the feet apart.

2a Start with your feet apart.

2b As you bring the rope over, jump in the air and click your heels together.

2c Land with your feet apart.

3a First jump the rope to land with your left foot crossed in front of your right foot.

3b Next land with your feet apart.

3c Then land with your right foot crossed in front of your left foot. Jump and land with your feet apart before repeating.

4a Jump over the rope and land with your knees together, your toes pointing in and your heels turned out.

4b Next time land with your knees and toes pointing out and your heels turned in.

4c Continue by alternating landing positions 4a and 4b.

4c

4b

4a

3c

3b

3a

©DIAGRAM

SOPHISTICATED EQUIPMENT

The preceding pages showed exercises using domestic articles and simple games equipment. There is also a growing market in sophisticated gadgets and specialized exercise equipment designed for use in the home, or, more commonly, in health clinics and gymnasiums.

Remember that no exercise machine will work wonders. The machines described here are all as good as the effort you put into them. Exercise machines do not provide an easy way to fitness, but they can be an efficient and convenient means of exercising your body and developing your muscle-power.

If you are considering buying your own exercise machine, do not be misled by pseudo-scientific sales technique and be sure you know how any machine works before you make your purchase. Perhaps the most important advantage of owning your own exercise equipment is psychological. Its visible presence in the home, combined with the often considerable expense involved, provides a constant reminder and incentive to exercise. When exercising with a machine, always avoid over-exerting yourself or straining your muscles — do not try to run before you can walk, even on the treadmill!

The increase in home equipment is paralleled by a growing number of gymnasiums and health centers, catering for everyone from the professional athlete to the figure-conscious businessman. Training gyms are really designed for the sportsman who wants to keep in peak condition, but health and exercise facilities are now available to everyone in hotels, offices, social centers or the main street sauna.

Joining a health gym has considerable advantages. Social and recreational aspects are very important in making the pursuit of fitness enjoyable, and the element of competition provides an added stimulus. Attending a gym makes available a wider variety of exercise equipment than most people would want to buy for themselves, but check that equipment is fitted with any recommended safeguards.

Every gym should give you a fitness test before you start an exercise program; good staff will be aware of this. Once enrolled at a gym, follow the instructors' directions strictly. Attention to these simple guidelines will mean that exercise with equipment will prove to be both good for you, and fun!

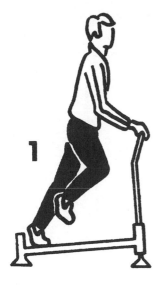

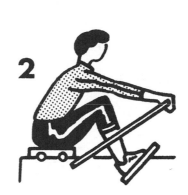

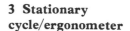

Indoor sport simulators
Although probably less enjoyable than the outdoor activities they simulate, these four exercise machines are, however, ideal for use in confined spaces and all kinds of weather.

1 Jogger or treadmill
This comprises a series of rollers and is used for on-the-spot jogging; the rollers can be inclined to make running more difficult. There is often a pulsometer to check your pulse rate, and many also have mileage meters. Use of this machine achieves the same ends as normal jogging, providing exercise for legs, heart, and lungs.

2 Rowing machine
Machines of this type adapt the movements used in rowing for use on dry land. There are two basic types available. The least satisfactory has a stationary seat so that the legs do not move during the exercise. The more advanced machines have a sliding seat like that in racing boats, which exercises the legs in a bending and pulling movement, as well as using the chest and arms for the actual "rowing." Many also have an adjustable resistance force.

3 Stationary cycle/ergonometer
Stationary cycling machines are often used in fitness tests to check the capacity of the heart and lungs. They are usually equipped with meters which enable you to find your working pulse rate and to work out a personal exercise program. Most makers recommend a daily routine of 15–20 minutes cycling. Exercise on these machines benefits the heart and lungs, and also improves the strength and endurance of the back and leg muscles. Most models have adjustable braking force and pedal resistance so that the effort involved in cycling can be increased as your fitness improves.

4 Combined exerciser
Combining a cycling leg action with a rowing arm action, this type of machine is designed to improve general fitness by providing exercise for the legs, arms, and cardio-vascular system. Fitted with adjustable controls, these machines can be adapted to suit most age groups.

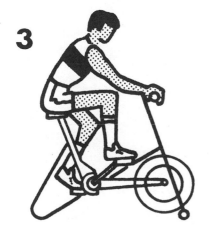

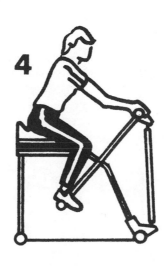

©DIAGRAM

Sophisticated equipment

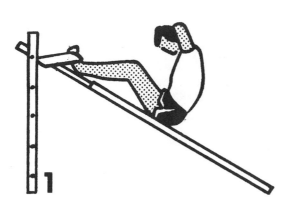

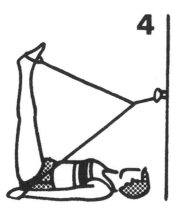

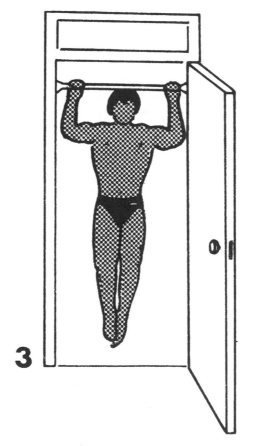

Indoor exercise equipment
The equipment included here provides exercise for the muscles mainly through pulling and stretching movements.

1 Incline bench
One use of this equipment is for a variation of the basic sit-up exercise. Lying on a sloping bench increases the difficulty of the pull-up and also the resulting exercise of the stomach muscles. As the incline is steepened, the exercise becomes more strenuous.

2 Leg press machine
This equipment involves lying on your back, and raising and lowering a weighted bar with your legs to increase the strength of the hip and leg muscles. As your strength grows, extra weight is added to the bar so that raising it is made more difficult.

3 Exercise bar
These often form part of large exercise units in gymnasiums; at home a bar wedged in a door-frame can be used. Reaching up to hold the bar with two hands you then raise and lower your body in order to exercise your arm, neck, stomach and back muscles. With practice you should be able to look over the bar.

4 Weights and pulleys
This machine uses opposing forces in the body itself, and also involves the force of gravity. It is often used in physiotherapy. First you use a pulley system to pull your legs into the air, so strengthening your arm muscles. Then you lower your legs again very slowly, making use of your thigh and stomach muscles.

A variety of sophisticated multi-purpose exercise units has been developed in recent years to meet a growing demand from offices, hotels, sports and health centers. Scientifically designed for maximum efficiency, these machines allow several people to exercise together.

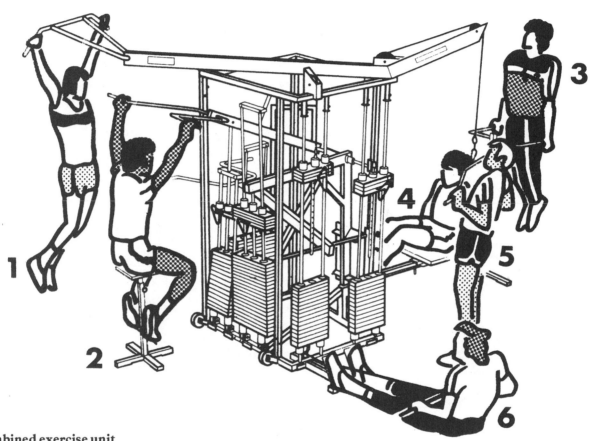

Combined exercise unit

The unit illustrated above is a typical example of the highly sophisticated exercise machines now available.

Different "stations" of the unit are designed to exercise different parts of the body, and users move around as part of a complete exercise program.

Adjustable weights and resistance factors make the units suitable for persons with widely varying degrees of fitness — everyone from tired executives to professional footballers!

Stations illustrated here include the following.

1 Chinning station The user raises his body with his arms, pulling himself up to rest his chin on the bar.

2 Press station While seated, the user moves the handles against the machine's resistance.

3 Dipping station The user holds the chest-level handles to raise and lower his body.

4 Leg press Sitting on a seat with a firm back, the user presses his legs against the machine's resistance.

5 Latissimus station The user strengthens his muscles by pulling the bar down against the weighted pulley.

6 Shoulder conditioner This is another weight and pulley system, for which the user sits on the floor with his feet resting on the blocks at each side of the pulley.

Chapter 6   EXERCISE AND SPORT

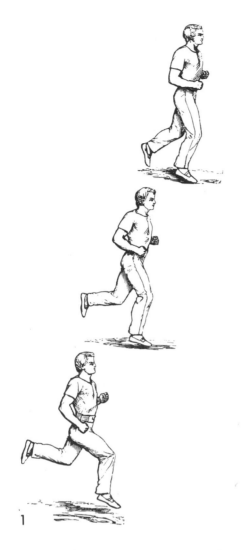

1

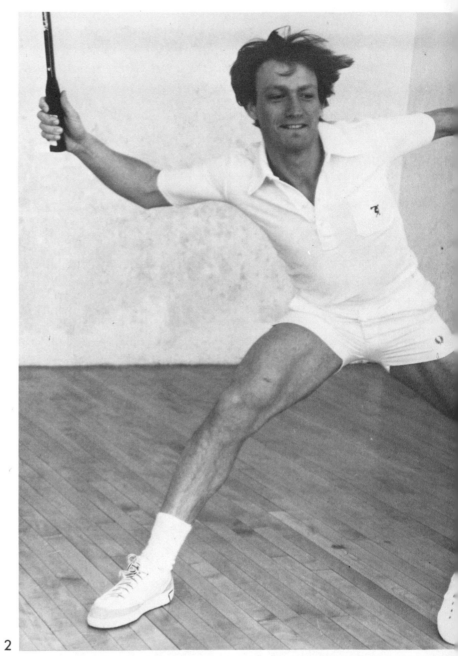

2

3.

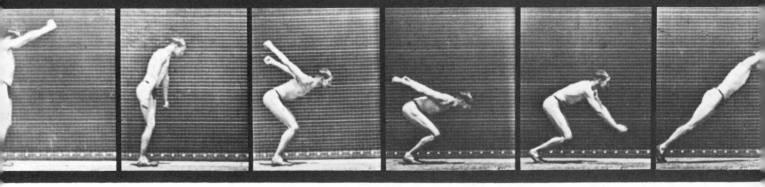

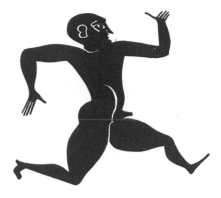

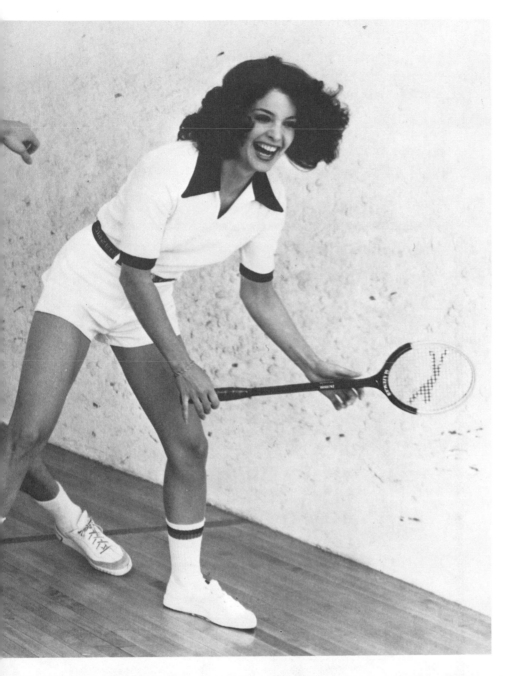

1 *Physical Education* by A. MacLaren
(Oxford 1869)
2 Squash players (Courtaulds Ltd)
3 *Animal Locomotion* by E. Muybridge
(USA 1887; by courtesy of Kingston-upon-
Thames Museum and Art Gallery)

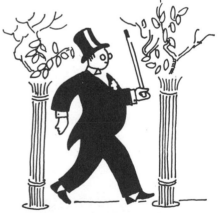

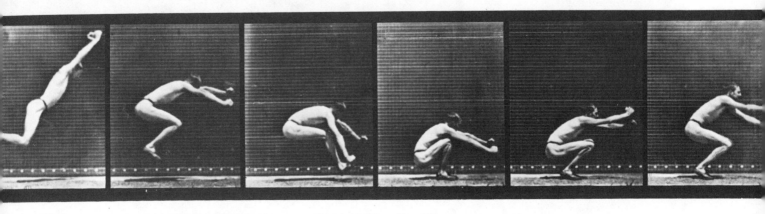

CHOOSING A SPORT

Sport provides many people with an extremely popular form of exercise. It is an integral part of our social structure, providing a dynamic expression of its values and an acceptable channel for the release of energy and aggression. Some sports, such as backpacking or climbing, also offer a positive means of escape from social pressures. Sport leads to physical fitness and develops mental discipline. Its aims provide incentives and motivation which, with the support of your colleagues, can help you overcome the laziness of depression and disillusionment.

Body types

There are three basic body types: ectomorphs, mesomorphs and endomorphs (see p. 54). Body type affects your physical capabilities and hence the types of sport that suit you best. You will gain more from a sport chosen to suit your personal body type than from struggling with a sport to which you are physically ill-suited. Ectomorphs are notable for their endurance and agility, making them good cross-country runners and basketball players. Mesomorphs are suited to many sports, their muscular frame being capable of developing strength, endurance, power and agility in equal lots. Endomorphs will find the most difficulty in sports, and are advised to concentrate on the less strenuous activities.

The table included here shows which sports are most suitable for the different body types.

A Ectomorphs
B Meso-ectomorphs
C Mesomorphs
D Meso-endomorphs
E Endomorphs

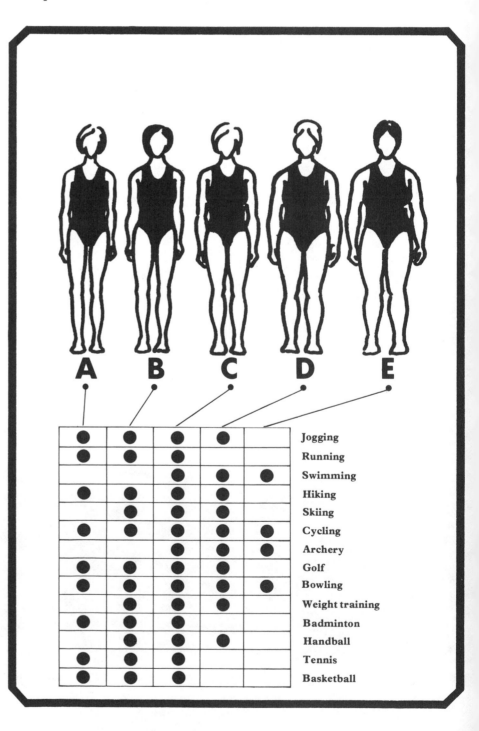

A	B	C	D	E	
●	●	●	●		Jogging
●	●	●			Running
		●	●	●	Swimming
●	●	●	●		Hiking
	●	●	●		Skiing
●	●	●	●	●	Cycling
		●	●	●	Archery
●	●	●	●		Golf
●	●	●	●	●	Bowling
	●	●	●		Weight training
●	●	●			Badminton
	●	●	●		Handball
●	●	●			Tennis
●	●	●			Basketball

The sport you choose should be the one that gives you the greatest benefits with the greatest enjoyment. First make sure that it is suited to your age — swimming, for example, is ideal for the older person whereas squash or American football are not. Your choice of sport will automatically be limited by the time and money you can afford, and by the facilities available. Other important factors are your body type, previous experience and current state of health. As your skills and fitness increase so will your enjoyment and confidence, and the range of sports open to you.

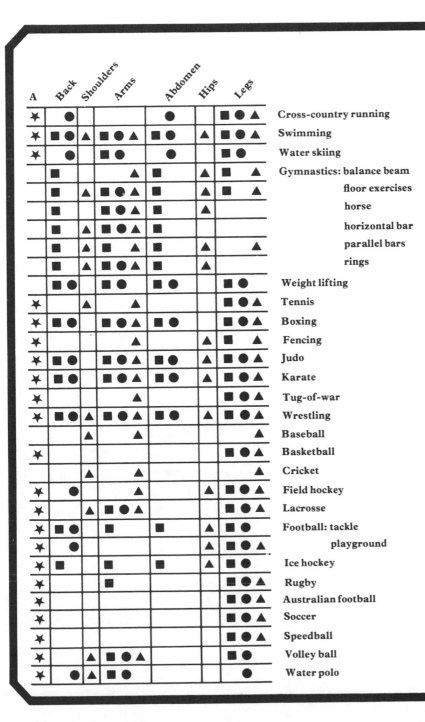

A	Back	Shoulders	Arms	Abdomen	Hips	Legs	
✷	●			●		■ ● ▲	Cross-country running
✷	■ ● ▲	■ ● ▲	■ ●	▲	■ ● ▲	Swimming
✷	●	■ ●	●		■ ●	Water skiing
	■		▲	■	▲	■ ▲	Gymnastics: balance beam
	■	▲	■ ● ▲	■	▲	▲	floor exercises
	■		■ ● ▲	■	▲		horse
	■	▲	■ ● ▲	■			horizontal bar
	■	▲	■	▲	■	▲	parallel bars
	■	▲	■ ● ▲	■	▲		rings
	■ ●		■ ●	■ ●		■ ●	Weight lifting
✷		▲	▲			■ ● ▲	Tennis
✷	■ ●		■ ● ▲	■ ●		■ ● ▲	Boxing
✷			▲		▲ ■	▲	Fencing
✷	■ ●		■ ● ▲	■ ●	▲	■ ● ▲	Judo
✷	■ ●		■ ● ▲	■ ●	▲	■ ● ▲	Karate
✷			▲			■ ● ▲	Tug-of-war
✷	■ ● ▲		■ ● ▲	■ ●	▲	■ ● ▲	Wrestling
		▲	▲			▲	Baseball
✷						■ ● ▲	Basketball
		▲	▲			▲	Cricket
✷	●		▲		▲	■ ● ▲	Field hockey
✷		▲	■ ● ▲			■ ● ▲	Lacrosse
✷	■ ●		■	■	▲	■ ●	Football: tackle
✷	●				▲	■ ● ▲	playground
✷	■		■	■	▲	■ ●	Ice hockey
✷			■			■ ● ▲	Rugby
✷						■ ● ▲	Australian football
✷						■ ● ▲	Soccer
✷						■ ● ▲	Speedball
✷		▲	■ ● ▲			■ ●	Volley ball
✷	●	▲	■ ●			●	Water polo

Physiological effects

Exercise develops the strength and endurance of muscles and increases the flexibility of both muscles and joints. It should also improve the capacity and endurance of the cardio-vascular and respiratory (CR) systems. To do this the heart rate of a fit adult should be raised to over 120 beats per minute for at least 10–15 minutes three or four times a week (with variations for age).

Most sports develop only one set of muscles, so you should participate in a variety of sports. But make sure that their effects are not too opposed. Weight lifting, for instance, tightens the muscles, giving explosive strength, whereas swimming relaxes and stretches them, giving endurance. The two sports, therefore, effectively work against each other. Swimming and running, on the other hand, are an excellent combination.

This table shows the effects on the body of different types of sport. Consulting it should help you to balance your sporting schedule.

A Cardio-respiratory endurance
■ Muscle strength
● Muscle endurance
▲ Flexibility

Choosing a sport

Learning a sport also means learning a new skill and widening your capabilities. This, with the combination of physical and mental effort and relaxation involved in sporting activities can also help cultivate a positive and happy attitude to other areas of life.

Joining a sports club or gymnasium will help you practice your sport more regularly. Adequate and safe facilities will be made available to you. Finding opponents or teammates will no longer be a problem, and the friendship of persons with a common interest will enrich your social life.

Calorie consumption
The table given here shows the number of Calories used by a 150lb (65kg) person during one hour in various sporting activities. (For Calorie consumption during domestic work and other daily activities see p. 47).

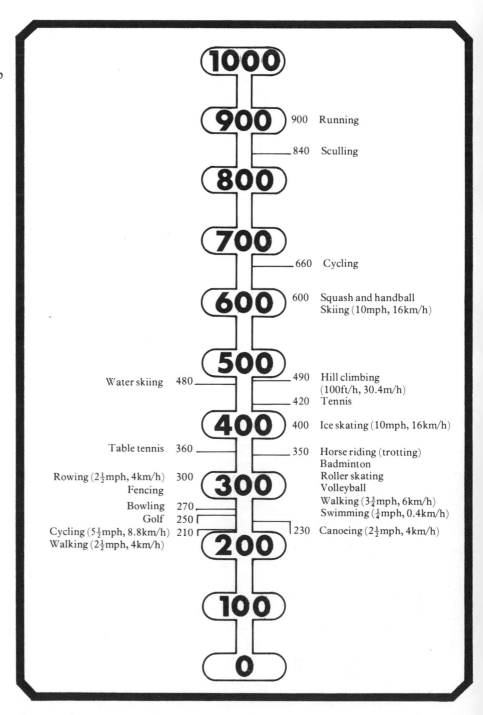

	Calories	Activity
	1000	
	900	Running
	840	Sculling
	800	
	700	
	660	Cycling
	600	Squash and handball / Skiing (10mph, 16km/h)
	500	
Water skiing 480	490	Hill climbing (100ft/h, 30.4m/h)
	420	Tennis
	400	Ice skating (10mph, 16km/h)
Table tennis 360	350	Horse riding (trotting) / Badminton
Rowing (2½mph, 4km/h) 300 / Fencing	300	Roller skating / Volleyball
Bowling 270		Walking (3¾mph, 6km/h) / Swimming (¼mph, 0.4km/h)
Golf 250		
Cycling (5½mph, 8.8km/h) 210 / Walking (2½mph, 4km/h)	230	Canoeing (2½mph, 4km/h)
	200	
	100	
	0	

People interested in reducing will find that sports are a valuable aid, increasing Calorie consumption (see page 204) and helping to trim and firm the figure.

Most important of all, remember that sporting activities of all kinds are intended to be an enjoyable means of getting necessary exercise. Enjoyment is the major factor in any choice. There is no need to choose a particularly demanding sport or to overdo your training. Indeed, to do so can be positively harmful. The quickest way to deter yourself from any sport is to injure yourself in your initial enthusiasm.

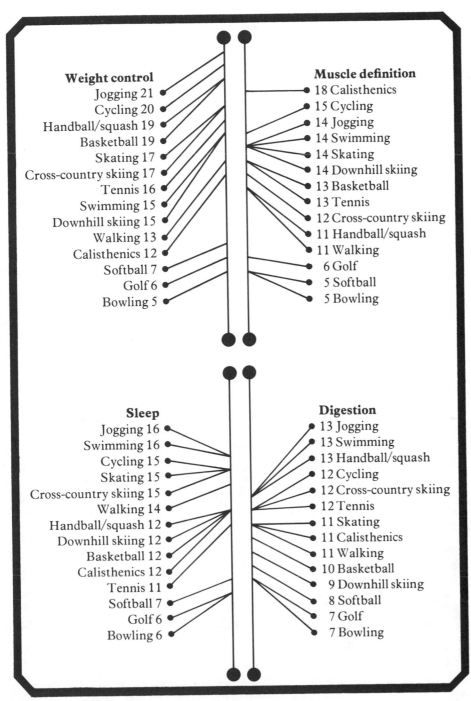

Weight control
Jogging 21
Cycling 20
Handball/squash 19
Basketball 19
Skating 17
Cross-country skiing 17
Tennis 16
Swimming 15
Downhill skiing 15
Walking 13
Calisthenics 12
Softball 7
Golf 6
Bowling 5

Muscle definition
18 Calisthenics
15 Cycling
14 Jogging
14 Swimming
14 Skating
14 Downhill skiing
13 Basketball
13 Tennis
12 Cross-country skiing
11 Handball/squash
11 Walking
6 Golf
5 Softball
5 Bowling

Sleep
Jogging 16
Swimming 16
Cycling 15
Skating 15
Cross-country skiing 15
Walking 14
Handball/squash 12
Downhill skiing 12
Basketball 12
Calisthenics 12
Tennis 11
Softball 7
Golf 6
Bowling 6

Digestion
13 Jogging
13 Swimming
13 Handball/squash
12 Cycling
12 Cross-country skiing
12 Tennis
11 Skating
11 Calisthenics
11 Walking
10 Basketball
9 Downhill skiing
8 Softball
7 Golf
7 Bowling

All-round effects
This table shows which sports offer the best all-round effects. Remember that the extent of the benefit of any sport depends on the effort you put into it. Also try to suit your sport to your own particular needs. Backpacking may not have the intense cardio-vascular benefits of running, but you may gain more from its relaxing and broadening effects. Cycling is very good for the legs and heart and is very enjoyable, but it is difficult to expand the lungs properly when you are bent over the handlebars.

In the table, sports are scored out of a maximum benefit of 21. Note that the golf ratings are based on the fact that many people use a caddy and/or a golf cart. However, if you walk and carry your clubs, the benefits are considerably greater.

©DIAGRAM

WALKING, RUNNING, SWIMMING

Jogging and running are excellent exercises, giving definite cardio-vascular, respiratory and figure benefits. Walking, if performed energetically enough, can produce the same benefits, but needs more time.

Golf is more useful as an enjoyable skill and social activity than as exercise. There is little, or no, heart and lung benefit, although walking around the course can be beneficial and the back and arms may be strengthened. Team games have the great advantage of providing good, regularized exercise in sociable conditions, but they do make great demands on time and perhaps on money, and usually depend upon special places and other people. Court games have the same advantages and drawbacks, although the personal aspects of the game make them more appealing to some. As in all exercise the physiological benefits depend upon the effort expended; usually the amount of running. Swimming is one of the best all-round activities, excellent for the heart and lungs, muscular strength and endurance, and the flexibility of the major joints. Breaststroke is the least demanding, followed by backstroke. The best stroke is the front crawl. Swimming is often recommended for convalescents and for sufferers of back pain.

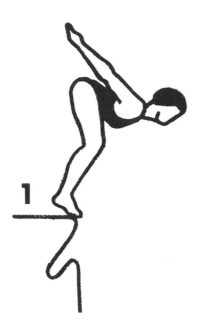

1 Swimming must be constant and energetic for at least 10 minutes to produce any positive results. A good target to aim for is 1000yd in 22–25 minutes (1km in 25–30 minutes), using mainly front crawl; anything down to half this distance in half the time is also excellent. Variety can be achieved by changing stroke and breathing rhythms, trying bursts of the very energetic butterfly stroke, and by using alternate sprint/slow in place of regular distance swimming.

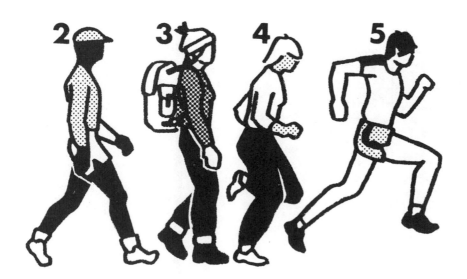

2 Walking at about 4mph (6.4km/h) for extended periods provides a rhythmical, unified exercise that does not strain the joints. It is an excellent form of exercise for the elderly.

3 Backpacking has the further advantages of involving longer distances with heavy loads over tougher terrain.

4, 5 Jogging and running
The human body is designed for running, and it is the best activity for providing the basic fitness needed for all sports. It exercises the arms and chest as well as the legs, strengthens the abdominal muscles and also exercises the internal organs.

Jogging should be used as an introduction to running. Covering 1 mile in 8 minutes (2km in 10 minutes) or 2 miles in 17–18 minutes (3km in 16 minutes) denotes a good standard of fitness.

SKATING AND SKIING

The low temperatures in which winter sports are performed have been proved to have an invigorating and stimulating effect. Skating is great fun and can provide very good all-round exercise providing it is sufficiently vigorous. Skiing is a highly enjoyable and vigorous sport that improves balance, coordination, agility, and often nerve. There are two main forms: Alpine and Nordic.

Alpine skiing includes regular downhill skiing and also slalom skiing, in which the skier negotiates a twisting course of gates. It provides great exercise for the legs, increasing their strength and endurance, but because of the short nature of the strenuous bursts of energy followed by rests and rides up the slope, it does not provide much cardio-vascular or respiratory stimulation.

Nordic skiing includes cross-country skiing, which provides much greater overall exercise than downhill skiing, exercising most of the muscle groups in the body. Skiing uphill and down provides constant, often strenuous effort over a longer period of time, making this form of skiing excellent exercise for the cardio-vascular and respiratory systems. It has the further advantages of allowing the skier a greater measure of freedom and solitude.

1 Skating is a sport of balance and grace. Exercise benefits depend on the degree of exertion, ranging from the mild exercise of "promenade" skating, through figure skating, to the intense physical efforts required for speed skating and hockey.

2 Downhill skiing provides very good exercise for the legs, but unless runs are of at least 10 minutes' duration it has the disadvantages of a high accident rate and of requiring a good level of fitness and periods of preconditioning.

3 Cross-country skiing is excellent for endurance and the major muscle groups. It is not as expensive or as dangerous as downhill skiing, requires only around a ½ hour of training, does not need slopes and can burn up to 1000 Calories an hour.

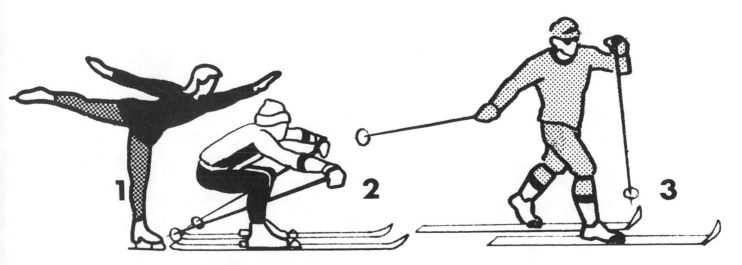

© DIAGRAM

CYCLING

Cycling is a healthy and highly enjoyable means of transport. It can also provide excellent exercise for the cardio-vascular system and the upper legs. It is also good for the lower legs and the lungs, although the sitting and often hunched position prevents the proper use of the diaphragm and can sometimes encourage shallow breathing with the upper chest instead of full diaphragmatic breathing. Cycling is the best way of traveling through the countryside, being clean, open and quiet. In cities bicycles can be useful to beat heavy traffic, but the danger of accidents is increased and there is the added drawback of increasing your lung ventilation in the clouds of city exhaust fumes. Leg injury is less likely than with running, but to be effective from an exercise point of view cycling must be done vigorously, usually at speeds over 10mph (16km/h). Cycling can aggravate back problems because of the hunched posture and strain on the lower spine, but should not cause problems for anyone with a healthy and flexible back. Styles of bicycle range from the usual 10-speed touring bicycle (though 15 gears are possible) to the gearless, brakeless, fixed-wheel, track-racing bicycle.

1 Everyday cycling usually consists of trips to and from the place of work. It is an excellent way to fit exercise into your daily routine. If the journey is short, it can be supplemented by 3–4 mile runs in the morning and evening.

2 Track and road racing both require a very high degree of fitness. Track racing needs a special bicycle and, usually, an angled track. For road racing, a lightweight 10-speed bicycle is usually used for distances up to 90 miles (150km) a day.

3 Cycle touring is becoming increasingly popular. Bicycles for touring must be stronger than road-racers with respect to the load carried.

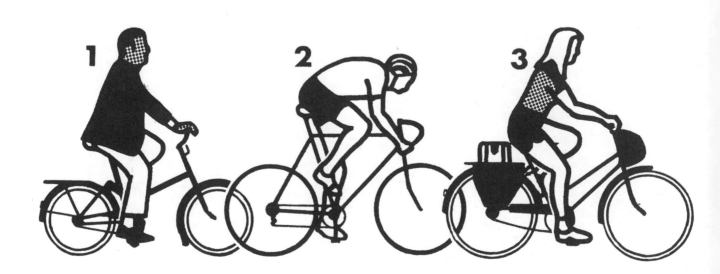

BOATING AND RIDING

Activities involving boats can be an effective and enjoyable way of taking exercise. Rowing is a vigorous sport providing excellent all-round exercise, and developing strength and stamina. There are, however, problems with facilities (or the nearness of flat water) and the availability of equipment, which can be expensive. Canoeing also provides good exercise, especially for the trunk and arms. Sailing, too, is an invigorating and exhilarating sport, though again the equipment is expensive. Ocean dinghy racing can provide good all-round exercise, but benefits are less in large boats or when sailing on lakes or rivers.

1 Canoeing provides good all-round exercise. Races are held on still water courses from 500m to 10,000m. There are individual, pair and team events for kayaks and Canadian canoes. Other events are held on wild, or white, water.

1

Riding horses remains an essential skill in certain areas but for most of its practitioners it is now a purely recreational activity. Buying and owning a horse is very expensive, and even the cost of hiring a horse at a riding school puts this activity out of many people's reach.

2 Horseback riding The physically beneficial effects of horseback riding vary with the particular activity. Apart from relaxation and enjoyment, the benefits of hacking and pony trekking are minimal, although they can be increased with long periods of trotting. Jumping, especially under show conditions, can be very energetic and provide good exercise. Hunting also provides good exercise, combining jumping and long, fast riding. Not everyone, however, agrees with the ethics of this sport.

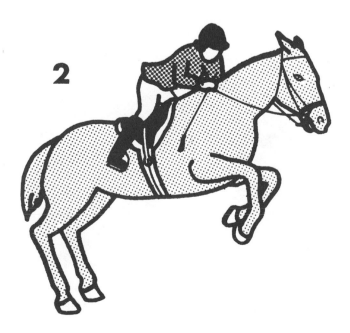

2

ATHLETICS

Athletics combines events which together lead to an all-round physical development of strength, speed, endurance, agility, coordination and flexibility. Facilities are found at schools, colleges and athletics clubs.

Within the broader categories of track and field there are four major groups of events: running, throwing, jumping and combined. All these require and promote a basic fitness, endurance and level of skill, but each specialization has its own needs and effects. It is here that the different abilities of body types and personal constitution are most visible. Running, especially middle and long distance, is best for endurance — top class runners often have a resting pulse rate of around 50 per minute, compared to an average man's 70 per minute. In sprinting and hurdling events leg strength is more important than endurance. Throwing requires weight and strength, especially in the arms and trunk, whereas jumping requires a greater degree of coordination and flexibility, with power in the legs.

Within the range of athletics an event can be found to suit almost everyone. Some people show good all-round ability and do best at combined events: the pentathlon for women and the decathlon for men. The pentathlon combines 100m hurdles, shot put, high jump, long jump and 200m. The decathlon combines 100m, long jump, shot put, high jump, 400m, 110m hurdles, discus, pole vault, javelin and 1500m. Both are two-day events in which competitors score points for individual performances.

Range of events
There are 25 athletics events in the Olympic Games, each requiring a slightly different skill and emphasizing a different aspect of fitness.
1 Sprints (100m, 200m, 400m) need powerful leg muscles for explosive speed.
2 Middle and long distance runs (800m, 1500m, 5000m, 10,000m) combine power with endurance.
3 Road races — marathon (42.195km) and walks (20km, 50km) — put emphasis on stamina and mental discipline.
4 Hurdles (100m, 110m, 400m) and steeplechase (3000m) combine running with jumping power.
5 Shot put, hammer, discus and javelin all need great strength, coordination, flexibility and, in all but the javelin, weight.
6 High, long and triple jump and pole vaulting (**7**) call for strong legs, flexibility and coordination.

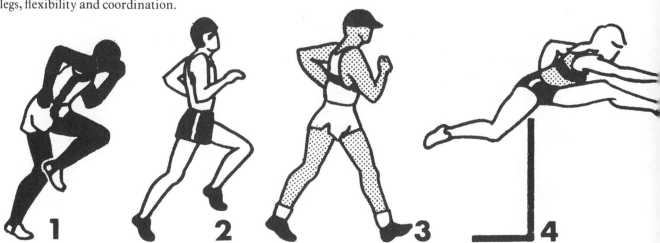

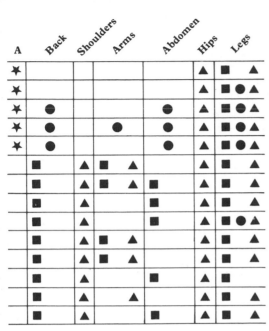

A	Back	Shoulders	Arms	Abdomen	Hips	Legs	
★					▲	■ ▲	**Sprints**
★					▲	■ ● ▲	**Middle distance**
★	●			●	▲	■ ● ▲	**Long distance**
★	●		●	●	▲	■ ● ▲	**Marathon**
★	●			●	▲	■ ● ▲	**Walking**
	■	▲	■ ▲		▲	■ ▲	**Shot put**
	■	▲	■ ▲	■	▲	■ ▲	**Pole vault**
	■	▲		■	▲	■ ▲	**Triple jump**
	■	▲		■	▲	■ ● ▲	**Hurdling**
	■	▲	■ ▲		▲	■ ▲	**Discus**
	■	▲	■ ▲		▲	■ ▲	**Hammer**
	■	▲		■	▲	■	**High jump**
	■	▲	▲		▲	■ ▲	**Javelin**
	■	▲		■	▲	■ ▲	**Long jump**

A Cardio-respiratory endurance
■ Muscle strength
● Muscle endurance
▲ Flexibility

Fitness benefits

This chart shows the fitness benefits, to the various parts of the body, of the major athletics events. Weight training aids all those muscle groups requiring strength and endurance, and professional dietary advice and special skill-development training should be followed by anyone taking part in competitions.

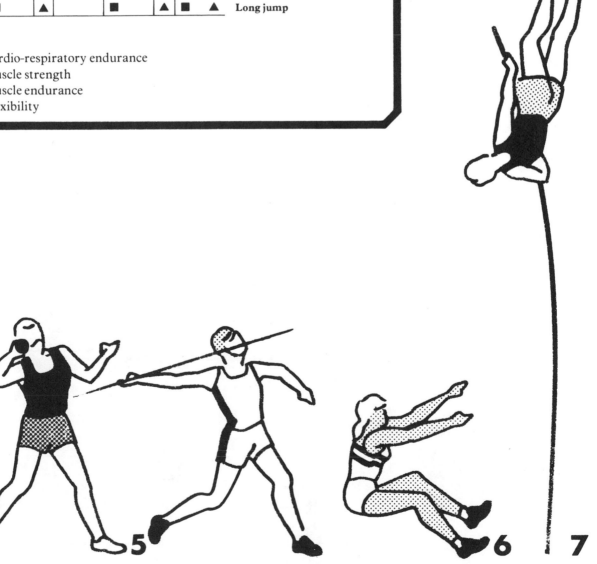

5 6 7

©DIAGRAM

GYMNASTICS

Gymnastics has been a popular sport from the days of ancient Greece to the current success of televised international competitions and displays. Its combination of strength, suppleness, beauty, grace and control make it a most demanding and rewarding sport. Performance requires a high degree of fitness and dedication in every form, plus confidence and courage. It is increasingly becoming a sport for the young, but once a basic level of competence has been acquired practice and enjoyment can be continued well into middle age.

Floor exercises (1) (women) are the most integrative exercises. The gymnast attempts to create an aesthetically unified image with a mixture of ballet, dance and acrobatic movements. This calls for a high degree of grace, flexibility, balance, strength, rhythm, creativity and imagination. Tumble jumps, spins, pirouettes, skips, jumps, handsprings, somersaults, dance steps, rolling, lying and kneeling positions must be combined into a flowing, harmonious and expressive sequence.
Floor exercises are performed on a mat 40×40ft (12×12m) and the entire area must be used during a combination of compulsory and optional exercises.

Apparatus work demands strength and muscle endurance, mainly of the arms and trunk, as well as overall flexibility and great skill. There are seven events.
Pommel horse (men) demands strength, balance and agility as the gymnast performs swings, circles, scissor and undercutting (where the legs pass under one raised arm) movements around the horse while supporting himself on the pommel with one or both arms. Great spinal flexibility and rhythm are necessary, as no part of the body is allowed to touch the horse.
Vaulting horse (men and women) demands balance, agility and control with some strength as the gymnast vaults over a plain horse.

Horizontal bar (men) is a simple, flexible bar suspended a maximum of 8ft 5in (2.55m) from the floor. Giant swings, circles and turns around the bar are performed with a wide variety of hand grips, one of which involves letting go of the bar and then grasping it again, each time with both hands at the same time.
Parallel bars (2) (men) are bars 1ft 4¾in (0.42m) apart and 5ft 3in (1.60m) off the ground. They require a combination of the skills and exercises of the pommel horse and horizontal bars.
Rings (men) hang 8ft 2in (2.50m) off the ground. Ring exercises show strength and flexibility with swings, handstands and hanging positions sometimes held for as long as 2 seconds.

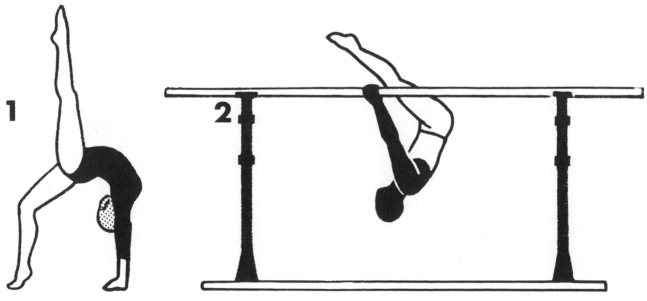

Certain gymnastic exercises can be used to supplement or add variety to all other forms of training. As a sport itself, gymnastics is best started young, and really needs a fair degree of fitness, strength and flexibility to begin, together with professional advice and training. Equipment may be a problem but is usually available at schools, colleges, private gymnasiums and clubs.

In competition, men perform on the pommel and vaulting horse, horizontal bar, parallel bars, rings and floor; women on the vaulting horse, asymmetric bars, beam and floor.

Beam (women) is only 4in (10cm) wide and is designed to test, primarily, the gymnast's balance and coordination as she performs turns, jumps, leaps, running and walking steps and even somersaults.

Asymmetric bars (women) are parallel bars of uneven height between which the gymnast swings, twists, turns and flies. This apparatus demands strength as well as agility, flexibility and coordination.

Gymnastique moderne (3) (women) is an international event not yet included in Olympic gymnastics. It is a floor event emphasizing grace and beauty of movement. The gymnast performs mainly dance and ballet movements with various kinds of hand apparatus including ribbon (see p. 188), ball, two skittles, rope and hula-hoop. The gymnast is judged on her precision of movement and direction, rhythm, elegance, coordination and musical and artistic interpretation, together with the complexity and originality of her performance.

Trampolining (4) helps to develop balance, rhythm, coordination, timing and endurance. Forward and backward somersaults, twists, turns and bounces from various positions should be performed in a synchronized, rhythmical routine. There should always be "spotters" stationed at each side of the trampoline ready to catch, or warn, the jumpers if they bounce too close to the edge.

Related activities include figure skating, dancing, diving and calisthenics, while gymnastic performance can also be aided by the controlled use of weights for strength and yoga for flexibility.

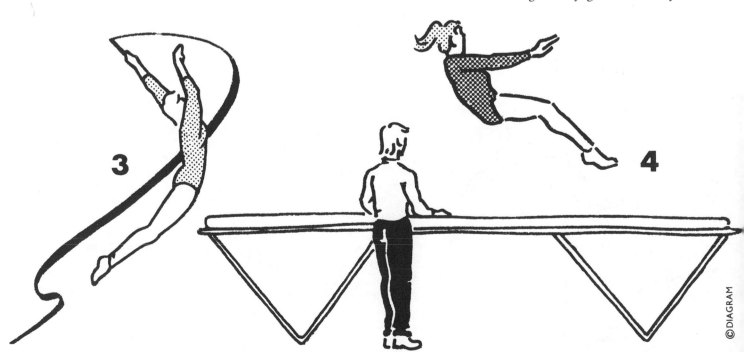

© DIAGRAM

FITNESS REQUIREMENTS

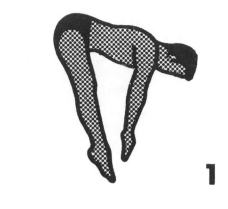

1 Swimming (pp. 202, 205, 206, 216)
Medium strength in arms, shoulders, back and abdomen.
Low to medium strength in legs.
High endurance in arms and shoulders.
Medium endurance in back, abdomen and legs.
High flexibility in all areas.
High CR (cardio-vascular and respiratory) endurance.

These categories assume that you swim for extended periods of time (15–30 minutes). Swimming is especially good exercise because the body weight is supported by the water, and shock to the tissues and joints is therefore avoided. It is an excellent form of exercise for back-sufferers, convalescents and the elderly.

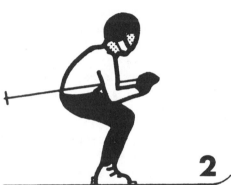

2 Skiing (pp. 205, 207, 217)
High strength in legs and back.
High endurance in legs.
High flexibility in knees, ankles and back.
Medium to high CR endurance.
The longer the actual skiing time the greater the fitness needs and benefits. Cross-country skiing requires high levels of fitness in all areas of the body.

3 Golf (pp. 202, 204, 205, 206, 218)
Low to medium strength in arms and shoulders.
Flexibility in arms, shoulders and back.
Little CR endurance needed, and even less if a cart or caddy is used.

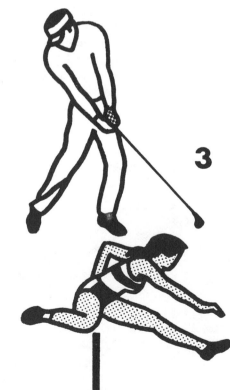

4 Athletics (pp. 210, 211)
Track events
High strength in legs.
High endurance in legs.
Medium flexibility in all areas.
High CR endurance.
Running in track events will tone and strengthen other areas of the body, which should also be exercised with complementary exercises.

Field events
High strength in legs and varying areas, dependent upon the event.
Medium endurance in all areas.
High flexibility in all areas, especially the back.
Low to medium CR endurance.

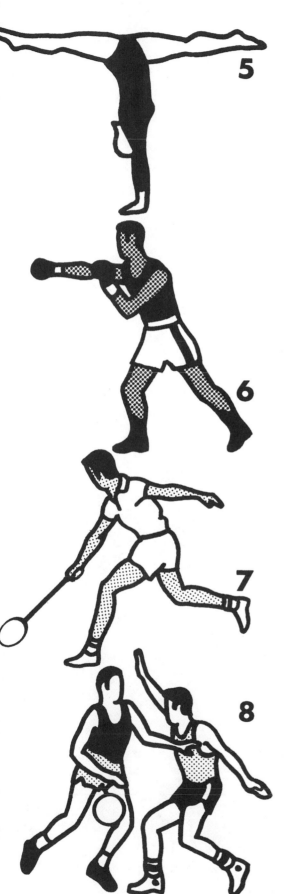

5 Gymnastics (pp. 203, 212, 213, 219)
High strength in all areas.
High endurance in all areas.
High flexibility in all areas.
Medium to high CR endurance.
Gymnastics also requires a high degree of development of balance, rhythm, coordination and concentration. It requires the highest degree of all-round physical competence of any sport.

6 Combat sports (pp. 203, 204, 220, 221, 247)
High strength in all areas.
High endurance in all areas.
Medium to high flexibility in all areas.
High CR endurance.
Oriental combat sports usually require more balance and coordination than other combat sports because of the greater range of movements.

The use of weights is for increasing strength, and "roadwork" (distance running) for CR endurance.

7 Racquet sports (pp. 202, 204, 205, 206, 222)
Medium strength in arms, shoulders, back and abdomen.
High strength in legs.
Medium to high endurance in all areas.
Medium to high flexibility in all areas.
Medium to high CR endurance.
Squash and handball are usually more demanding than, for

example, tennis. The powers of endurance necessary vary with how vigorously the game is played.

8 Team sports (pp. 203, 205, 206, 223)
Medium to high strength in all areas depending upon the game being played.
High endurance in the legs and all other areas involved.
Medium to high endurance in all areas.
High CR endurance.
Most team games require the ability to run for often extended

periods of time, and the other areas of the body should be kept proportionally exercised.

FOR SWIMMERS

EXERCISES

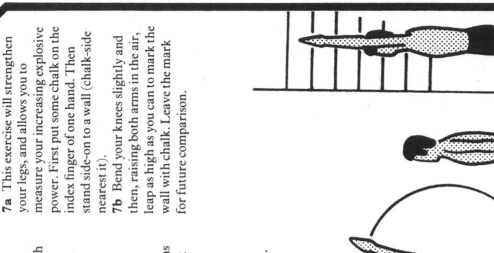

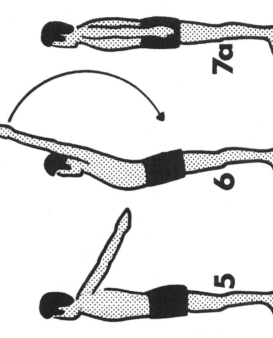

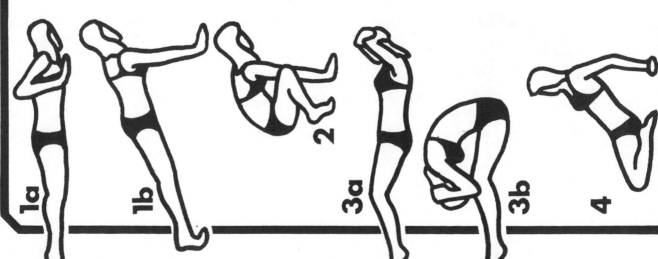

Exercises for swimmers
Although there is no need to be fit to enjoy a swim, power and efficiency in the water can be much improved by exercises done on dry land. Weight training and other strength exercises can be used to build up muscles and to increase stamina. Also very helpful are mobility exercises using movements similar to those involved in swimming.

1a Lie facedown with your legs together, your toes tucked under, and your hands, palms down and fingers forward, directly under your shoulders.

1b Keeping your back and legs rigid, straighten your arms to raise your body to balance on your hands and toes. Lower yourself gently down again and repeat. This exercise will strengthen arm and shoulder muscles; if it is too difficult, see p. 286 for easier versions.

2 From position 1b, jump forward to squat as shown, balancing on your toes with your palms flat on the ground. Then kick your feet back to return to the starting position. Repeat.

3a Lie on your back, with legs together, knees slightly bent, hands linked behind your neck.

3b Use your stomach muscles to sit up and then lean forward until your forehead touches your knees. Slowly return to the starting position, and repeat.

4 Ankle flexibility will improve your swimming kick; this exercise should help. Sit on the ground with your knees bent and your feet tucked under your buttocks. With your hands on the ground behind you, lean back, raising your knees to stretch your ankles.

5 Stand with your arms raised to shoulder height in front of you, palms together. Keeping your arms at shoulder height, pull them back hard to the sides. Repeat.

6 Stand with your arms raised to shoulder height in front of you, palms down. Swing them up and back in as large a circle as you can. Repeat. ✍

7a This exercise will strengthen your legs, and allows you to measure your increasing explosive power. First put some chalk on the index finger of one hand. Then stand side-on to a wall (chalk-side nearest it).

7b Bend your knees slightly and then, raising both arms in the air, leap as high as you can to mark the wall with chalk. Leave the mark for future comparison.

FOR SKIERS

Exercises for skiers

Skiing is a very demanding sport, requiring overall fitness and stamina. To make the most of your time on the slopes you should start a training program several months in advance. Dry ski runs are available in many areas for practicing, but pre–ski exercises are still essential.

The action of skiing involves swinging your arms, twisting your trunk, and flexing your knees and ankles. It also needs good coordination, rhythm and balance. General posture and breathing are also important, as is relaxation.

Running, jogging, jumping and skipping rope, climbing stairs, balancing on one leg, and flexing your feet will all help prepare your body for skiing.

The following exercises are recommended for use in the months before you go skiing and also for limbering up before a run.

1 Stand erect with your arms by your sides. Keeping your feet flat on the ground, raise your arms as high as you can for a count of 5. Lower them slowly.

2 This exercise will increase the flexibility of your waist and develop your arm swing. Stand with your arms raised above your head. Moving from the waist up, swing your arms as far to the left as possible. Then swing them over to the right. Repeat from side to side.

3 Stand erect with your arms raised to the sides to shoulder level. Swing your arms back as far as you can. Then swing them forward. Repeat several times.

4 Stand erect with your feet together and your arms raised behind you, palms up. Then bend your knees as far as you can, keeping your upper body straight and your legs together. Slowly straighten up. Repeat.

5 Stand erect with your feet together. Keeping your body straight and your feet flat on the ground, bend your knees while at the same time twisting them to the left. Straighten up, and then repeat the exercise twisting your knees to the right. Repeat from side to side.

6 Stand erect with your feet together and a bottle placed by your right heel. Bend your knees and swing to the right to pick up the bottle with your left hand. Repeat with the bottle by your left heel, picking it up with your right hand.

7a Stand with your feet together and your knees bent. Then jump up, turning 90° left in the air before landing, on your toes, facing the side.

7b Crouch down again and jump 90° to the right so that you end up facing the direction in which you started.

8 Stand with your feet together and your knees bent. Jump as high as you can to the left, as though clearing a fence. Then jump to the right. Repeat from side to side.

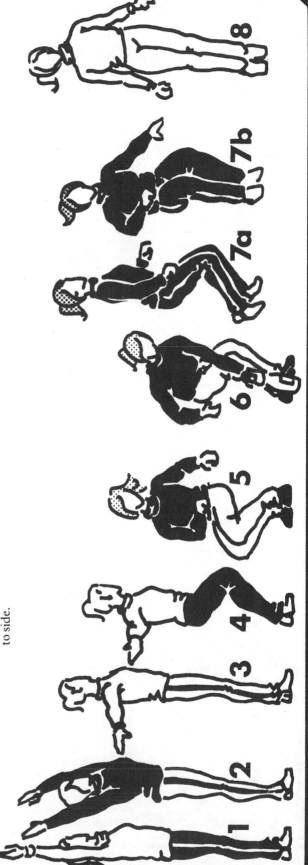

EXERCISES

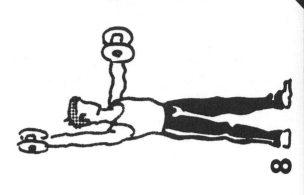

Exercises for golfers

Requirements for a golfer include good posture, coordination, balance, fluidity of movement and a sense of rhythm. You also need to be reasonably supple to enable you to pivot smoothly to follow through a stroke. Training with weights, or improvised equipment, will help improve your swing by increasing the strength of your arm and shoulder muscles. Grip will be improved by strengthening your wrists and fingers.

1 Stand about 2ft (60cm) behind a chair, your hands resting on its back. Raise your left leg as high as you can behind you. Bring it back beside the other leg. Then repeat the action with your right leg.

2 Grip a golf ball in each hand and stretch your arms behind you. Swing them forward, up, back and round in a circle. Then swing them in the opposite direction.

3 Hold a weight in each hand in front of your thighs. Then swing your arms and upper body as far as you can to the left. Swing back to face forward, and then swing to the right. Repeat.

4 Stand with your feet apart, holding a golf club across your back. Turn as far as you can to the left, keeping your hips to the front. Repeat to the right.

5 This exercise will strengthen your knees and legs. Stand with your feet apart, holding a barbell across your shoulders. Keeping your feet flat on the ground and your back straight, squat down, breathing out. Straighten up, breathing in. Repeat several times.

6 Hold a barbell across your thighs. Keeping your back straight, bend your arms and bring it up to your chest. Repeat several times.

7 Stand with your feet together, holding a barbell across your thighs. Keeping your legs straight, bend over slowly to lower the barbell to the ground. Straighten up slowly. Repeat.

8 Stand with your feet slightly apart, a weight in each hand. Raise your right arm straight up and extend the left arm forward. Reverse your arm positions, repeating several times.

EXERCISE

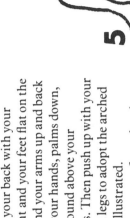

5

6a **6b**

7a **7b**

8c

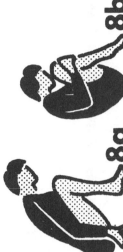

8b

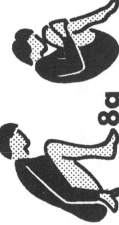

8a

1

2a

2b

3

4

Exercises for gymnasts

A gymnast must be both strong and supple, and preliminary exercises are designed to develop these qualities. Strength can be increased with bodybuilding exercises. Here we describe a number of mobility exercises, which should be performed daily, if possible, to extend your range of movement and to keep you generally supple. They can also be used to warm up gradually before apparatus work in the gym — absolutely essential if serious muscle injury is to be avoided.

1 Stand with your back to a wall and raise your left leg as high as you can. Then get a partner gently to push it still farther. Repeat with your right leg.

2a Lie flat on your back and lift your right leg as high as you can.

2b Keeping the rest of your body flat, grasp your raised leg with both hands and pull it toward your face. Repeat with your left leg.

3 Sit on the ground with your legs in the "splits" position. Then with your right arm raised above your head and your left arm held across your body, lean over toward your left foot. Change arm positions and repeat to the other side.

4 Sit with your legs wide apart. Bending from the base of your spine, lean forward to touch each foot with the corresponding hand.

5 Lie on your back with your knees bent and your feet flat on the floor. Bend your arms up and back to place your hands, palms down, on the ground above your shoulders. Then push up with your arms and legs to adopt the arched position illustrated.

6a Lying on your front, bend your knees and reach back with both hands to clasp your ankles.

6b Pull hard so that your chest and thighs are raised as shown.

7a Kneel down with your buttocks resting on your feet, and your hands out to the sides.

7b Lie back to adopt the position shown, and then press down with your hands in order to return to the starting position.

8a Sit with your knees bent close to your body.

8b Grip your knees and bring them up to your chin.

8c Roll back and balance as in the illustration.

FOR COMBAT SPORTS

EXERCISES

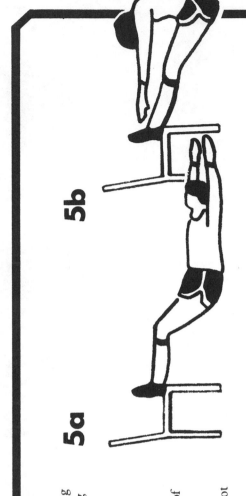

1

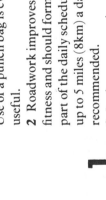
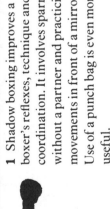
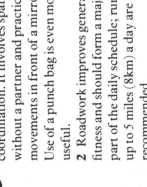

4

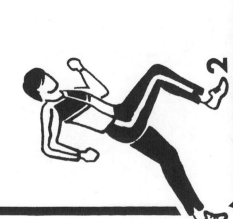

3

2

Exercises for participants of Western combat sports

Boxing and wrestling call for a combination of strength, stamina, coordination, speed and agility. Training must reflect all these aspects. Weight training (p. 234) and exercise machines (p. 196) are invaluable. Here we describe several other types of training.

1 Shadow boxing improves a boxer's reflexes, technique and coordination. It involves sparring without a partner and practicing movements in front of a mirror. Use of a punch bag is even more useful.

2 Roadwork improves general fitness and should form a major part of the daily schedule; runs of up to 5 miles (8km) a day are recommended.

3 In the gym, running on the spot or on a treadmill will increase stamina and strengthen the leg muscles.

4 Jumping rope is good training for participants of combat sports (see p. 190). This type of exercise increases muscular strength, endurance, cardio-respiratory fitness, speed, flexibility, agility, balance and footwork.

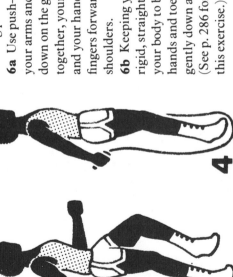

6a
6b

5b
5a

5a Use this exercise to strengthen your stomach muscles. Lie on your back with your heels on a chair seat and your arms stretched overhead behind you.

5b Pulling from your stomach muscles, raise yourself into a sitting position and then lean forward to touch your ankles. Hold for a count of 5 and then slowly lower yourself back to your starting position. Repeat.

6a Use push-ups to strengthen your arms and shoulders. Lie face-down on the ground, with your legs together, your toes tucked under, and your hands, palms down and fingers forward, under your shoulders.

6b Keeping your back and legs rigid, straighten your arms to raise your body to balance on your hands and toes. Lower yourself gently down again, and repeat. (See p. 286 for easier versions of this exercise.)

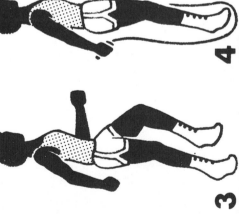

EXERCISES

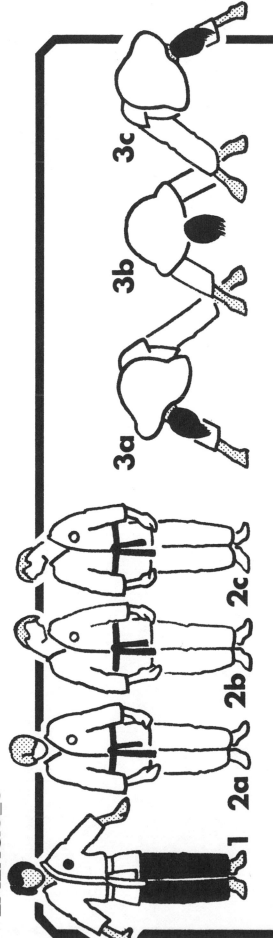

3c

3b

3a

2a 2b 2c

1

Exercises for participants of Oriental combat sports

Judo, Karate and Kung Fu are all ancient forms of self-defense. Speed, agility and flexibility are more important than strength. Relaxation, grace and self-control are also vital. Exercises for participants are designed to develop the various physical and mental qualities required for most Oriental sports.

1 Let your arms hang at your sides. In turn, shake your hands, your lower arms, and finally your entire arms until they feel loose.
2a Let your head hang forward.
2b Roll your head to the left.
2c Roll your head back, then to the right. Repeat in reverse.
3a Stand with your legs wide apart. Keeping them straight, bend from the waist and touch your forehead to your right knee.
3b Bend between your legs.
3c Touch your left knee with your forehead. Straighten up. Repeat.

4a From a standing position, squat down, bending your right knee and extending your left leg forward and to the side as shown, while at the same time bending your right arm across your chest and pressing your left hand on your left leg.
4b Repeat, reversing your arm and leg positions.

5a Stand with your hands on your hips. Bend your right knee to rest your right foot on your left knee. Balance in this position.
5b Repeat, raising your left leg.
6 With your arms out to the sides, raise your left leg straight in front of you as high as you can, leaning back to balance. Repeat, raising the other leg.

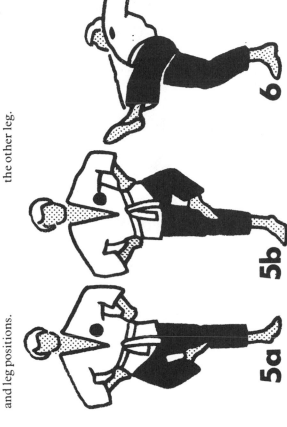

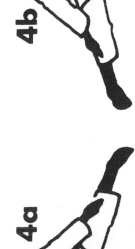

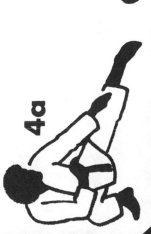

5a

5b

6

4a

4b

FOR RACQUET SPORTS

EXERCISES

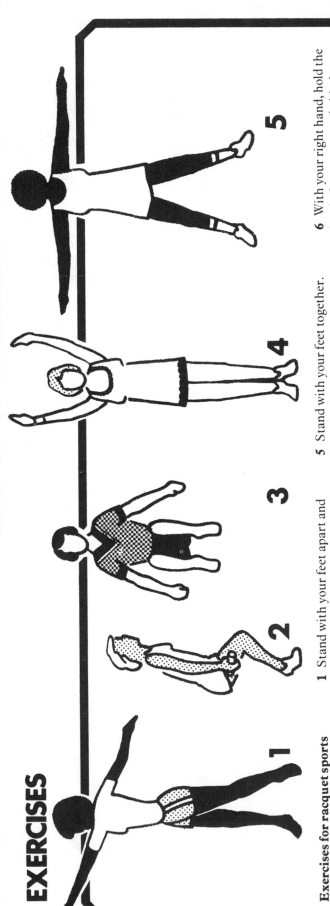

Exercises for racquet sports
These sports call for a combination of speed, agility and strength. Jogging, running and swimming are ideal all-round conditioners. Clasping exercises, such as squeezing a tennis ball, will strengthen your grip. Arm and shoulder muscles can be developed with the aid of weights and pulleys. Much of a player's control over the ball lies in his capacity to stretch, pivot or jump and then to recover instantly. Jumping exercises will strengthen your legs and improve balance and coordination, while stretching exercises will greatly increase your ability to return a well-placed ball.

1 Stand with your feet apart and your arms raised to shoulder level to the sides. Pivoting from the hips, swing as far as you can to the right and then to the left. Continue swinging from side to side.

2 Stand with your feet apart, holding a light weight in each hand. Raise your heels and bend your knees to sink to a half-squat. Then lean back and try to touch your heels with the weights.

3 Stand with your feet together. Jump as high as you can, bringing your knees up to your chest as you jump. Straighten up and land on your toes. Repeat.

4 Stand with your feet together. Jump as high as you can, stretching your arms above your head. Land on your toes and bend your knees to sink into a squat, bounce, and leap up again.

5 Stand with your feet together. Jump in the air to turn through 90°, raising your arms and legs out to the sides and then lowering them again during the course of your jump. Carry on jumping in this way to make a complete circle. Continue round and round, as fast as you can.

6 With your right hand, hold the head of your racquet behind your neck. Reach round with your left hand to grasp its handle. Pull hard with both arms. Repeat, reversing your arm position.

7 Stand with your legs apart and your arms raised to the sides at shoulder level. Pull your arms back as hard as you can.

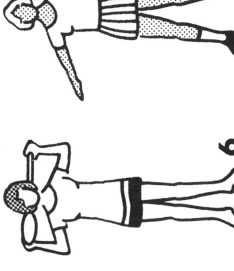

EXERCISES

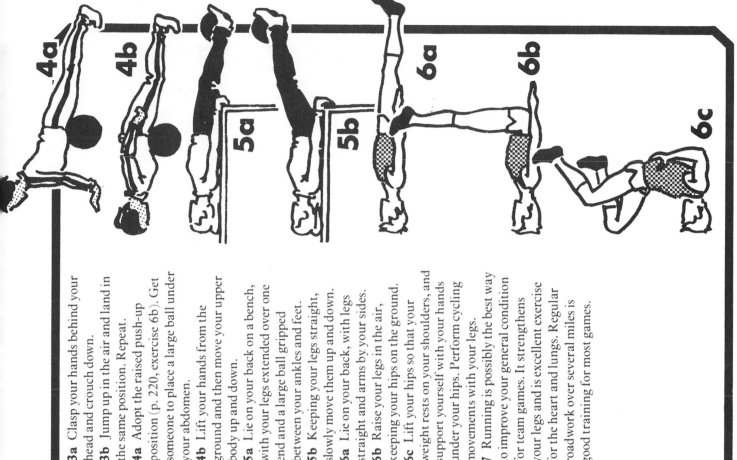

Exercises for team games

A team must practice together to develop quick reflexes and skill in passing or tackling. But these actions also depend on individual fitness. All team games demand strength, mobility and stamina. Arms and legs must be strong for running and tackling, while heart and lungs must be in very good shape to work extra hard to provide for sudden spurts of speed.

1a Stand with hands on hips.
1b Keep your back straight as you lunge forward onto your right leg. Then jump up in the air and quickly reverse your leg positions. Continue jumping and reversing legs.

2 Start with one foot on a bench. Jump in the air and return that foot to the ground while putting your other foot on the bench. Continue changing feet.

3a Clasp your hands behind your head and crouch down.
3b Jump up in the air and land in the same position. Repeat.

4a Adopt the raised push-up position (p. 220, exercise 6b). Get someone to place a large ball under your abdomen.
4b Lift your hands from the ground and then move your upper body up and down.

5a Lie on your back on a bench, with your legs extended over one end and a large ball gripped between your ankles and feet.
5b Keeping your legs straight, slowly move them up and down.

6a Lie on your back, with legs straight and arms by your sides.
6b Raise your legs in the air, keeping your hips on the ground.
6c Lift your hips so that your weight rests on your shoulders, and support yourself with your hands under your hips. Perform cycling movements with your legs.

7 Running is possibly the best way to improve your general condition for team games. It strengthens your legs and is excellent exercise for the heart and lungs. Regular roadwork over several miles is good training for most games.

©DIAGRAM

Chapter 7   SPECIALTY EXERCISES

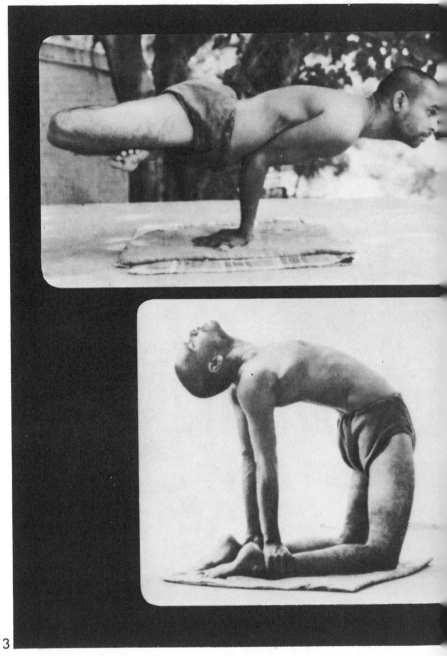

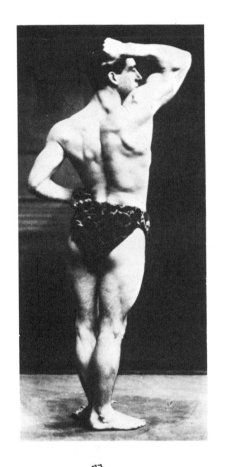

3

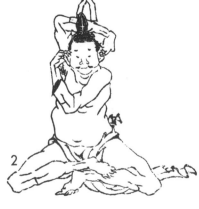

2

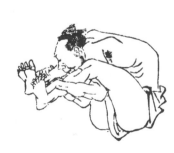

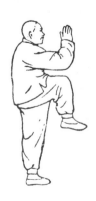

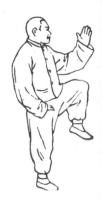

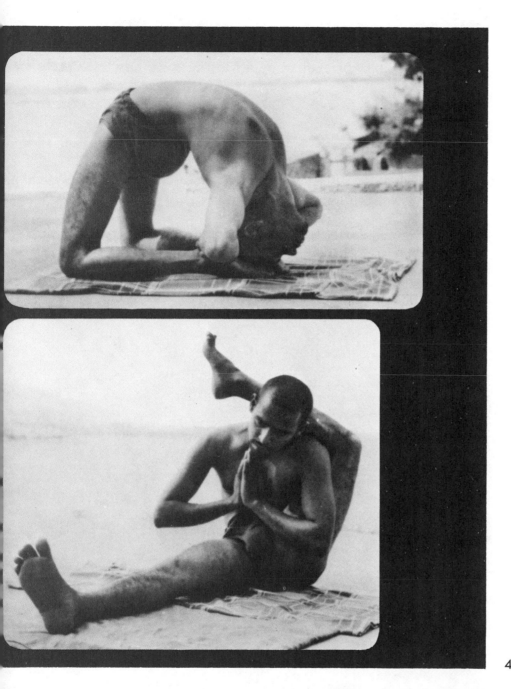

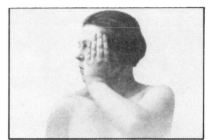

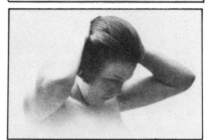

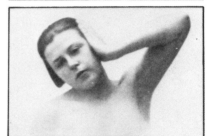

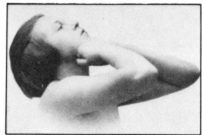

4

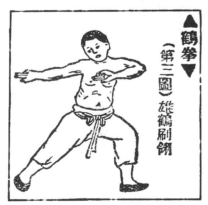

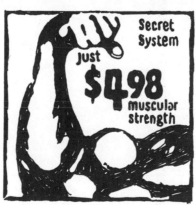

1 Circus performer (Radio Times Hulton Picture Library)
2 *Hokusai Manga:* sketchbooks of Hokusai (Tokyo 1814)
3 *Yoga Asanas* by Louis Frederic (Thorsons Publishers, UK 1970)
4 *The Body Beautiful* by Alice Bloch (The Bodley Head, London 1933)

ISOMETRICS

Isometric exercises are exercises without movement, in which one group of muscles exerts pressure against an immovable object or an opposing group of muscles. This means that the muscles involved in the exercise are put into a state of "static contraction," with no movement at the joints and no change in the length of the muscles (hence the name "iso"-"metric," meaning same length). This is in contrast to "isotonic" exercises, which involve the lengthening and shortening of the muscles and the moving of joints, as for example in weight lifting.

Isometric exercise
This form of exercise calls for maximum muscular exertion. Since our daily routine uses only 20–30% of our potential muscle strength, isometric exercises which use up to 100% of this strength can obviously have very significant results.

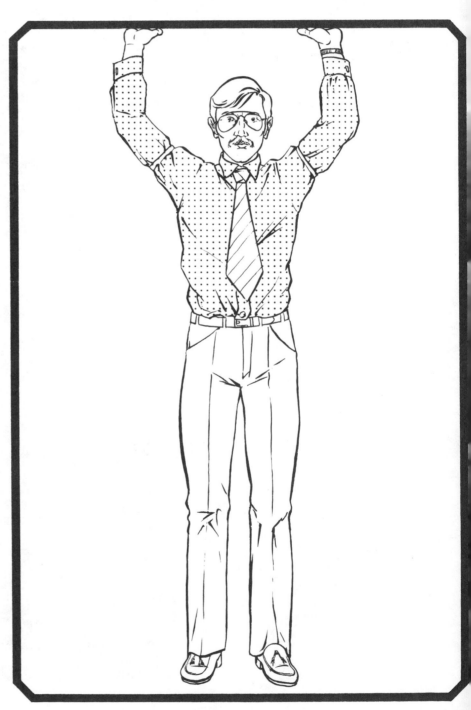

Isometrics increase the strength and improve the muscles' tone and shape, and one of their main advantages is the speed with which this is accomplished. A single exercise takes up surprisingly little time, being based on the exertion of maximum muscle force for a recommended period not exceeding 6 seconds. It is argued that a comprehensive program of only 15 exercises will exercise the whole body — and this in only 90 seconds! Since the muscles are used to maximum efficiency in isometric exercises, it is further argued that an isometric program will bring results within days rather than weeks or months.

Isometric exercises can easily be done by the busiest housewife or office worker. As well as requiring very little time, isometric exercises can be done without special equipment in the home, the office, the car or a bus. Many exercises use no equipment at all, force being exerted against opposing groups of muscles. Others use walls, door frames, chairs, tables and other easily available objects like telephones and waste baskets. Use whatever is at hand, but make sure that furniture is sufficiently sturdy. For variety some people may like to make the bar and rope device used in some of the exercises included in this book, but other equally effective exercises can be easily substituted.

There are, however, a number of drawbacks to isometrics, especially if they are a person's only form of exercise. Their main disadvantage is that they do not exercise the circulatory or respiratory systems. To compensate for this they should be done in conjunction with, and as an aid to, one or more of the many forms of aerobic exercise (see pages 20 and 320). Also the lack of movement in isometrics can lead to a shortening of muscle length and provides no improvement in joint flexibility. Carelessly done, isometric exercises can place undue strain on the joints and can damage them if they are weak. Because isometrics can place a strain on the heart they should most definitely be avoided by anyone suffering from high blood pressure or heart trouble. As with any form of exercise the usual warning applies — if it hurts while you are doing it, or in any way other than "muscle stiffness" afterward, stop without delay! There is such a wealth of different types of exercise that there is no need for anyone to persevere with an activity for which they are unsuited.

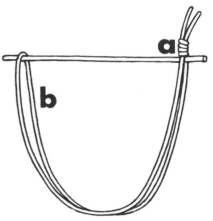

Bar and rope
Some of the exercises in this section make use of a bar and rope. This piece of equipment is easily made with a stout broom handle and a length of rope. Double up the rope to make a large loop, fastening the ends together with a slip knot(**a**). The loop is then placed over the broom handle as shown(**b**), and the slip knot can be used to adjust the size of the loop to suit the different exercise positions.

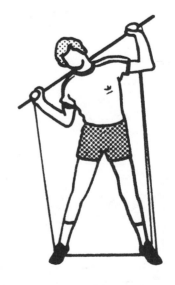

©DIAGRAM

Isometrics

EXERCISES

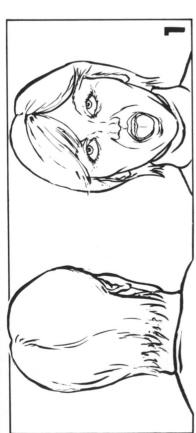

1

2

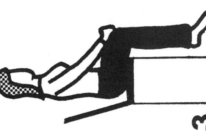

3

4

WARNING

Isometric exercises are more powerful than you may think. In each case the exercising activity should last for a maximum of 6 seconds. Do not do the same exercise more than once a day.

Exercises for the face

Our normal expressions use only a few of our facial muscles. These isometric exercises will tone up your face, neck and throat muscles and help to combat the formation of wrinkles. Try them in front of a mirror.

1 Open your mouth and eyes very wide as though screaming silently. Hold this position for 6 seconds. Then relax.

2 This exercise is a good follow-up to the previous one. Screw up your eyes and mouth, trying to make your face as small as possible from top to bottom. Hold for 6 seconds. Then relax.

General exercises

3 This exercise relieves tension and tiredness in the muscles. Sit up straight on a chair and place your hands on your knees. Press down hard, using the muscles of your arms, shoulders and chest. At the same time push up from your toes against this force, using the muscles of your thighs and abdomen. Push for 6 seconds. Then relax.

4 This exercise helps to relieve tension and low spirits. Stand about 2ft (60cm) away from a wall, with your arms in front of you at shoulder level and your palms flat against the wall. Rise onto your toes and bend your knees to crouch slightly. Lean forward against the wall, pushing against it with your arms, shoulders, back and legs. Push for 6 seconds. Then relax.

EXERCISES

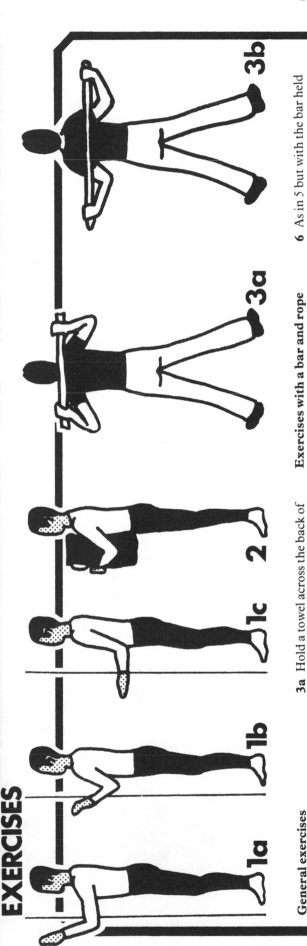

3a **3b**

1a **1b** **1c** **2**

General exercises

1a Place your hands at eye level one on each side of a doorjamb. Then push your hands toward each other as hard as you can for 6 seconds. Lower your arms and relax.

1b Repeat the pushing action with your hands at chest level.

1c Repeat the exercise with your hands at waist height.

2 Put your arms around a large bag or pillow and squeeze it as hard as you can against your body for 6 seconds. Then relax.

3a Hold a towel across the back of your neck, as shown. Pull it outward for 6 seconds. Relax.
3b Hold the towel across your back and over your upper arms. Pull outward for 6 seconds. Relax.

Exercises with a bar and rope

See p. 227 for how to make this.

4 Lie on your back with your knees bent. Hold the bar over your chest with the rope under your shoulders and your elbows bent. Push the bar up for 6 seconds.

5 Stand with the rope under your feet and the bar on your shoulders behind your neck. Push the bar up for 6 seconds.

6 As in 5 but with the bar held across the forehead to start.

7 Push up for 6 seconds with the rope under a chair seat and the bar across your forehead.

8 Stand on the rope and for 6 seconds pull the bar up from waist level.

9 Pull the bar up with your feet on the rope and your bottom out.

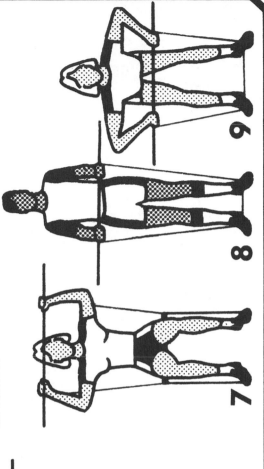

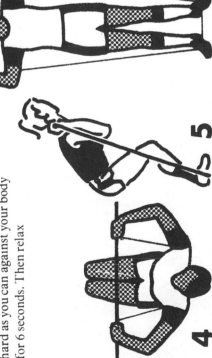

4 **5** **6** **7** **8** **9**

© DIAGRAM

Isometrics

EXERCISES

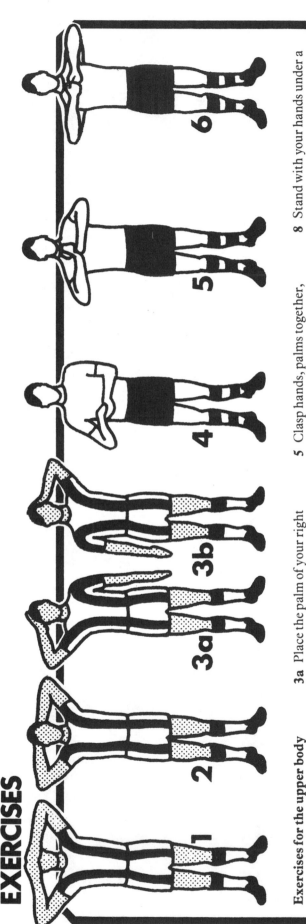

Exercises for the upper body

In each case the exercising action should be for 6 seconds.

1 Interlace your fingers across your forehead; push forward hard with your head and press back with your hands.

2 Interlace your fingers behind your head; push back with your head and pull forward with your hands.

3a Place the palm of your right hand against the right side of your head; push with your hand as you resist with your head and neck.

3b Repeat with your left hand.

4 Bend your left arm, palm up, across your stomach and lay your right palm on the left one as shown; press up with the left palm and down with the right. Reverse hands to repeat.

5 Clasp hands, palms together, close to your chest; press your hands hard against each other.

6 With elbows raised and hands close to your chest, link hands by curling the fingers of one hand up and the other down; try to pull your hands apart.

7a While seated, spread your fingers on a table or desk top and press down hard.

7b Repeat while standing.

8 Stand with your hands under a very heavy desk or table; pull upward and try to lift it.

9 Sit on an armless chair and grip the seat; try to lift it.

10 Sit with your knees together and your hands on the outside of them; push out with your knees and in with your hands.

11 Spread out your fingers as far as you can and then try to spread them even further.

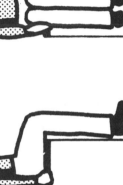
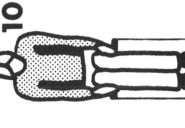
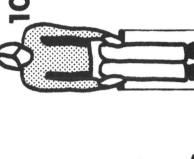
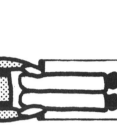
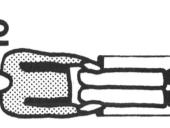
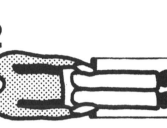

EXERCISES

Exercises for the upper body

In each case the exercising action should be for 6 seconds.

1 Stand with your back to a wall, with your arms by your sides and your palms facing the wall. Keeping your arms straight, press back hard against the wall.

2 Stand facing a wall, with your feet a few inches away from it, your arms straight down, and your palms turned toward the wall. Press your hands against the wall as hard as you can.

3 Stand in a doorway with your hands resting against the inside of the door frame as shown; push out as hard as you can.

4 Stand facing a wall, with your feet about 1ft (30cm) away from it and your hands, fingers pointing up and palms against the wall, raised above your head. Then push with your hands as though trying to lower them through the wall.

5 Stand in a doorway and raise your arms to push your palms up against the top of the door frame

(if your arms are insufficiently bent for you to be able easily to push up against the door frame, find a box that will raise you to a more comfortable height).

6 Stand with your left side a few inches away from a wall. Without bending your elbow, raise your left arm to the side so that the back of your hand is against the wall; continue pushing your hand against the wall as though to raise your arm still higher. Repeat, changing sides.

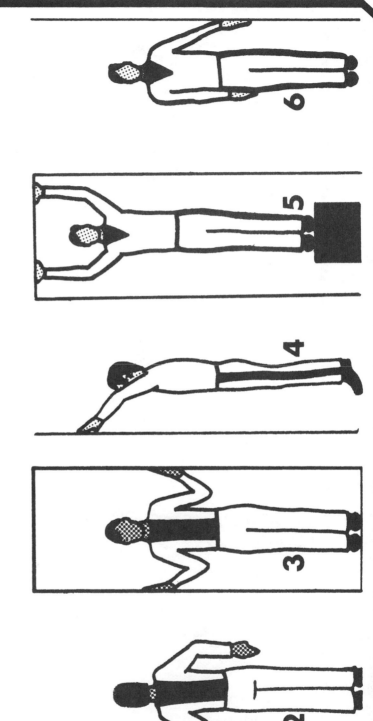

©DIAGRAM

EXERCISES

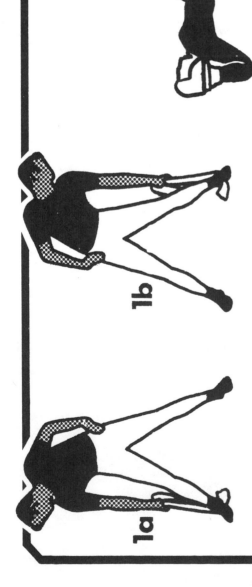

1a

1b

2a

2b

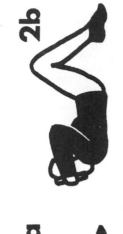

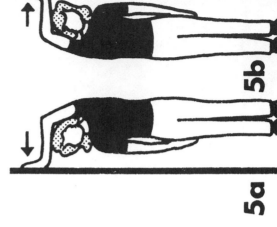

5a

5b

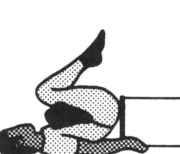

4

3a

3b

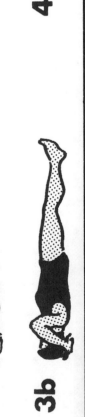

Exercises for waist and sides
In each case the exercising action should be for 6 seconds.

1a With one end of a towel in your right hand and with your left hand on your hip, stand with your feet apart and your right heel on the other end of the towel. Pull strongly on the towel, keeping your head, shoulder, arm and foot in a vertical line.

1b Repeat, holding the towel in your left hand.

2a Lie on your back with your knees raised, using both hands to hold a book behind your neck.

2b Try to sit up, bending but not arching your back. Pull up as high as you can and then hold this position for 6 seconds.

3a Lie on your back with your legs straight out, your feet together and your arms folded behind your head.

3b Pull your stomach in as hard as you can, as if trying to flatten it against your backbone.

4 Sit near the front of a strong chair and rest a pillow on your thighs. Gripping either the sides of the chair seat or the top of its back legs, raise your knees to crush the pillow between your thighs and stomach.

5a Stand with your right side about 18in (40cm) away from a wall. Raise your left hand above your head to push hard against the wall, bracing your left leg as you push.

5b Repeat, changing sides.

EXERCISES

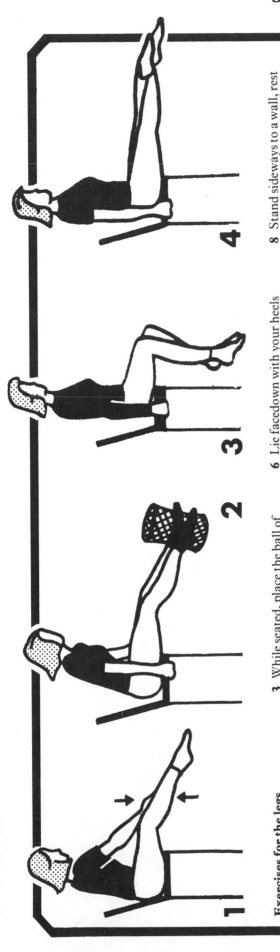

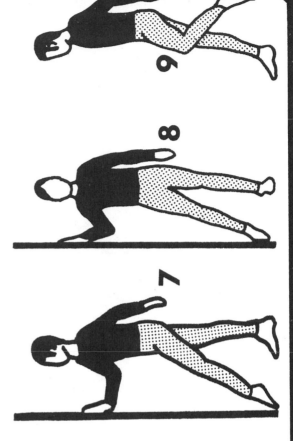

Exercises for the legs
Actions to be for 6 seconds.
1 Sit well back in a chair with your legs raised and your hands resting on the top of your shins; push up with your legs and down with your hands.
2 Holding onto the sides of your chair seat, grip a waste basket between your legs and raise them as shown; squeeze the basket as hard as you can.

3 While seated, place the ball of your left foot on the toes of your right foot; push down with your left ankle and up with your right. Change feet.
4 Gripping the sides of your chair seat, raise your feet straight in front of you with your left ankle crossed over your right; push the inside of your left foot and the outside of your right foot hard against each other. Change feet.
5 Lie facedown with one leg raised under a table as shown; push your foot hard against the table. Change legs to repeat.

6 Lie facedown with your heels under a low bed; push your heels up, keeping your legs straight.
7 Stand facing a wall with your right hand and left toes against it; push your foot against the wall. Change sides to repeat.

8 Stand sideways to a wall, rest your right hand and right foot against it as shown; push your foot against the wall. Change sides.
9 Face away from a wall, resting your forearms and left leg against it as shown; push your foot hard against the wall. Repeat with your other foot.

©DIAGRAM

BODYBUILDING

Few of the people who read this chapter will want to develop massive biceps or to become a future Mr or Ms Universe, although even the professionals begin with the basic exercises included here. For sportsmen and office workers alike a good bodybuilding program will certainly increase physical strength; it may also improve physical appearance. It does not really matter at what age you begin bodybuilding but many experts feel that the best time is adolescence, when body growth is greatest.

The "ideal" physique
People come in all shapes and sizes and there is no one ideal physique. The aim of bodybuilding is to produce a firm, strong, healthy body with proportions that are right for the body's size and type. The table included here gives an indication of the physical proportions that a man of 5ft 8in (172cm) might aim for, depending on his frame size.

Frame	Small	Medium	Large
Height	5ft 8in (172cm)	5ft 8in (172cm)	5ft 8in (172cm)
Weight	154lb (69.9kg)	161lb (73.0kg)	176lb (79.8kg)
A Chest (expanded)	43in (109cm)	45in (114cm)	47in (119cm)
B Waist	29in (74cm)	30in (76cm)	31in (79cm)
C Thigh	23in (58cm)	24in (61cm)	25in (64cm)
D Calf	14in (36cm)	15½in (39cm)	16in (41cm)
E Neck	14½in (37cm)	15½in (39cm)	16½in (42cm)
F Upper arm	14in (36cm)	15in (38cm)	16in (41cm)
G Wrist	6½–6¾in (17.0–17.2cm)	7in (18cm)	7½–7¾in (19.1–19.7cm)

Bodybuilding works on the principle of progressive resistance — the more resistance your muscles have to work against the stronger and firmer they become. Exercises may be isometric, calisthenic, isokinetic, or may involve weight training. Unlike weight lifting, which is a competitive sport, weight training is concerned more with repetitions than with lifting heavy weights. For the exercises described here the weights are quite light — about 3–5lb (1.4–2.3kg) for beginners.

Bodybuilding exercises can be carried out in a gym or in the home. The room should be well ventilated but quite warm, with a temperature of at least 65–70°F (18–21°C). It is a good idea to work in front of a mirror to check that you are doing the exercises correctly. For most people, a sensible bodybuilding program consists of 15 minutes exercise on alternate days. This gives muscle tissue, which is broken down by exercise, a chance to rebuild. Always limber up with some simple exercises before using weights, and after your workout take a warm shower. Never exercise straight after a meal; wait an hour or two. Also don't eat straight after exercising; wait a half hour. A well-balanced, nutritious diet is an essential part of bodybuilding. High-quality proteins, carbohydrates, vitamins, minerals and plenty of liquids and roughage are all needed. If you are weight training about 1g of protein per 1lb of bodyweight is recommended daily — this means lots of meat, fish, eggs, milk and cheese.

Safety If you have any doubts about fitness consult a doctor before you start. Bodybuilding injuries are not uncommon, especially the pulling or straining of muscles or tendons. More serious injuries include back strain, torn muscles or ligaments, and even hernias. Almost inevitably injuries occur because a person tries to rush too fast into bodybuilding. You must ease yourself gently into your training program, and take care not to over-reach your capabilities. It is a great temptation to try using heavy weights before you are ready; instead you should start with the lightest weights and the simplest exercises. Start with 8 or 10 repetitions and gradually build up to 20 or 30, later using heavier weights. Also start by taking long rests between exercises, reducing these as your stamina grows.

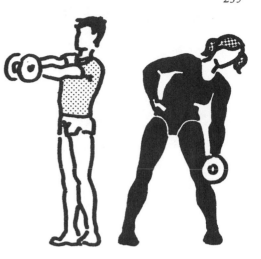

Women too!
Bodybuilding is suitable for women as well as men. Fears that women might develop huge muscles have proved unfounded — muscle bulk depends on the male hormone testosterone, of which women have very little.

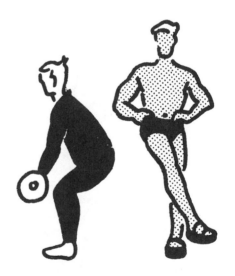

Clothing
Warm clothing such as a track suit is recommended at the start of a bodybuilding session. Muscles respond better to exercise when they are warm, making them less prone to injury. Top clothing can be stripped off as the session proceeds.

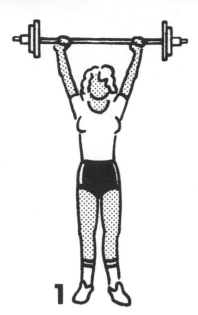

Bodybuilding

There are three main categories of bodybuilding equipment: weight, isotonic, resistance. All the apparatus shown here would be found in a gym; most of it can also be used at home.

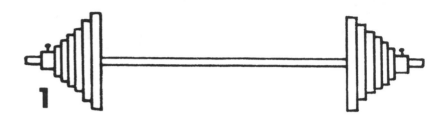

Weights

1 The barbell helps to develop the entire body; it is a traditional and essential piece of equipment. A set consists of a long bar and an assortment of adjustable weights. If you buy a set, choose one that contains $2\frac{1}{2}$lb (1.1kg) plates so that weight can be gradually increased.

2 The swingbell is a compact piece of apparatus, consisting of a short bar with a weight in the middle.

3 Dumb-bells are generally used for arm and shoulder exercises. They consist of a short bar on which are fixed two weights. You can use one or two at a time. A dumb-bell is gripped, in one hand, between the weights.

4 A wrist roller is used for strengthening the wrist and forearm. The weight is attached by a cord to a short bar. You can improvise by tying a brick or heavy object to a piece of string attached to a length of wood.

5 The neck developer consists of a head harness to which is attached a steel chain and weight.

6 Iron boots or leg bells are used for developing thigh and calf muscles.

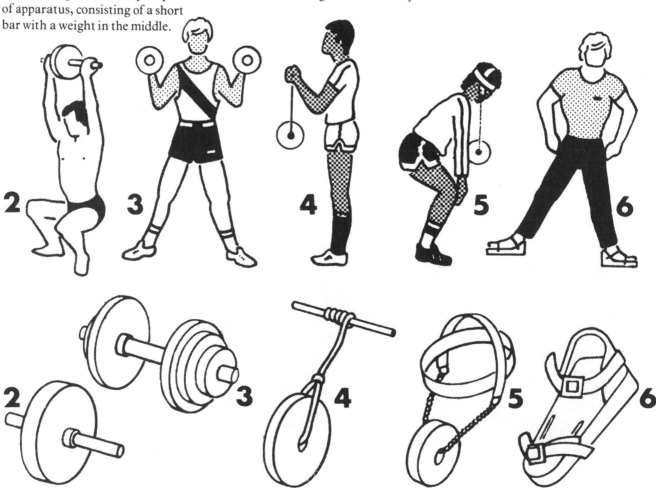

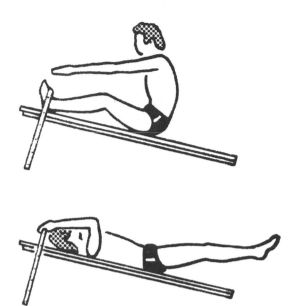

Isotonic equipment

The inclined bench or board is a very useful piece of equipment. Fitted with an adjustable foot or head strap it can be raised or lowered to any height. The purpose of the strap is to exert resistance to the bodybuilder's efforts in such exercises as sit-ups or leg raises; it is a particularly good way of developing the abdominal muscles. There are other pieces of equipment, such as the leg press machine, which work on the same principle.

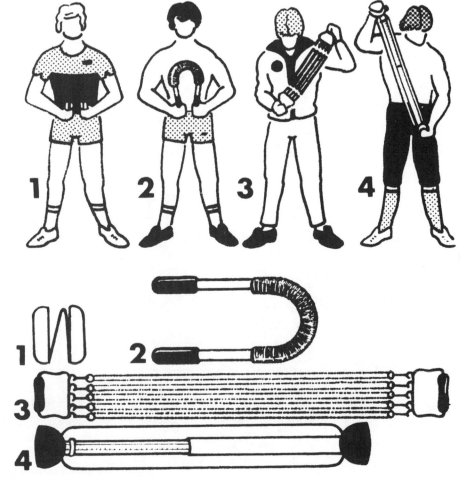

Resistance equipment

Resistance objects of one sort or another help to strengthen muscles, tendons and ligaments. This sort of apparatus is quite compact and good for training at home.

1 Hand grips are used for developing wrist power.

2 This curved expander is used for strengthening the arms.

3 Expanders are used for developing the chest and whole of the upper abdomen.

4 The bullworker is now probably one of the best-known expanders.

©DIAGRAM

Bodybuilding

EXERCISES

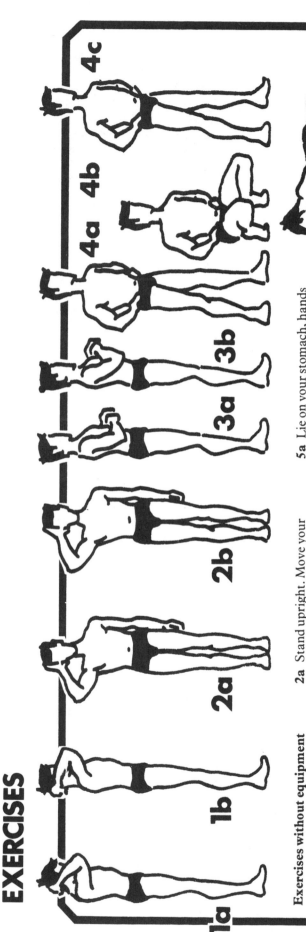

Exercises without equipment
These are simple bodybuilding exercises that you can do without equipment.

1a Stand erect and lower your chin to your chest. Clasp your hands firmly behind your head.
1b Force your head back, resisting the pressure with your clasped hands. Repeat 10 times; gradually increase to 15.

2a Stand upright. Move your head down toward your right shoulder, resisting with your right hand against the right side of your head.
2b With your right hand push your head upright and to the left, resisting this movement with your head. Repeat to the other side.

3a With your right arm down at your side, make a fist with your right hand. Then grasp this fist with your left hand.
3b Raise your right hand toward your shoulder, resisting with your left hand. Repeat, this time clenching your left fist. Repeat the entire exercise 10 times; gradually increase to 15.

4a Stand feet apart, hands on your hips. Breathe in deeply.
4b Squat down.
4c Stand up and breathe out. Repeat 10 times, building up to 20 repetitions.

5a Lie on your stomach, hands clasped behind your head.
5b Raise your head and body up from the floor, breathing in as you do so. As you return to your original position, breathe out. Repeat 5 times, gradually increasing to 15 repetitions.

6a This is the classic push-up or press-up. Lie facedown on the floor, with your hands, palms down, near your shoulders, and the balls of your toes ready to take your body weight.
6b Push your body off the ground until your arms are straight. Breathe in, bend your arms and lower yourself again. Push up and breathe out. Repeat 5–10 times.

7a Lie on your back, hands behind your head. Breathe in.
7b Sit up, breathing in.
7c Stretch your palms out toward your toes. Return to your original position, breathing in.

EXERCISES

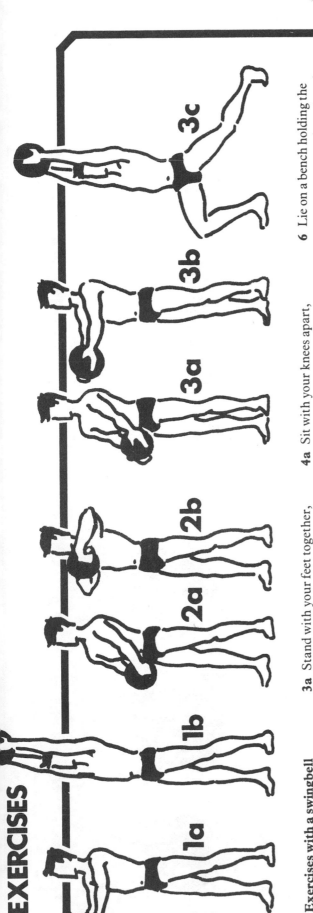

Exercises with a swingbell

1a Stand with your legs astride, arms in front of your body. Swing the weight forward.

1b Swing the weight up and breathe in. Lower the weight and breathe out. Repeat 10–20 times.

2a Grip the swingbell with your knuckles facing forward.

2b Raise the weight up to your chin, keeping your elbows bent and high. Lower the weight again.

3a Stand with your feet together, holding the swingbell down in front of you.

3b Swing the weight forward to arms' length.

3c Keeping your trunk upright, swing the weight upward and lunge forward onto your right leg. Repeat the exercise lunging onto your left leg. Repeat 12 times, lunging onto alternate legs.

4a Sit with your knees apart, leaning slightly forward. Hold the swingbell with your palms facing forward.

4b Breathing in, bend your arms and bring the weight up to your chest. Lower the swingbell and exhale. Repeat 12 times.

5a Sit upright with your knees apart, holding the swingbell behind your head.

5b Straighten your arms so that the weight is fully stretched above your head. Lower the weight. Repeat 8 times.

6 Lie on a bench holding the swingbell on your chest. Keeping your arms bent, move the weight up over your head and then down behind your head as far as possible. Bring it back the same way. Repeat 8 times.

7 Lie on a bench holding the swingbell straight above your chest. Keep your arms straight and bring the weight as far behind your head as possible. Repeat 12 times.

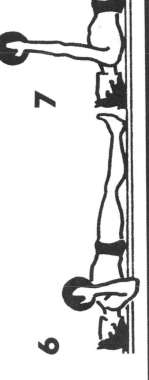

Bodybuilding

EXERCISES

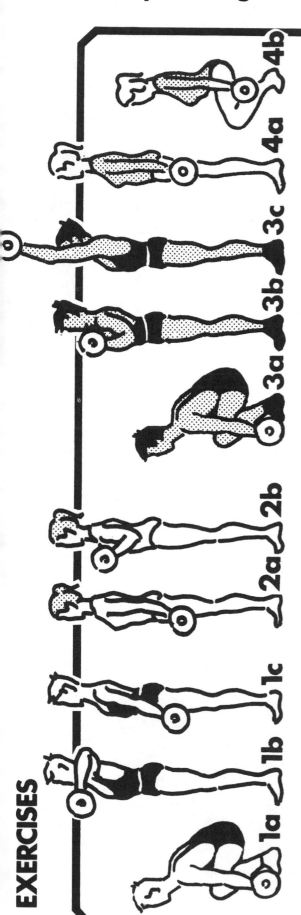

1a 1b 1c 2a 2b 3a 3b 3c 4a 4b

Exercises with dumb-bells
Use one or two dumb-bells to vary your program.

1a Crouch down with a dumb-bell in each hand, knuckles uppermost.

1b Straighten your body, pulling the dumb-bells up to your chin.

1c Keep your back straight and slowly lower the dumb-bells. Repeat 10 times.

2a Stand facing forward, with the dumb-bells by your thighs.

2b Bend your arms and raise the dumb-bells up to your chest. Lower them again. Repeat 10 times.

3a Crouch down with the dumb-bells resting on your toes and your knuckles uppermost.

3b Straighten up, bend your arms, and lift the dumb-bells in to your shoulders.

3c Push the dumb-bells to arms' length above your head. Then lower them to the floor.

4a Stand upright, holding the dumb-bells at arms' length by your sides.

4b Crouch down toward the floor. Then straighten up again.

5a Stand with your feet apart, right hand on your hip, and left hand holding a dumb-bell.

5b Bend to the left.

5c Bend to the right. Bend 10 times alternately to left and right. Repeat with the right hand.

6a Lie on your back, with the dumb-bells on your thighs.

6b Bring your arms straight up above your head.

6c Stretch your arms behind your head. Keeping your arms straight, return the dumb-bells to your thighs. Repeat 10 times.

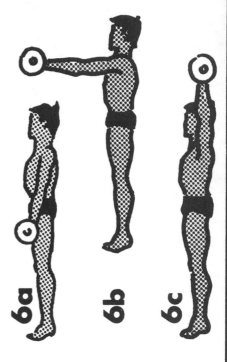

6a 6b 6c

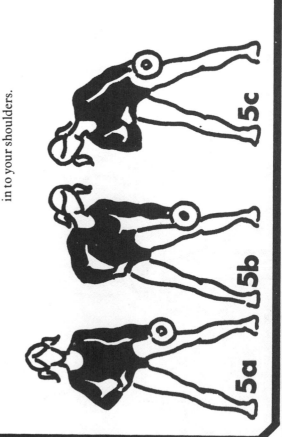

5a 5b 5c

EXERCISES

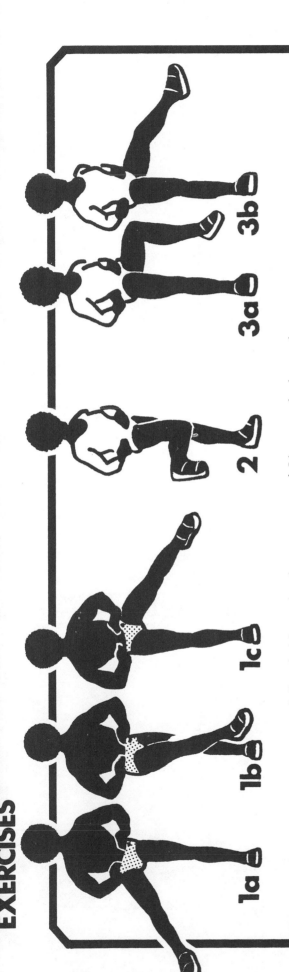

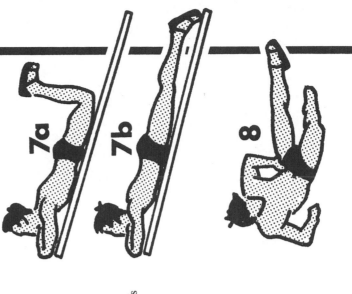

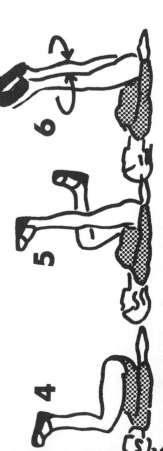

Exercises with leg weights
Use iron boots or leg-bells for these exercises.

1a Stand with your hands on your hips and your right leg stretched out to the side as far as possible.

1b Lower your right leg down and in front of your left leg. Point your toes as far left as possible.

1c Repeat with your left leg. Then repeat the entire exercise 12 times.

2 Stand with your hands on your hips and your feet together. Bend your right knee to raise your foot behind you, pointing your toes toward the ground. Return to the starting position. Repeat 12 times with alternate legs.

3a Stand with your hands on your hips. Bend your left leg.

3b Straighten your leg forward and stretch it out firmly. Repeat 12 times, stretching alternate legs.

4 Lie on your back, arms by your sides and legs up in the air. Bend and stretch both knees vigorously 12 times.

5 Lie on your back. Raise your feet as high as possible. Keeping your toes pointed, "cycle" with your legs.

6 Lie on your back with your arms by your sides. Raise your legs. Keeping your legs straight and your toes pointed, make a circle with both legs. Bring your legs down again. Repeat 8–12 times.

7a Lie facedown on a table or sloping board. Bend your knees and bring your feet up.

7b Stretch your legs out again. Repeat 12 times.

8 Lie on your right side with your right knee bent. Raise your left leg as high as possible. Change sides and repeat 12 times.

© DIAGRAM

Bodybuilding

EXERCISES

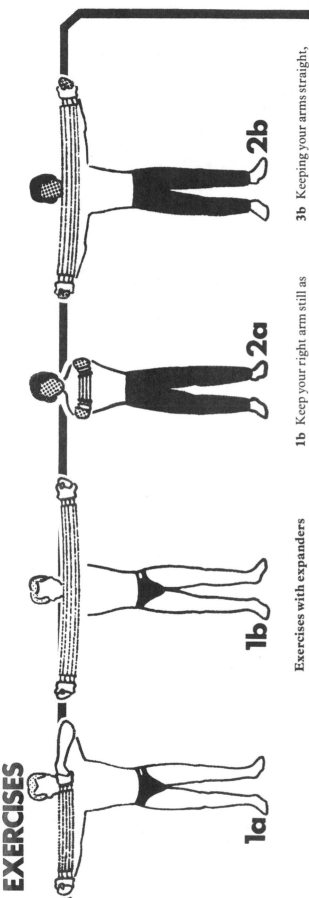

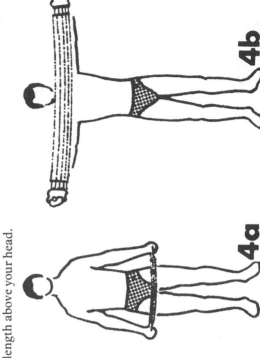

1a   **1b**

2a   **2b**

3a   **3b**   **3c**

4a   **4b**

Exercises with expanders
Stand with your feet together or apart, as you prefer.

1a   Hold the expander with your right arm, palm forward, to the side, and your left arm, knuckles forward, across your chest.

1b   Keep your right arm still as you bring your left arm out to the left side. Repeat several times. Then repeat with arms reversed.

2a   Hold the expander at arms' length in front, knuckles forward.

2b   Keeping your arms straight, pull them back to the sides so the expander touches your chest.

3a   Hold the expander at arms' length above your head.

3b   Keeping your arms straight, pull them down and out so the expander is across your chest.

3c   Alternatively, pull the expander down behind your neck.

4a   Hold the expander in front of your thighs, keeping your knuckles outward.

4b   Raise your arms out to the sides to stretch the expander.

EXERCISES

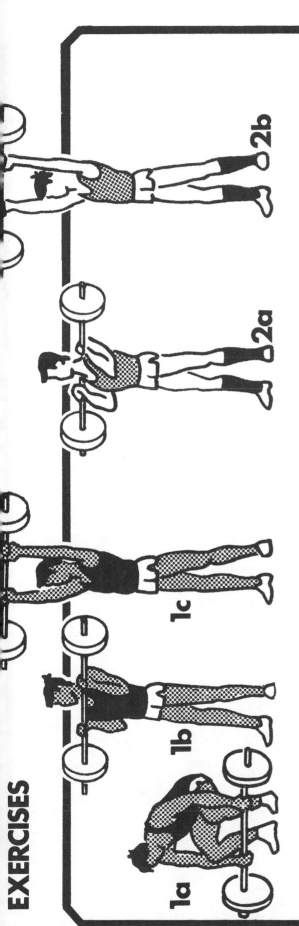

1a

1b

1c

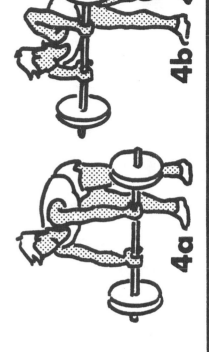

2a

2b

3a

3b

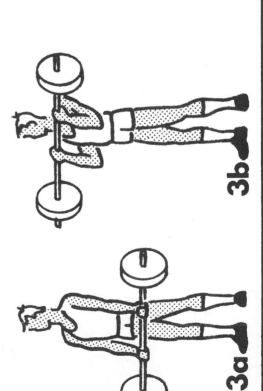

4a

4b

Exercises with a barbell

1a Stand with your feet about 15in (38cm) apart under the bar. Keeping your back flat and chest and head well up, bend your knees to grasp the bar, with your knuckles up and your hands just over shoulder-width apart.

1b Breathe in and straighten your legs, pulling the bar up until it is under your chin, touching your upper chest; then twist your hands so they are now palms up, and breathe out. (Beginners should practice only this first part of the exercise — called the "clean.")

1c Breathe in again and "press" (raise) the weight to arms' length above your head. Bring the bar back down to chest level and breathe out. Repeat 10 times.

2a Stand erect with your feet apart, holding the barbell behind your neck so that it rests across your shoulders.

2b Breathe in and "press" the weight to arms' length above your head. Return the bar to behind your neck and breathe out. Repeat 10 times.

3a Stand erect with your feet apart and the bar held down at arms' length, palms forward.

3b Keeping your elbows in the same position, bend them to bring the bar up to your chest. Pause and then lower the bar again. Repeat 10 times.

4a Using a fairly wide grip, knuckles forward, let the bar hang down as you stand feet apart with your body bent forward at right angles to your legs.

4b Keeping your body still, lift the bar up to your chest. Then slowly lower it again. Repeat 10 times.

© DIAGRAM

Bodybuilding

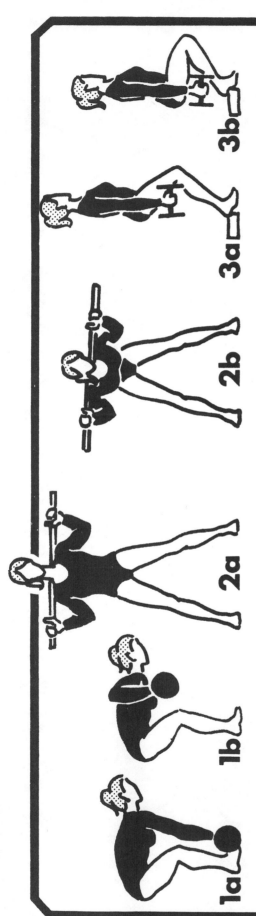

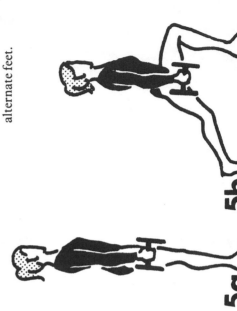

Exercises for women

A selection of simple but effective bodybuilding exercises for women is included here. Always warm up before using weights. Start gently, using only light weights. Repeat each exercise about 10 times.

1a Stand with your feet slightly apart under a barbell. Bending your knees slightly, lean forward to grasp the barbell.

1b Still bending over, and with your knuckles forward, lift the barbell up to your chest. Pause, and return to position 1a.

2a Stand feet apart, holding a light bar so that it rests on your shoulders behind your neck.

2b Breathe in and bend forward until your upper body is parallel to the floor. Breathe out and straighten up.

3a With a dumb-bell in each hand, stand with your heels on a wood block and your knees bent.

3b Keeping your back straight, lower yourself into a squat, pause, and then straighten up.

4a Grasp one dumb-bell in both hands. Feet apart, bend to swing the dumb-bell between your legs.

4b Swing the dumb-bell up above your head, rising onto your toes as you straighten your body.

5a Stand straight, holding a light dumb-bell in each hand.

5b Keeping your back straight and upright, lunge onto your left foot. Step back. Repeat with alternate feet.

EXERCISES

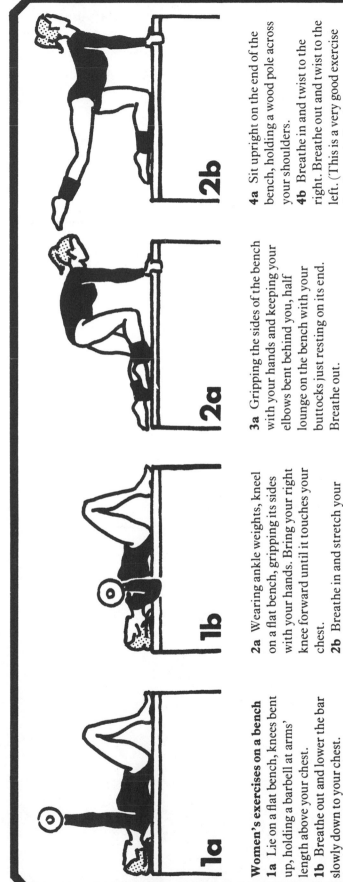

1a **1b** **2a** **2b**

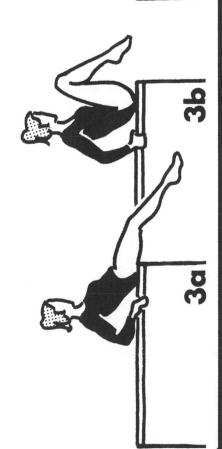

3a **3b** **4a** **4b**

Women's exercises on a bench
1a Lie on a flat bench, knees bent up, holding a barbell at arms' length above your chest.
1b Breathe out and lower the bar slowly down to your chest. Breathing in, push the bar up again. (This is an excellent exercise for building up the pectoral muscles.)

2a Wearing ankle weights, kneel on a flat bench, gripping its sides with your hands. Bring your right knee forward until it touches your chest.
2b Breathe in and stretch your right leg back as far as you can, pointing your toes. Bring your legs back together again. Then repeat the exercise with alternate legs.

3a Gripping the sides of the bench with your hands and keeping your elbows bent behind you, half lounge on the bench with your buttocks just resting on its end. Breathe out.
3b Bring your knees up and into your chest, at the same time raising your upper body slightly. Breathe in. Return to the starting position and repeat.

4a Sit upright on the end of the bench, holding a wood pole across your shoulders.
4b Breathe in and twist to the right. Breathe out and twist to the left. (This is a very good exercise for the waistline.)

ORIENTAL EXERCISES

Increased cultural interaction between East and West and the desire of many Westerners to find a more meaningful view of life have in recent years resulted in a big increase in the popularity in Western countries of the philosophy and practices of the Orient.

Traditional methods of exercise in the East are very different from those of the West, each style being an expression of underlying cultural attitudes. Western materialism has produced exercise programs of a purely physical and essentially practical character; exercises are

Benefits of T'ai Chi

T'ai Chi is a graceful, total form of exercise. It is suitable for persons of any age, sex or state of health, since the amount of effort made is regulated by yourself for yourself. Developed to cultivate Chi (life energy), T'ai Chi can lead to an all-round increase in health and vitality. When combined with K'ai Men and Ch'ang Ming (Taoist diet and herb therapy), its benefits are further enhanced. Specific areas of benefit include the following.

1 Concentration
2 Self-awareness and control with mind/body unity
3 Relaxation through concentration and exercise
4 Breathing
5 Heart and circulation
6 Posture
7 Relief from stiff muscles and joints
8 Coordination and balance

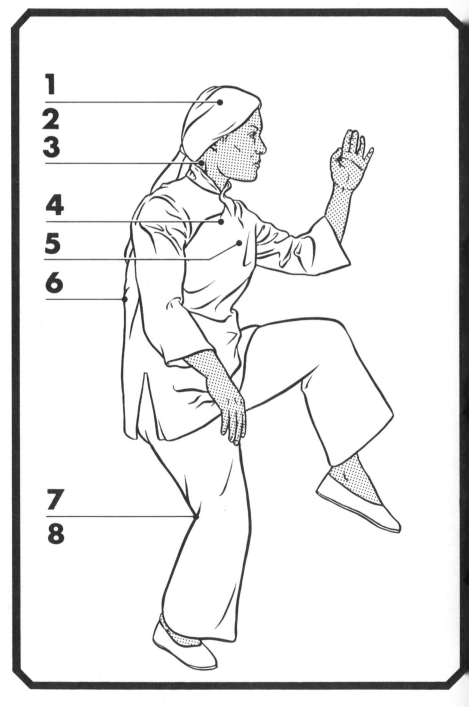

designed to develop muscles, strength, speed, efficiency and competitiveness. In the East, exercise forms an integral part of the religious philosophies; it involves self-conquering and self-betterment for union with a higher reality. Eastern exercises aim at the harmonious development of strength, suppleness and dexterity together with mental clarity and control.

In this section we concentrate on exercises of the Eastern Orient, which are primarily Chinese in origin. They differ from Indian exercises (for yoga, see page 256) in their emphasis on continuous flowing movement designed to allow the life energies to flow freely instead of being stopped by holding the breath or by holding a set position.

Origins and development Although ancient Chinese followers of the Taoist religion had already experimented with movement for thousands of years, Oriental exercise systems as we know them today began to develop only after Bodhidharma, a monk, arrived from India at the Shaolin temple in about 200BC. Bodhidharma was responsible for the development of a system of movement that came to be known as Shaolin temple boxing; from it many other Oriental arts were to develop. The martial arts of the Eastern Orient developed when the monks modified the system for self-defense. *T'ai Chi Ch'uan* is a dynamic meditation, a "soft" (interior, flowing, energy-oriented) form of the "harder" (exterior, emphasizing physical force) system of Chinese boxing called *Wu Shu* (literally translated as martial arts). In Okinawa, Shaolin boxing was combined with the native form of self-defense to give *Kempo* or *Karate* ("China hand"). Japanese martial arts comprise *Kendo*, the sport of sword-fighting (the deadlier art of which is called *Ken-Jutsu. Kyndo* is the art of archery. With the introduction of Shaolin boxing, *Aiki-jujitsu* was developed. This, coupled with Buddhist meditation, produced *Aikido*, and was adapted to give the sporting *Judo*.

Shotokan, Wado Ryu, Gojo Ryu and *Kyokushinkai* are all late Japanese forms of *Karate*. In Korea there arose *Soo Bahk*. Under further Chinese influence *Tang Soo Do* and *Hapkido* were developed. These were later combined into *Tae Kwon Do* (hand/foot art).

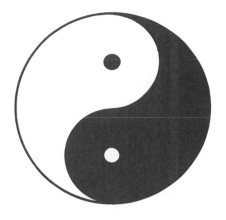

Unity in duality
Shown here is the Chinese symbol for unity in duality, the combination of the opposites Yin and Yang needed to form a whole as, for example, with dark and light, inner and outer, male and female. All Chinese arts aim to create a harmonious balance of Yin and Yang.

Chi
Chi is the essential life energy of the body, and depends for its quality and strength on the balance of Yin and Yang. Chinese medicine promotes this balance, or, as with acupuncture (see p. 118), removes a blockage that is obstructing the flow of Chi around the body, so restoring harmony and energy — in Western terms, health.

Oriental exercises

Chinese arts of movement were originally based upon the movements of animals. Shaolin temple boxing had five styles: of the dragon, the snake, the tiger, the leopard and the crane. Each was meant to develop and harmonize one of the five essences of spirit, bone, strength, Chi and sinew, and to synthesize hard and soft, internal and external, substantial and insubstantial. T'ai Chi and K'ai Men retain the original objectives, symbolized by the use of animal and bird names in the terminology of stances.

Recommendations

In the case of both T'ai Chi and K'ai Men correct teaching and perseverance are essential. T'ai Chi is a Yang exercise, with outer movement and inner stillness. K'ai Men is a Yin exercise, with outer stillness and inner movement. They are complementary. Remember that everybody goes through Yin and Yang phases and these will affect your performance. Do not become dispirited if you do not seem to be making progress for a while. Do what you feel you can. The following recommendations apply for both T'ai Chi and K'ai Men.

1 Use mental concentration on the movements to achieve mental and physical relaxation.

2 Breathe through the nose.

3 Breath fully and naturally, using the diaphragm and abdomen. The energy of your body depends on your breathing.

4 Dress should be loose and light. There is traditional dress for all the arts.

5 Make your movements soft and gentle. Move like a cat.

6 Make movements with careful deliberateness and even, slow, flowing continuity. Never hold a posture as this blocks the flow of Chi. Use "sentiment not force."

7 Act with all your body.

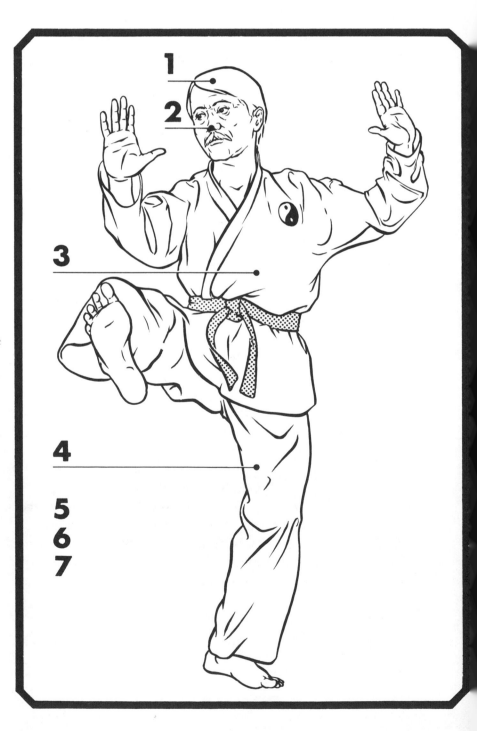

T'ai Chi ("Supreme Ultimate") aims to exercise the muscles, to integrate mind and body and to ease the internal flow of Chi. The "form" of T'ai Chi popularly performed as exercise in the West is, in fact, only one-eighth of the complete art which, as well as including disciplines for mental and physical control and the storage of energies, includes T'ai Chi dance, sword and stick. These last reveal T'ai Chi's base in, and still possible use as, a form of self-defense. When exercising, imagine yourself to be "swimming in air." This will aid continuity and muscle tone. T'ai Chi consists of 37 basic postures, expanded to a form of 108 to 128 complete movements, depending on the school of T'ai Chi followed.

K'ai Men (Chinese yoga) is based on the concept of "movement with stillness," in which each gentle exercise produces a series of mild muscle changes which, in effect, perform an internal massage of the channels along which Chi flows. The practice of K'ai Men aids mental and physical growth, and the development of consciousness, Chi and Li (the external energy of the body). Each separate posture is a series of movements performed gently and continuously. No posture is held at any time, as this would stop the flow of Chi.

Ch'ang Ming (Taoist long-life therapy) is a system of eating and herbal medication that will add to the benefits of T'ai Chi and K'ai Men. Ch'ang Ming aims to balance the Yin and Yang of the body; it is characterized by subtle prevention and not by drastic cures. The ancient Chinese used to pay their doctors when they were well, not when the doctor failed and they were ill!

Despite its ancient origins the eating recommendations of Ch'ang Ming sound extremely modern, with its emphasis on eating only natural, whole foods free from chemical additives. White bread and refined or processed foods, coffee, alcohol, tobacco, chocolate, sweets and fried food are not allowed. Nor are spices, rock salt, mustard, pepper, vinegar, pickles, curry, pork or red meats, red or blue fish, sugar, tropical fruits, potatoes, tomatoes, aubergines, dairy products (except cottage cheese), and products containing animal fat.

EXERCISES

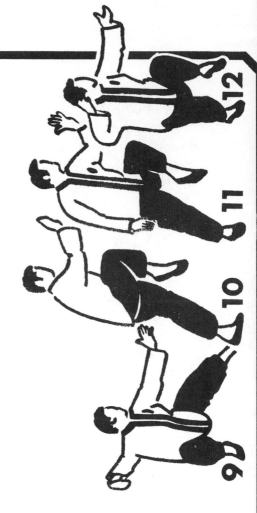

T'ai Chi

A full T'ai Chi sequence includes as many as 128 postures with linking movements. Here we include a short sequence made up of examples designed to give you a "feel" of this type of exercise. The illustrations should be followed as though looking in a mirror. In keeping with Chinese tradition, instructions refer to compass points; take East as the direction you face to begin. Proceed slowly; remain relaxed.

1 Stand relaxed with your feet about shoulder-width apart.

2 Bend your elbows slightly and lift your arms slowly to shoulder height in front, hands and fingers to be horizontal and relaxed. Concentrate awareness on your forearms.

3 Slowly lower your hands to your thighs, fingers of your right hand pointing down, and your left palm facing down.

4 Raise your arms to shoulder height, left elbow slightly bent.

5 Turn your left foot out to 45°, then bend your knees until they are over your toes. Lower your left arm until the palm is under and facing your right palm.

6 Move your left leg forward one step. Straighten your right arm, palm down, and raise your left arm so that the palm faces your breastbone.

7 Turn your left foot 45° inward. Turn to the West and take one step West with your right leg; keep body weight on your left leg. Slightly bend your left arm and turn the palm upward. Move left palm, facing downward, over the center of your left forearm.

8 Move your weight onto your right leg, bending it until the knee is over your toes. Move your arms slightly forward.

9 Return weight to left leg. Bend your left leg, keeping your right leg straight. Extend your right arm over your right leg, palm facing North. Extend your left arm and draw it back slightly over shoulder height, hand limp.

10 Move to stand on your right leg. Simultaneously lift left arm and left leg forward, bent at elbow and knee. Left elbow is to be over the knee, toes pointing down and fingers up; right arm should hang by your side palm toward your thigh.

11 Lower your left leg and stand on it. Repeat action 10, with reversed sides.

12 Bend your left leg. Draw left hand up so that the palm faces your left ear and extend your right arm, palm up.

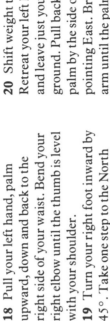

13

14

15

16

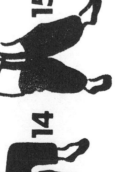

17

18

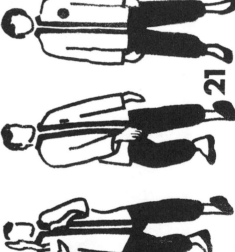

19

20

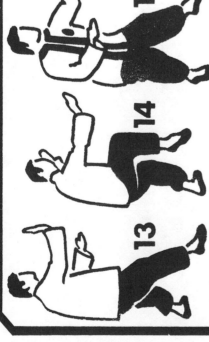

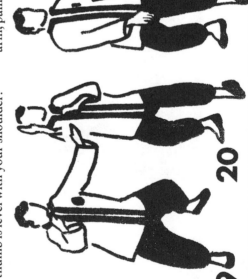

21

22

T'ai Chi

13 Place your right foot on the ground one step behind your left foot. Transfer your weight to your right foot, bending the knee a little. Push your left hand forward, palm forward and fingers up. Lower your right elbow until the hand is near your waist.

14 Lift your left leg and turn your left palm upward. Pull your right hand back and up until the palm faces your right ear.

15 Step on your left leg one step behind the right, and repeat action 13 with reversed sides.

16 Lift your right leg. Move your left hand up until the palm faces your ear. Turn your right palm up.

17 Step back onto your right leg and repeat 13. Then pull your left hand, palm upward, down and back to the right side of your waist. Bend your right elbow until the thumb is level with your shoulder.

18 Pull your left hand, palm upward, down and back to the right side of your waist. Bend your right elbow until the thumb is level with your shoulder.

19 Turn your right foot inward by 45°. Take one step to the North with your left leg and face North. Bend your left leg and extend your left arm, palm upward, forward to shoulder height. Extend your right arm, palm downward, to the side.

20 Shift weight to right leg. Retreat your left leg by half a step and leave just your heel on the ground. Pull back your left arm, palm by the side of your face, pointing East. Bring in your right arm until the palm faces your left elbow.

21 Drop your right arm to the side and drop your left arm down in front.

22 Return to starting position.

Oriental exercises

EXERCISES

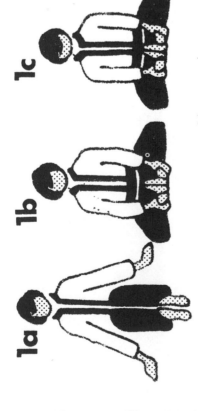

1a 1b 1c 1d 1e

K'ai Men

There are 42 basic postures and over 400 exercises in K'ai Men. Here we are able to describe only a few of them, but it is hoped that by trying these you will gain an impression of the ease and gentleness of this form of exercise. All K'ai Men exercises are split into two parts: sequence and extension. During the first year of practice, teachers recommend that you perform the sequence twice and then the extension twice. Never perform the extension without having done the sequence. In all K'ai Men exercises remember always to move fluidly and never to hold any position.

Lotus leaf (sequence)

1a Sit on the floor with your legs extended in front of you.

1b Bend your knees, place your soles together, grip your ankles and gently pull your legs toward you.

1c Straighten your body. Then tilt your head slightly forward. Straighten up again, and return to the starting position.

Lotus leaf (extension)

Start by repeating 1a, b, c as in the sequence, except in 1b pull your feet as close to your body as possible.

1d Lean forward as far as possible and then lift your head back as far as you can.

1e Straighten your body. Then bend your head forward until your chin touches your chest.

Fish (sequence)

2a Lie on your right side, with your legs straight, your raised head resting on your right hand, and your left hand on the ground in front of you for balance.

2b Raise your left leg, keeping it straight. Lower it and roll over onto your left side. Repeat with your right leg. Roll back.

Fish (extension)

2c Start as in 2a. This time raise your left leg as high as you can while at the same time lifting your right hip and thigh off the ground. Roll over and repeat with your right leg and your left hip and thigh.

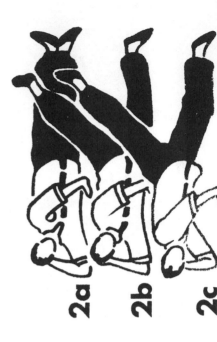

2a 2b 2c

EXERCISES

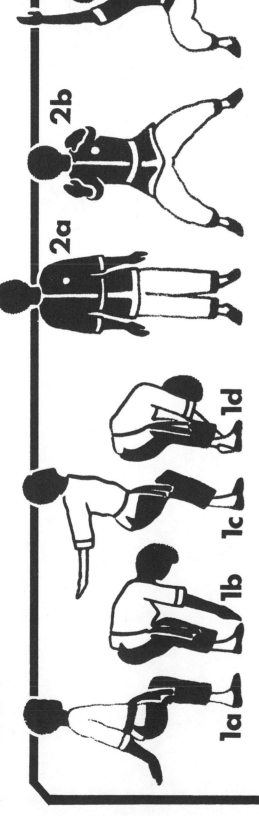

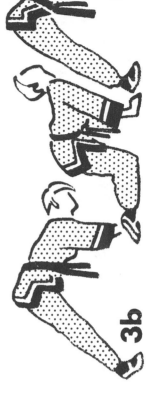

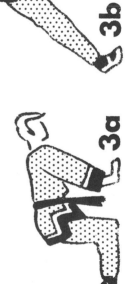

K'ai Men

Riding horse (sequence 1)

1a Start by standing with your feet together and your arms hanging loosely by your sides. With your left foot take a step to the side. Bend your knees until your thighs are parallel with the floor. Then swing your arms back.

1b Swing your arms forward, and bend so that your fingers touch the floor. Return to the starting position, and repeat the sequence, stepping to the right.

Riding horse (extension 1)

1c Start and step to the left as for the sequence. Swing your arms back, and then slowly raise them as far back as you can while also tilting your head back.

1d Swing your arms forward to grip your ankles on the inside and then pull your shoulders down as far as possible. Return to start and repeat to the right.

Riding horse (sequence 2)

2a Stand feet together with your arms hanging by your sides.

2b Step to the left and bend your knees until your thighs are parallel with the floor. Raise your arms to shoulder level in front of you. Lower your arms. Return to starting position. Repeat, stepping to the right.

Riding horse (extension 2)

2c As for the sequence, except raise your arms straight up and lower your buttocks as close as possible to the floor. Return to the starting position and repeat the extension to the right.

Turtle (sequence)

3a Start by sitting on your heels. Next kneel on all fours, with your toes pointing to the rear and your arms and thighs at right angles to the floor. Without moving your hands and knees, lean forward until your shoulders are in front of your wrists. Now move back so that your arms and thighs are again at right angles to the floor.

3b Raise your buttocks in the air and straighten your legs. Next lower your knees onto the floor and then sit back on your heels.

Turtle (extension)

3c As in 3a except this time tilt your head back when you are leaning forward with your shoulders over your hands.

3d As in 3b but bend your head down to look between your arms.

©DIAGRAM

Oriental exercises

EXERCISES

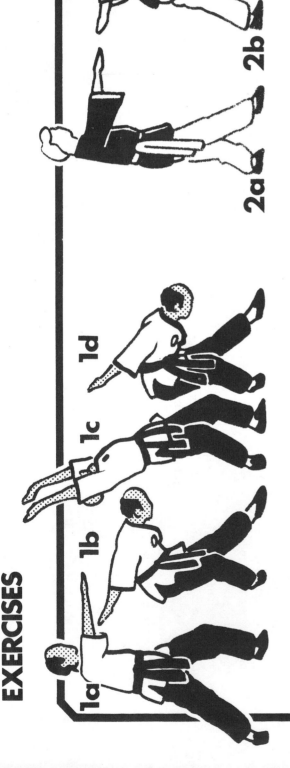

1a **1b** **1c** **1d**

2a **2b**

K'ai Men

Dragon (sequence)

1a Stand with feet together and arms loosely by your sides. Step forward with your left foot. Keeping your right leg straight, transfer your weight onto your left foot and bend your left knee while at the same time raising your arms to shoulder level in front of you.

1b Transfer your weight to your right leg, bend your right knee, and straighten your left leg, raising the toes of your left foot. Swing your arms back and bend your body forward. Return to starting position. Repeat, changing legs.

Dragon (extension)

1c As in 1a except raise your arms up and as far back as possible, bend your head back, and keep your weight on your forward leg.

1d As in 1b, but bend your body so that your head touches your forward knee, and lift your arms up and forward as far as you can.

Monkey (sequence)

2a Start with your feet together and your arms hanging by your sides. Step back with your left foot. Put your weight onto this foot and bend your knee, while at the same time swinging your arms up and forward to shoulder level.

2b Transfer your weight onto your right leg, lift your right heel off the ground and swing your arms back. Return to your starting position. Repeat the sequence, changing legs.

Monkey (extension)

The movements for the extension are the same as those for the sequence, but this time push down on whichever foot is taking your weight.

Chicken (sequence)

3a Stand with your feet just over shoulder-width apart, and your arms hanging by your sides. Now turn completely to the left, pivoting on the balls of your feet. Keeping your body erect, bend your right knee until it is about 1in (2.5cm) off the ground. Straighten your legs to turn and face the front. Repeat to the right.

Chicken (extension)

3b As in 3a except place both your hands on your left thigh, lean your head back as far as possible, and push your abdomen forward. Then, as you straighten your legs, push strongly on both hands. Repeat to the right, with both hands on your right thigh.

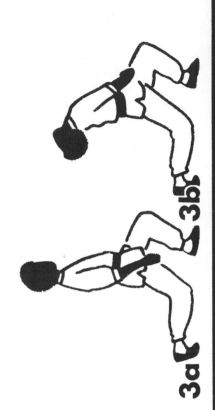

3a **3b**

K'ai Men

Eagle (sequence)
1a Stand straight but relaxed.
1b Turn your body slowly to the right, letting your arms swing with your body.
1c Repeat to the left.

Eagle (extension)
1d, e As for the sequence, but twist your body and turn your head as far as possible without moving your feet.

Praying mantis (sequence)
2a Start by kneeling down and sitting on your heels, with your toes pointing backward and your hands on the floor by your feet. Then lean slightly backward, pushing on your fingers and raising your knees slightly off the ground.
2b Return to the starting position and then lean forward, putting your hands on the floor in front of your knees so that your arms and legs are parallel. Return to the starting position.

Praying mantis (extension)
2c As in 2a, but for the extension raise your knees as far as possible and then bend your body forward and try and touch your knees with your chin.
2d As in 2b, but this time raise your feet as far as possible and tilt your head back as far as you can. Return to the starting position.

Drunkard (sequence)
3a Lie relaxed on your back, feet together, and palms down.
3b Keeping your legs straight, raise feet about 1ft (30cm).
3c Raise feet until legs are perpendicular. Return to position 3b and then 3a.

Drunkard (extension)
3d As in 3b but with your right leg crossed over your left.
3e As in 3c but then open your legs wide. Then close them.
3f As in 3d but with your left leg crossed over your right. Then back to 3a.

©DIAGRAM

YOGA

Many people think of yoga, with its Indian origins, as a form of religion, but it need not be by any means. Hatha yoga is the branch that concentrates on the physical side, based on the achievement of physical and mental control and relaxation, and it is on Hatha yoga that we concentrate here.

Hatha yoga is not a series of exercises, but of postures or poses known as asanas; it is the stages toward assuming the postures that really constitute the exercise, the final achievement being the asana. Some are easy to assume;

Tadasana
This is the basic standing pose used in yoga. Its characteristics are:
1 Back and neck pulled up
2 Chin slightly tucked in
3 Throat relaxed
4 Chest open
5 Shoulders back
6 Arms hanging loose
7 Stomach pulled in
8 Hands loose
9 Knees pulled up
10 Weight evenly on heels and toes
11 Feet together

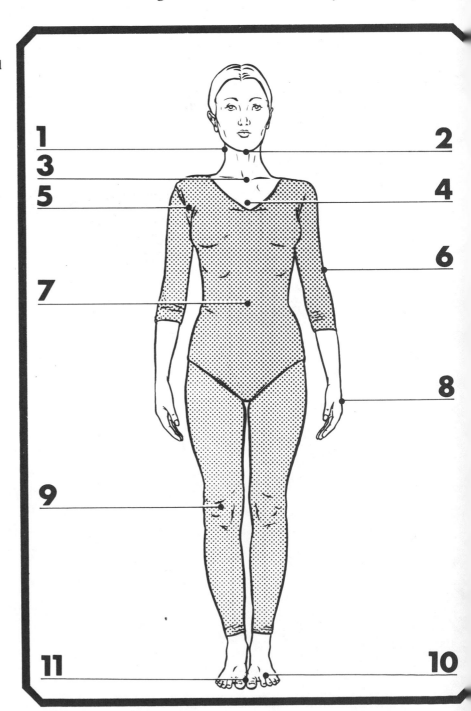

others require much practice before the muscles and limbs are supple enough. Each asana has a purpose, and very often a name easily identified with the pose, such as the bow, the lotus, etc. At the end of this section is a useful picture glossary of asanas. Because of the precise nature of yoga poses and because some poses are unsuitable for persons with physical conditions such as high blood pressure or back trouble, anyone who is considering taking up yoga is recommended to attend classes for at least a year.

There are two important points to remember when assuming the poses. First, make every movement slowly and gracefully, avoiding all strain and remembering that a good deal of practice is needed before some of the more advanced poses can be achieved. You are seeking for poise and suppleness, and a consequent relaxation of body and mind, so do not exhaust yourself or attempt advanced poses before you are ready. Second, correct breathing is vital to yoga, and exercises to help with this are given on page 264; remember that the achievement of proper breath control may also require considerable practice.

A great advantage of Hatha yoga is that no equipment of any kind is required; even a mat, though convenient, is not essential. The poses can be assumed anywhere and at any time, although always wait for at least an hour after a meal. Clothes should be light and loose around the waist; shoes should be removed. Hatha yoga, with its emphasis on physical well-being, is a good preparation for other, more mystical forms of yoga, which involve far more meditation or seeking after wisdom, such as Jnanayoga, Karma yoga, Bhakti yoga and Raja yoga. Closely related to these other forms is transcendental meditation, which is now being taken more seriously by the medical profession; through concentration this induces a relaxed, tensionless state of mind, and can be very helpful in counteracting psychosomatic disorders. Transcendental meditation is usually practiced in the lotus position of Hatha yoga. But even without entering these higher realms, the practice of Hatha yoga can have results that are not only easily discernible but also rapid. You will soon experience its physical benefits, if only in a general feeling of well-being, and some people who have practiced yoga regularly even claim that it has helped them to overcome overindulgence in eating, drinking or smoking. In everyone it will tone up the muscles, increase suppleness and improve the circulation.

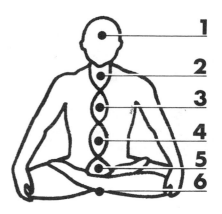

The six chakras
Yoga is designed to stimulate these traditionally particularly sensitive points of the body:
1 Ajna
2 Vishudda
3 Anahata
4 Manipuraka
5 Swadhisthana
6 Muladhara

Yoga

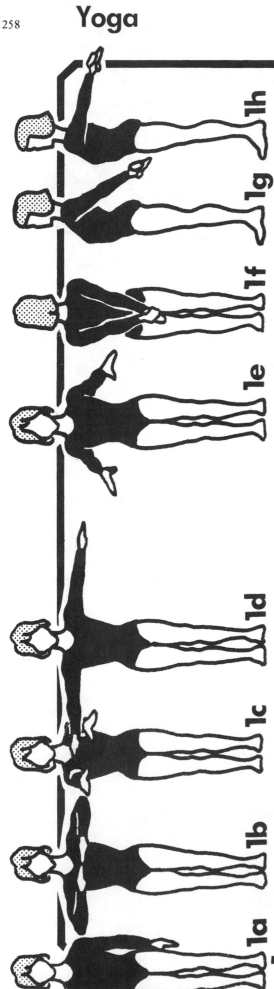

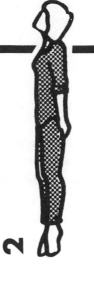

2

Relaxing and recuperative poses

1a Stand with your back straight and your feet together.
1b Bring your hands flat and level across your chest.
1c Stretch out your arms in front.
1d, e Pushing your chest out, bring your arms around at shoulder level behind your back.
1f Clasp your hands at the base of your spine.

1g, h Straighten your arms and lift them as high as you can; hold for a count 5.
2 This posture, the corpse, is one of deep relaxation. Lie flat on your back with your arms at your sides and your feet together. Let your arms and legs go limp, and allow your feet to fall gently apart. Raise your chin, close your eyes, and breathe in deeply and regularly.

3a Sit with your feet on opposite thighs, hands on your knees.
3b, c, d Roll your head to the left, around to the back, and then to the right.
4a Turn your face to the right and raise your chin, then lower it to your chest.
4b Bring your head to the front and allow it to hang down completely for several seconds.

1a **1b** **1c** **1d** **1e** **1f** **1g** **1h**

3a **3b** **3c** **3d** **4a** **4b**

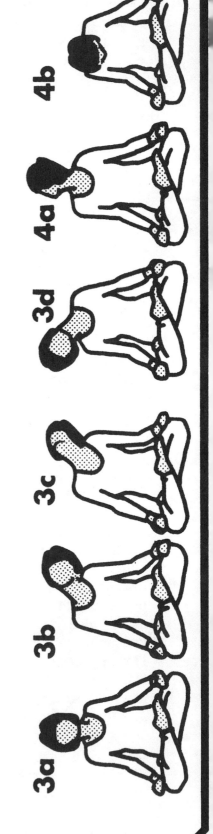

POSES

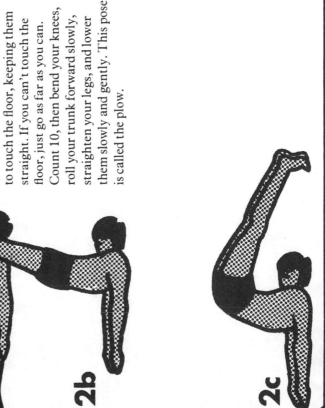

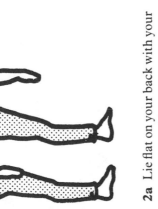

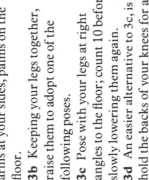

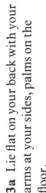

Relaxing poses

1a Stand with your feet apart, arms at your sides.

1b, c, d With your head and arms hanging, let your body bend forward as far as it will go. Count 10 then slowly straighten up. With practice, your body will bend until your hands touch the floor.

2a Lie flat on your back with your arms at your sides.

2b Press your palms against the floor and slowly raise your legs to an upright position, resting on your head and shoulders.

2c Take your legs over your head to touch the floor, keeping them straight. If you can't touch the floor, just go as far as you can. Count 10, then bend your knees, roll your trunk forward slowly, straighten your legs, and lower them slowly and gently. This pose is called the plow.

3a Lie flat on your back with your arms at your sides, palms on the floor.

3b Keeping your legs together, raise them to adopt one of the following poses.

3c Pose with your legs at right angles to the floor; count 10 before slowly lowering them again.

3d An easier alternative to 3c, is to hold the backs of your knees for a count of 10.

3e If you wish to go on to a more advanced position, raise your trunk, leaving only your head and shoulders on the floor, and slowly bring your straight legs over your head, supporting your back with your hands. Hold for a count of 10.

3f Then slowly bend your knees, keeping your feet well tucked in. Straighten your legs, and then lower them slowly to the floor without lifting your head.

©DIAGRAM

POSES

Standing poses

1a Stand with your feet well apart and your arms stretched sideways from the shoulders.

1b Slowly bend to the left from your hips, keeping your right arm in line with your shoulder, and holding your left knee with your left hand. Both arms should be straight.

1c, d Bring your right arm, still straight, as close to your head as possible, and hold for a count of 5. Repeat on the other side.

As this exercise is repeated you will find that you can bring your arm over a little farther so that eventually it is parallel to the floor.

2a Stand with your heels together and raise your arms, palms inward, above your head.

2b Keeping them parallel, bend your head and trunk a little way to the left. Count 10, straighten up, and bend to the right.

2c Each time you repeat, increase the distance of the bend.

3a Stand with your heels together.

3b Stretch your arms out to the front.

3c Swing them right back at shoulder level and link your fingers.

3d Bend back slightly and count 5.

3e Keeping your arms straight and fingers linked, very slowly bend forward so that your trunk is at right angles to your legs. Return to starting position.

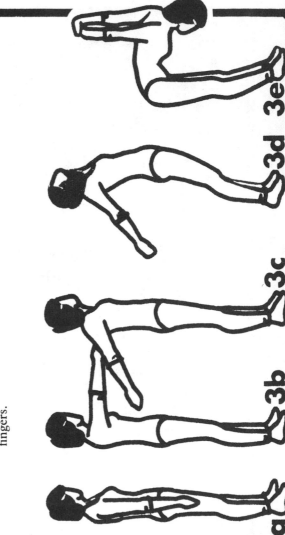
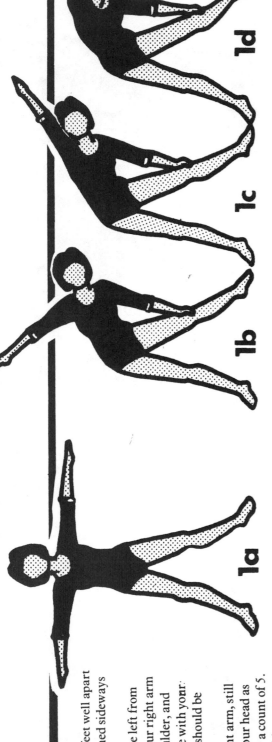
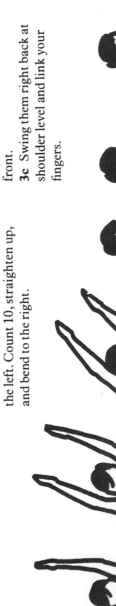

POSES

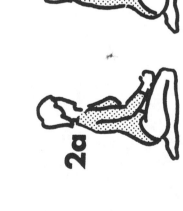

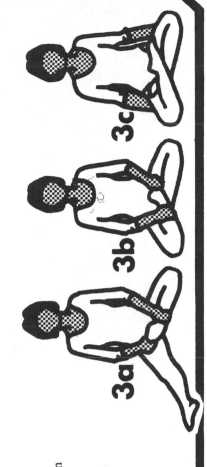

Sitting poses

1a Sit with your legs straight in front, arms above your head.
1b Bring your arms down so that your hands lie on your thighs.
1c Hang your head down.
1d Exhaling, lean forward as far as you can to touch your feet.
1e If possible, grip your toes with your fingers and pull your head down onto your knees, extending your spine and trying to keep your back concave.

2a This exercise must be done with care. Kneel with your knees together and your toes stretched back. Then lower yourself gently to sit, if possible, on the floor between your feet (otherwise sit on your feet). Link your fingers and rest your hands on your knees.
2b Stretch your arms above your head, your fingers still linked and your palms upward; hold for 30 seconds, breathing normally. Return your hands to your knees.

2c Place the palms of your hands on the soles of your feet. Bend forward from the hips, breathing out. Hold this pose for about 60 seconds, breathing normally. Then sit up, breathing in.
2d For this advanced pose, begin by holding your feet with your hands. Then gently lower your body backward to rest first your elbows and then your back and head on the floor. Stretch your arms above your head, and hold this position for as long as possible, breathing deeply. Take hold of your feet again, push up onto your elbows and sit up, breathing out.

3a Sitting on the floor with your legs straight and apart, first place your left foot on your right thigh.
3b Then place your right foot on your left thigh.
3c Hold this classic lotus pose. (A good deal of practice will be needed before you are flexible enough to attain this pose.)

© DIAGRAM

POSES

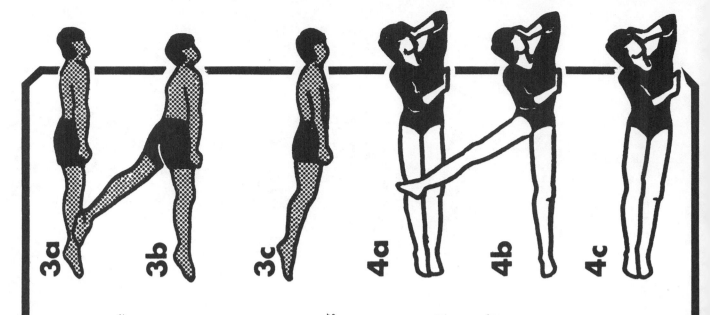

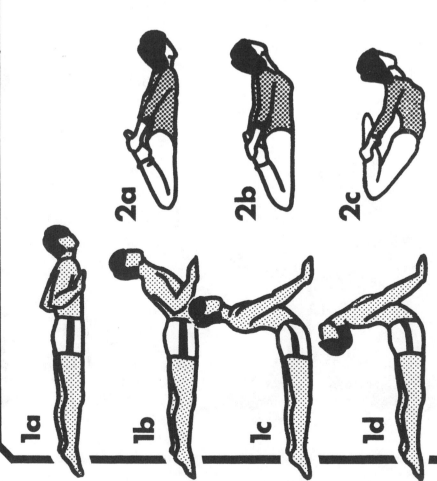

3a Lie facedown with your chin on the floor and your arms by your sides. Clench your fists and press them, thumbs underneath, on the floor.

3b Press hard and slowly raise one leg as high as you can, keeping it straight. Hold for a count of 10; lower, and repeat with the other leg.

3c Pushing on the floor, and with your chin still resting on it, raise both legs together as high as you can. Hold for a count of 5. Exhale, and lower your legs. (Practice will increase the height to which you can raise your legs.)

4a Lie on your left side with your left arm bent and your head resting on your left palm. Bend your right arm and place your right palm flat on the floor in front of your chest.

4b Raise your right leg as high as you can, at the same time pressing against the floor with your right hand. Count 10. Change sides, and repeat with the other leg.

4c As a variation to 4b, start as in 4a but then raise both legs together a few inches from the floor.

2a Lie facedown with your legs straight and your toes pointed back. Then bend your knees as far as you can, reaching back to catch hold of your feet to pull them even farther, as shown.

2b Slowly raise your head.

2c Pulling on your feet, raise your trunk and knees from the floor (bringing your knees together if you are an advanced student). Hold this pose as long as you can.

Lying down poses

1a Lie facedown with your legs and toes stretched back. Put the palms of your hands under your shoulders on the floor.

1b Inhaling, raise your head and shoulders from the floor.

1c Straighten your arms to raise your head and shoulders higher.

1d Keeping your hips on the floor and your shoulders square, put your head back to look up.

POSES

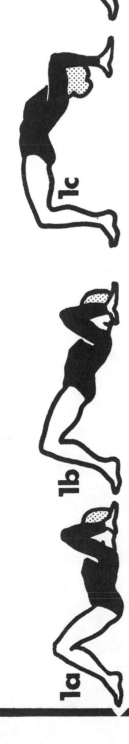

1a

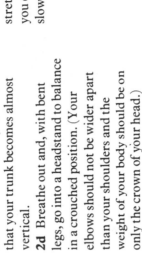

1b

1c

1d

Upside-down poses

1a Lie on your back with your knees bent and your feet flat on the floor. Place the palms of your hands on the floor by the sides of your head.

1d, c, d Breathe in and then raise your body gradually to form an arch, keeping your feet flat on the floor. Hold 5–10 seconds. Slowly lower yourself back to the starting position.

2a When trying this headstand for the first time enlist the aid of a friend, or try it near a wall for support.
With a folded towel or blanket, make a pad for your head. Kneel near the pad.

2b Link your fingers to cup your hands. Use your cupped hands to support the back of your head and place your crown on the pad. Straighten your legs and raise your bottom to form an arch.

2c Walk forward on your toes so that your trunk becomes almost vertical.

2d Breathe out and, with bent legs, go into a headstand to balance in a crouched position. (Your elbows should not be wider apart than your shoulders and the weight of your body should be on only the crown of your head.)

2e Slowly straighten your legs and stretch them up. Hold as long as you can, then bend your knees and slowly lower your legs.

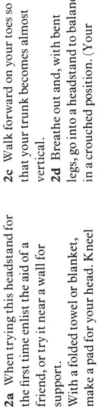

2a

2b

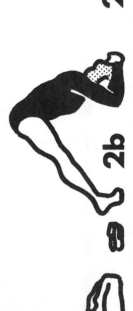

2c

2d

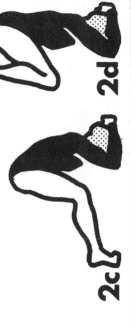

2e

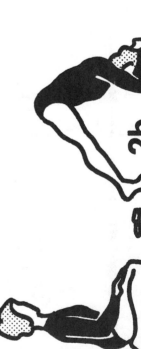

Yoga

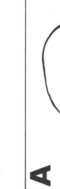

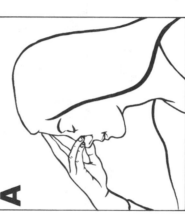

A

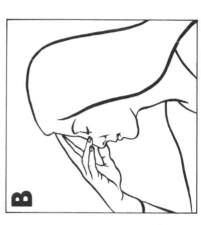

B

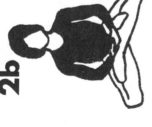 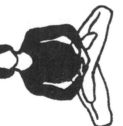 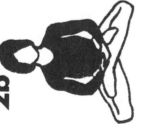 **1**

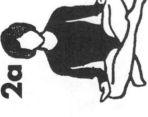 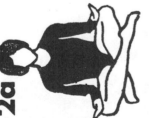 **2a**

 **2b**

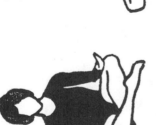 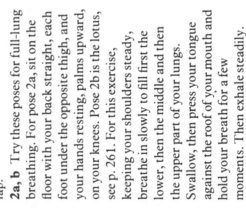 **3**

3 Adopt a comfortable sitting or kneeling pose to practice alternate nostril breathing. The theory that one nostril plays a positive role while the other plays a negative one lies behind this important yoga breathing exercise.

A Place the first and second fingers of your right hand on your forehead with your thumb against the right nostril and your third and fourth fingers against the left. Counting 4, breathe in through the right nostril, closing the other with your fingers.

B Now use your thumb to close the right nostril so that you are holding your breath for a count of 4. Then lift your third and fourth fingers to enable you to exhale, counting 4. With your lungs empty, count 4 again. Then repeat the exercise, reversing nostrils and hands.

Yoga breathing principles

Correct and regular breathing is an essential feature of all yoga poses and sequences. Most people do not breathe deeply enough, and this is one of the first shortcomings that the student of yoga needs to overcome. There are many different exercises, but the general principles are to breathe out deeply to empty the lungs, and then to expand the chest as you inhale deeply. Continue to breathe in and out deeply and rhythmically, pulling in your stomach muscles as you inhale. The nostrils should be relaxed (i.e. not contracted) and you should be conscious of the movement of your chest and stomach.

Poses and exercises

1 This pose (Virasana) is ideal for practicing deep breathing. Kneel with your knees together, your feet well apart with the upper parts down on the floor, your body resting on your legs, your back straight, and your hands held loosely, palms upward, on your lap.

2a, b Try these poses for full-lung breathing. For pose 2a, sit on the floor with your back straight, each foot under the opposite thigh, and your hands resting, palms upward, on your knees. Pose 2b is the lotus, see p. 261. For this exercise, keeping your shoulders steady, breathe in slowly to fill first the lower, then the middle and then the upper part of your lungs. Swallow, then press your tongue against the roof of your mouth and hold your breath for a few moments. Then exhale steadily.

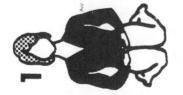

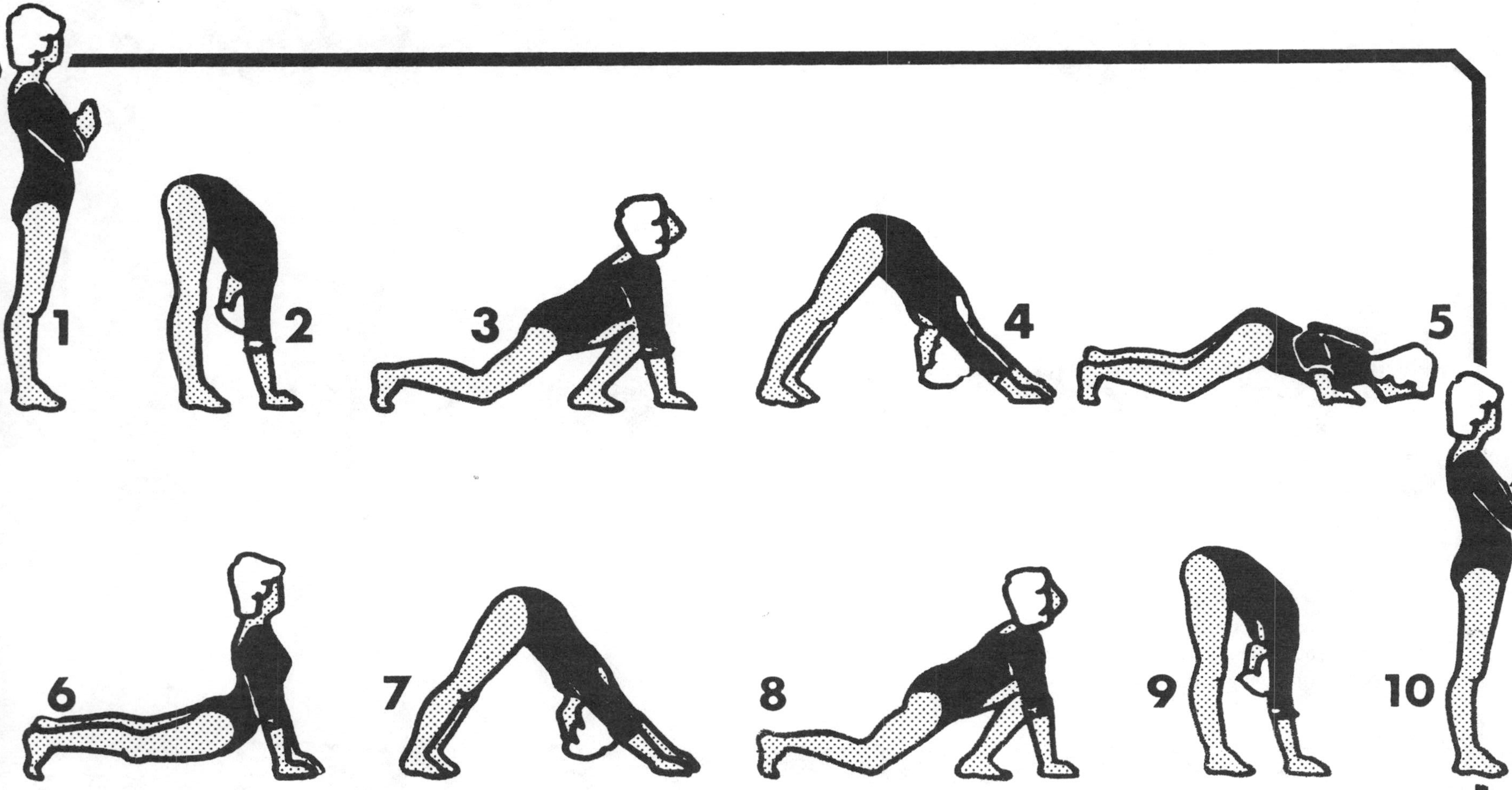

Salute to the sun

This is a sequence of yoga poses performed in a strict order; appropriately, the best time to make the salute is early in the morning. Perform the sequence rhythmically, breathing in and out as you change positions.

1 Stand erect with straight legs and with your hands in front of your chest, palms together.

2 Breathe rhythmically, and as you exhale, still keeping your legs straight, bend over so that your hands are on the floor.

3 Inhale as you stretch one leg behind you, bending the other leg; lift your head back.

4 Straighten the other leg beside the first. With your feet flat on the floor, drop your head through your outstretched arms to touch the floor.

5 Bend your arms and lower your body so that your knees, chest and head touch the floor.

6 Straighten your arms and legs so that your body is supported by your toes and hands.

7 Straighten your legs to raise your bottom and allow your head to fall through your arms to the ground.

8 Bend your knees and bring one knee forward so that you are again in position 3.

9 Bring your back foot forward, level with the other, and tuck your chin well in.

10 Return to the starting pose. Repeat the sequence at least once more, alternating leg positions in stage 3.

©DIAGRAM

Yoga

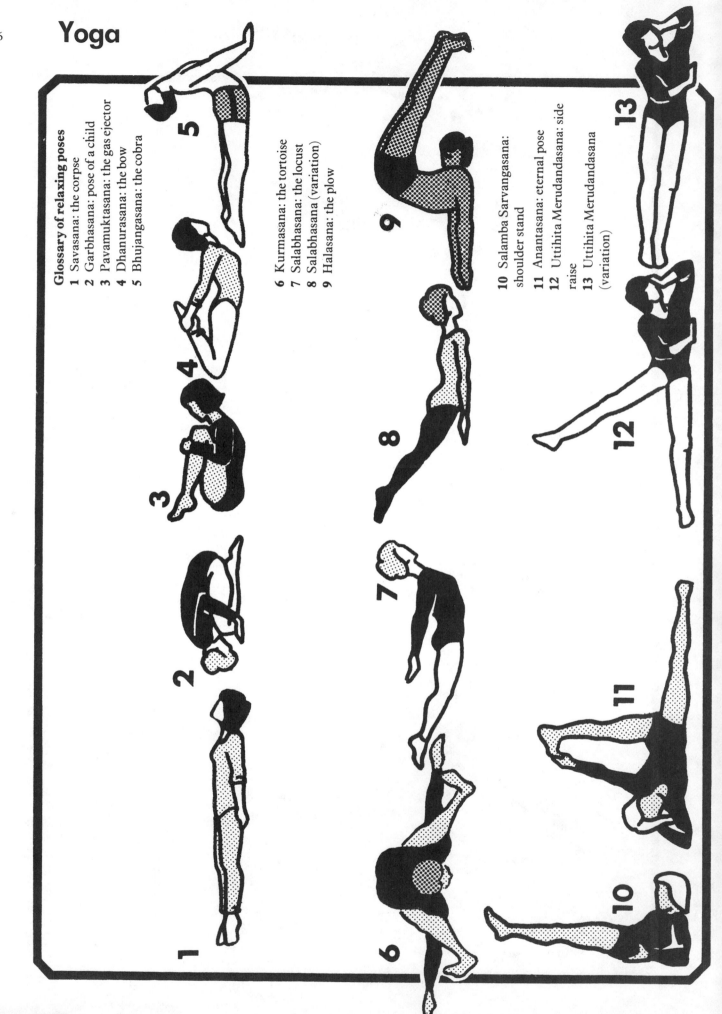

Glossary of relaxing poses

1 Savasana: the corpse
2 Garbhasana: pose of a child
3 Pavamuktasana: the gas ejector
4 Dhanurasana: the bow
5 Bhujangasana: the cobra

6 Kurmasana: the tortoise
7 Salabhasana: the locust
8 Salabhasana (variation)
9 Halasana: the plow

10 Salamba Sarvangasana: shoulder stand
11 Anantasana: eternal pose
12 Uttihita Merudandasana: side raise
13 Uttihita Merudandasana (variation)

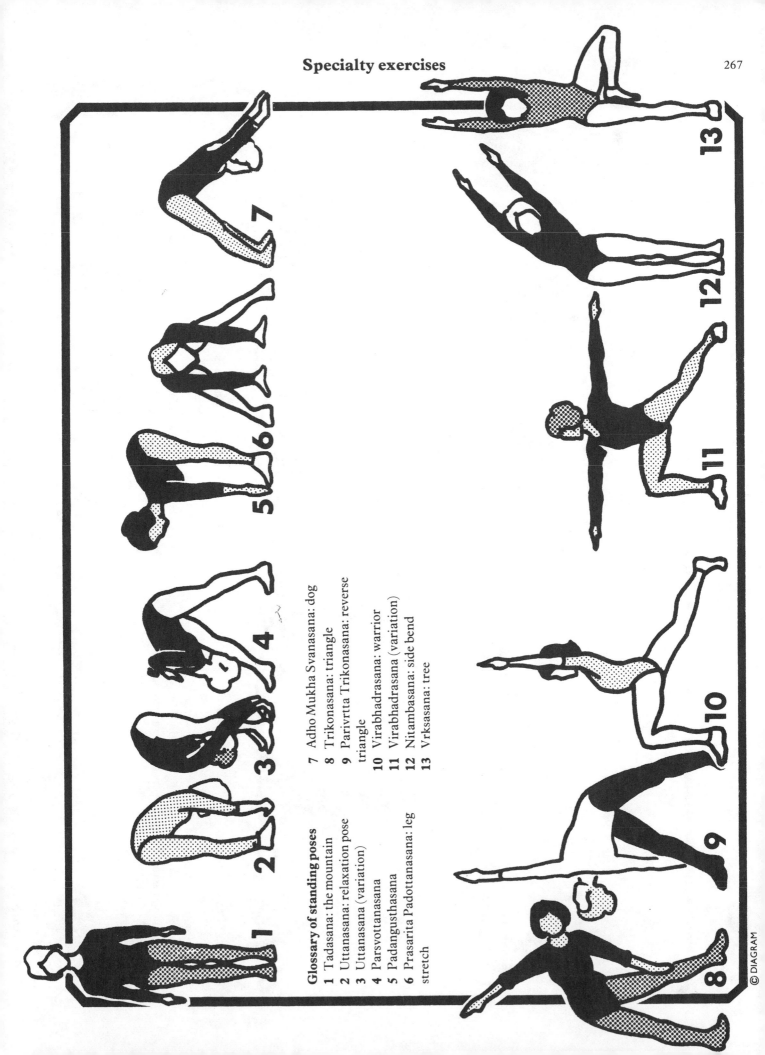

Glossary of standing poses

1 Tadasana: the mountain
2 Uttanasana: relaxation pose
3 Uttanasana (variation)
4 Parsvottanasana
5 Padangusthasana
6 Prasarita Padottanasana: leg stretch
7 Adho Mukha Svanasana: dog
8 Trikonasana: triangle
9 Parivrtta Trikonasana: reverse triangle
10 Virabhadrasana: warrior
11 Virabhadrasana (variation)
12 Nitambasana: side bend
13 Vrksasana: tree

© DIAGRAM

Yoga

POSES

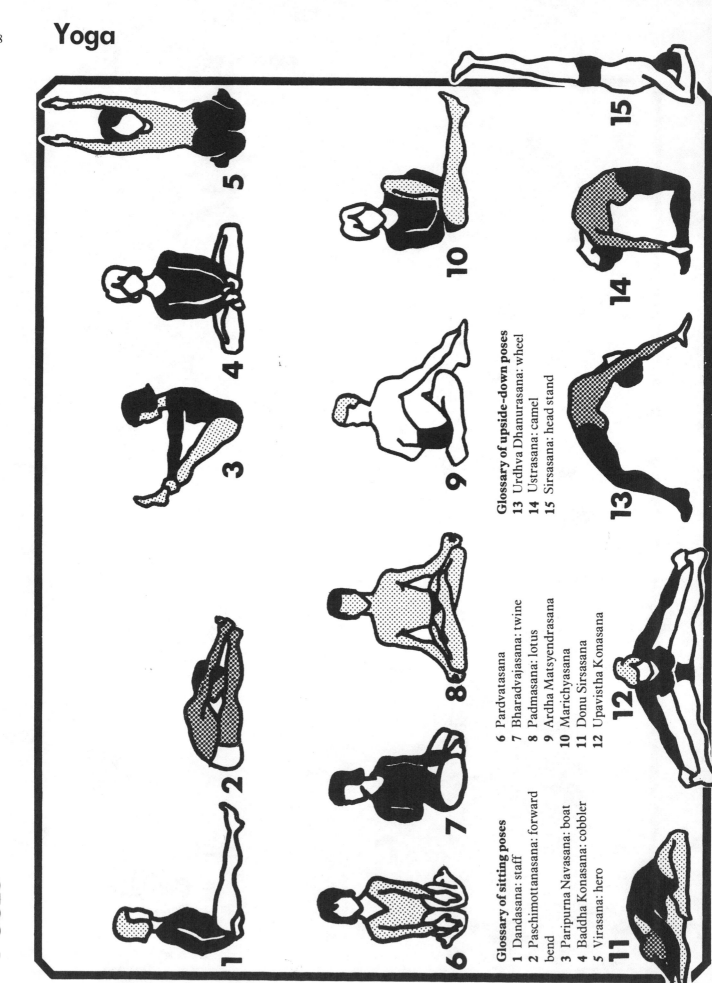

Glossary of sitting poses

1 Dandasana: staff
2 Paschimottanasana: forward bend
3 Paripurna Navasana: boat
4 Baddha Konasana: cobbler
5 Virasana: hero
6 Pardvatasana
7 Bharadvajasana: twine
8 Padmasana: lotus
9 Ardha Matsyendrasana
10 Marichyasana
11 Donu Sirsasana
12 Upavistha Konasana

Glossary of upside-down poses

13 Urdhva Dhanurasana: wheel
14 Ustrasana: camel
15 Sirsasana: head stand

POSES

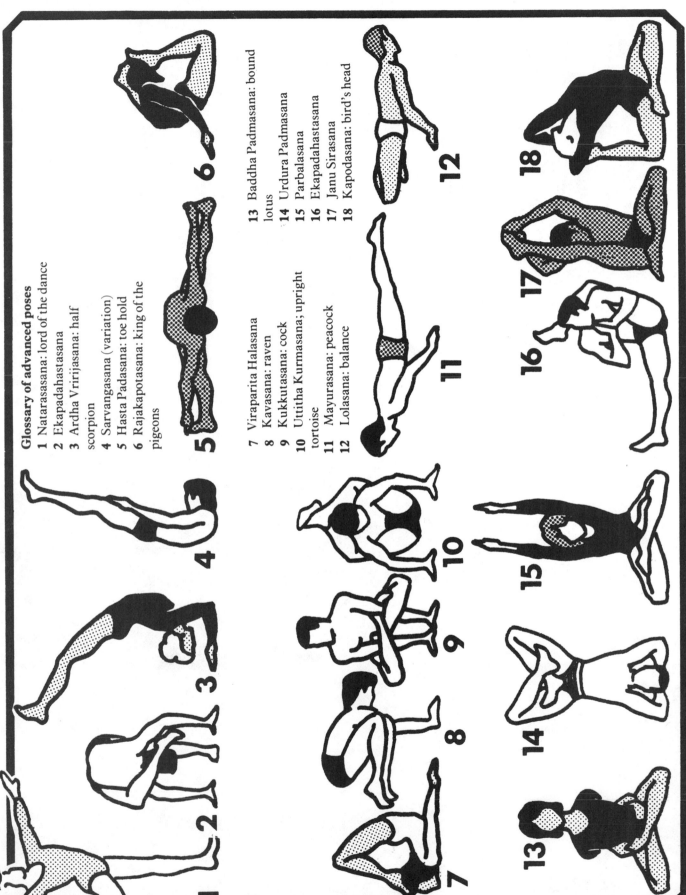

Glossary of advanced poses

1 Natarasasana: lord of the dance
2 Ekapadahastasana
3 Ardha Virirjasana: half scorpion
4 Sarvangasana (variation)
5 Hasta Padasana: toe hold
6 Rajakapotasana: king of the pigeons

7 Viraparita Halasana
8 Kavasana: raven
9 Kukkutasana: cock
10 Uttitha Kurmasana; upright tortoise
11 Mayurasana: peacock
12 Lolasana: balance

13 Baddha Padmasana: bound lotus
14 Urdura Padmasana
15 Parbalasana
16 Ekapadahastasana
17 Janu Sirasana
18 Kapodasana: bird's head

© DIAGRAM

Chapter 8   EXERCISE PROGRAMS

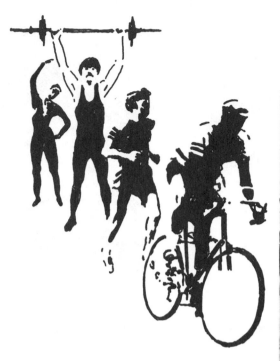

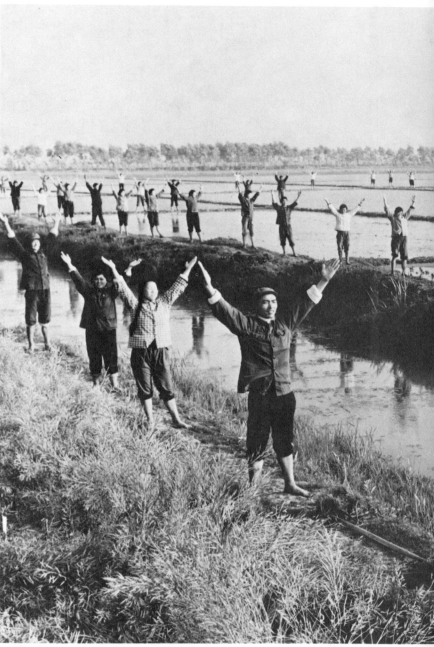

1 Seven Miles Walk (The Mansell Collection)
2 Exercising in the fields (Anglo-Chinese Educational Institute)

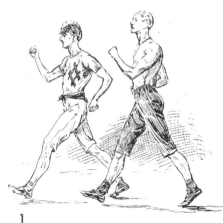

1

2

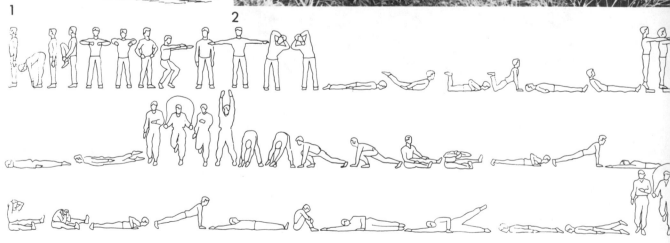

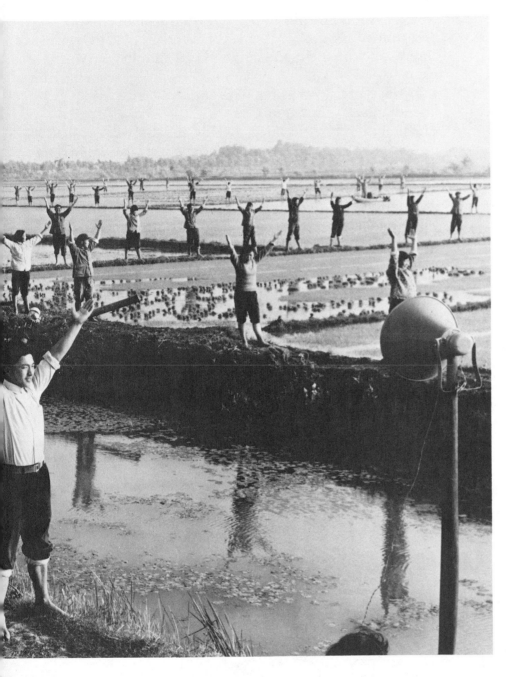

CHOOSING A PROGRAM

Obviously it is possible to build up your own exercise program by assembling a series of exercises of your own choice, and other chapters in this book should give you plenty of ideas. Many people, however, prefer to embark on a formal exercise program, with carefully planned ingredients, levels and targets.

The first exercise programs of modern times were probably those of J.C.F. Guts Muths. His *Gymnastik für die Jugend* was published in Germany in 1793 and became very popular in Europe and North America. It included instruction in jumping, running, throwing, wrestling, climbing, balancing, lifting, carrying, pulling, dancing, walking, military exercises and swimming.

Today, organizations both public and private offer their techniques for transforming you into an office athlete with the minimum of effort; from "get big quick" programs that appeal to the imagined physical inadequacy of the lean adolescent, to official programs designed for members of armed forces and secret services.

During the 1960s the Royal Canadian Air Force 5BX and XBX programs acquired considerable popularity. These are still widely available in other publications and have

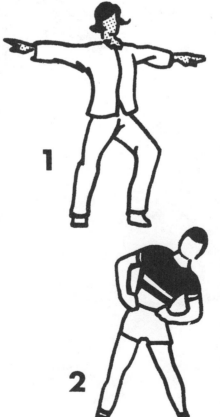

1 The Chinese program
This provides a good all-round calisthenic program with more development of muscle control and coordination than most Western systems. Since it does not provide any CR exercise, it is recommended to be used in conjunction with some form of aerobic exercise. It is ideal for joggers who want to exercise other parts of their body.

2 The UK program
Including exercises of three different types — mobility, strength, and heart and lung (CR) — this program aims at all-round fitness. It begins with exercises for the very unfit, and at all levels places particular emphasis on gradual improvement at your own pace. The advanced schedule uses weight training for strength and CR exercise.

therefore not been included in this book. Also, concentrating as they do on 11–12 minutes of calisthenic exercises, the Canadian programs do not reflect the more recent emphasis in fitness programs on exercising the circulatory-respiratory (CR) system. A major influence in this change in emphasis toward CR exercise was Dr Kenneth Cooper's book *Aerobics*, published in the late 1960s and aimed almost exclusively at CR development by means of walking, swimming, running, stationary running, cycling and selected sports. His points system is still very commonly used.

It is now believed that to be most effective, an exercise program should aim for 15–30 minutes of aerobic CR exercise, with warming-up and cooling-down exercises, and also movements for increasing strength and mobility. The emphasis you give to the latter will depend upon your individual needs and wants.

We have selected four government-sponsored exercise programs for inclusion in this chapter: a calisthenic program from China, an all-round program from the UK, and a general and an aerobic program from the USA.

3 The US general program
Developed by the President's Council on Physical Fitness, this is the most comprehensive of the programs offered. It affects all aspects of fitness in steadily increasing grades. If possible try to do the jog/run or swimming CR exercises as it has been argued that the skipping or running-on-the-spot alternatives are less effective.

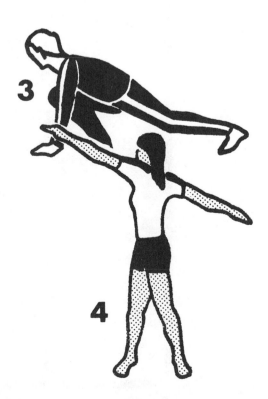

4 The US aerobic program
Also devised by the President's Council, this can be used as an alternative or complement to the above program, or any other program that does not provide sufficient aerobic exercise. It is designed for the very unfit, and is part of a series of programs that will take you through to, and keep you at, an advanced stage of fitness.

CHINESE PROGRAM

"Promote physical fitness and build up the people's health," was Chairman Mao's instruction that led to the creation of calisthenic exercise programs to be performed throughout China by its population of over 822 million. The most recent of these programs was introduced in 1971 by the Peking Physical Culture Institute. Like its four predecessors, this program was devised to make physical culture serve the needs of the Chinese people. It consists of seven sets of three to five exercises, each set designed to meet the specific needs of a particular group of workers. Groups catered for in this

Chinese exercise programs
The exercise programs of modern China are rooted in a tradition dating back to Shaolin temple boxing and T'ai Chi Ch'uan (see p. 246). Modern programs consist of calisthenic exercises, which are usually performed in groups early each morning to music broadcast over the radio.

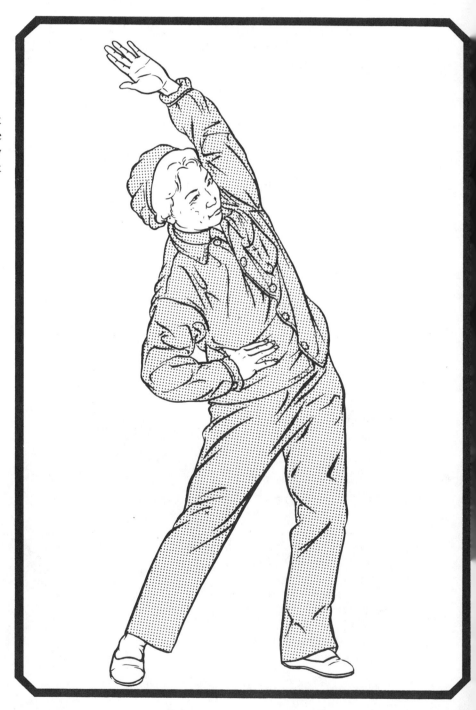

latest program are iron and steel workers, drivers, coal miners, masons, textile workers, electronics workers and persons working in stores.

Each set of exercises has similar aims: to reduce fatigue, to relieve strain on those parts of the body that are most used in a particular occupation, to provide exercise for parts of the body that are insufficiently used, and to help prevent occupational illnesses. How these aims can best be met obviously varies from group to group, and this is reflected in the different sets of exercises. For drivers, the exercises concentrate on the legs. For people such as miners who must do a lot of bending, the emphasis is on the back, chest, shoulders and arms. For electronics workers, eye massage is included to relieve fatigue from long concentration. On subsequent pages we describe the sets of exercises designed by the Chinese for workers in stores and for schoolchildren. Each involves more or less the whole body and is therefore also suitable for more general use.

Eye massage from the exercises for electronics workers
1 Clench both fists and put one thumb on each sun tsubo (marked on the diagram by dots). Use the second joints of your forefingers to rub outward along the lines indicated in the diagram by arrows. Rub once above your eyes and once below them. Repeat 4 times.

Drivers' leg exercise
2a Stand upright.
2b Pull your left knee to your body with your hands.
2c Repeat with the other leg.
2d Bend your body forward and place your hands on your knees.
2e Bend your knees and squat, face forward and elbows out.
2f Return to position 2d.
2g Stand upright.

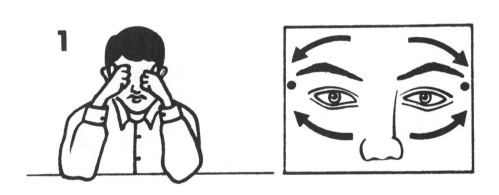

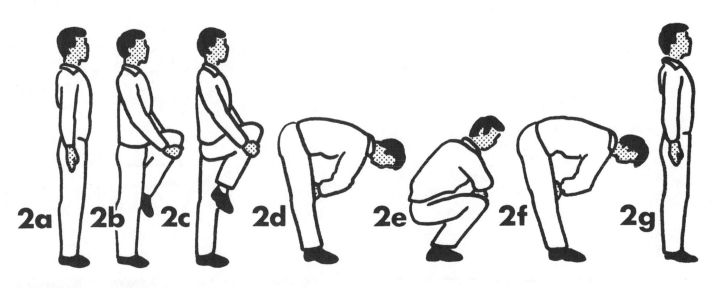

Chinese program

FOR SALESPEOPLE

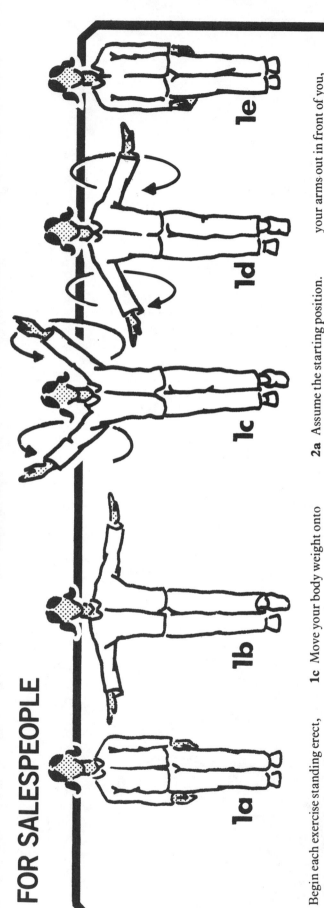

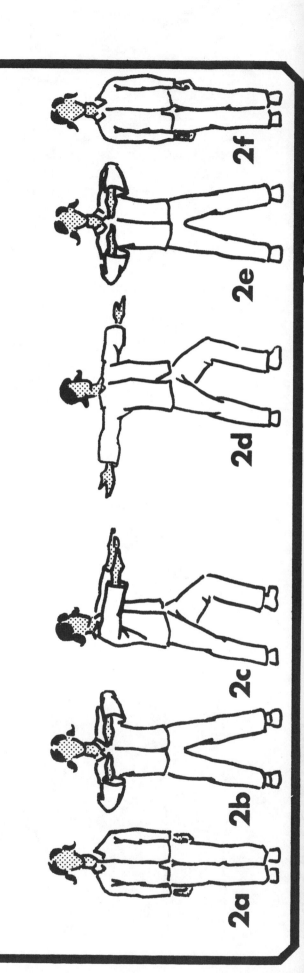

Begin each exercise standing erect, with your feet together and arms by your sides.

1a Assume the starting position.
1b Point your left foot forward, raising both your arms to the sides at shoulder level.
1c Move your body weight onto your left foot, raising your right heel. Make a forward circle with your arms.
1d Circle your arms backward.
1e Return to the starting position. Then repeat, changing sides.

2a Assume the starting position.
2b Take one step to the left, raising your arms as shown, with elbows at shoulder level and palms facing down.
2c Bending the left leg, turn your body 90° to the left; straighten your arms out in front of you, palms upward.
2d Move your arms out to the sides, palms upward.
2e Return to position 2b.
2f Return to the starting position and repeat to the right.

FOR SALESPEOPLE

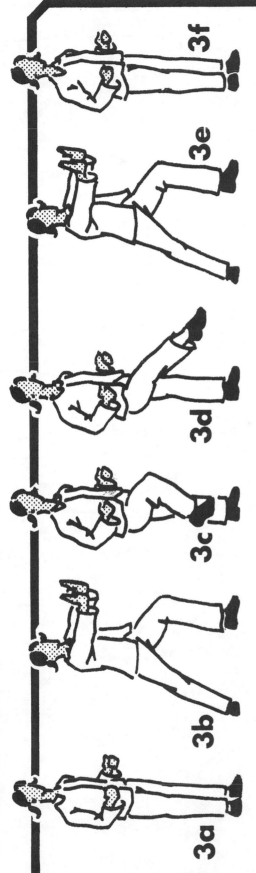

3a From the starting position raise your clenched fists to your waist, palms upward.
3b Step forward onto your left leg; bend the knee and push both arms forward, palms to the front.
3c Moving onto your left foot, bend your right leg as shown and again clench your hands to your waist.
3d Kick your right leg forward.
3e Return to position 3b.
3f Return to position 3a and repeat with the other leg.

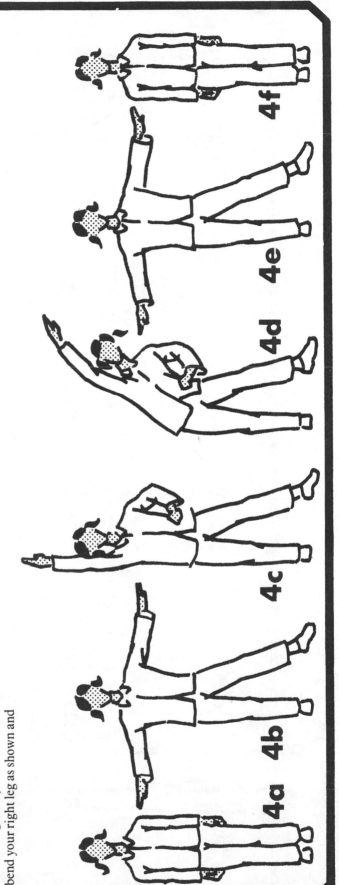

4a Assume the starting position.
4b Point your left foot to the side and raise your arms sideways to shoulder level.
4c Place your left hand on your waist and raise your right arm above your head, palm facing left.
4d Bounce twice to the left, bending at the waist.
4e Return to position 4b.
4f Return to the starting position and repeat to the right.

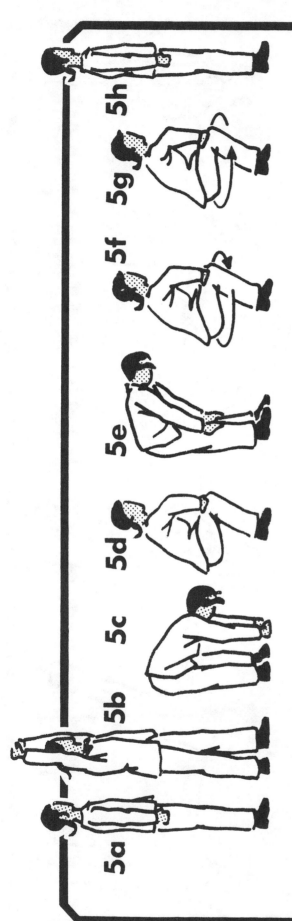

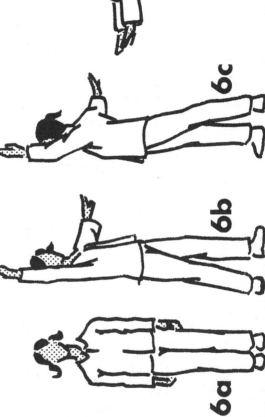

5a Assume the starting position.
5b Move your left foot one step to the side. Lock your fingers above your head, palms down. Turn the palms up and straighten your arms, bending your back slightly and looking up.
5c Bend your body forward and try to touch the floor with your palms, keeping your legs straight.
5d Bring your feet together and crouch on your heels, putting your hands on your knees and pushing your elbows out.
5e Straighten your knees.

5f Bend your knees again slightly and circle them clockwise.
5g Circle your knees counter-clockwise.
5h Return to the starting position and repeat to the right.

6a Assume the starting position.
6b Take one step to the left and turn your body 90° to the left without moving your feet. Raise your right arm forward and over your head, and your left arm out to shoulder height, palm down.
6c Twisting on the balls of your feet turn 180° to the right, reversing the position of your arms.
6d Raise both arms above your head. Then bend forward from the waist and move your body as far as you can in a counterclockwise circular movement.
6e Return to starting position and repeat to the other side.

FOR SALESPEOPLE

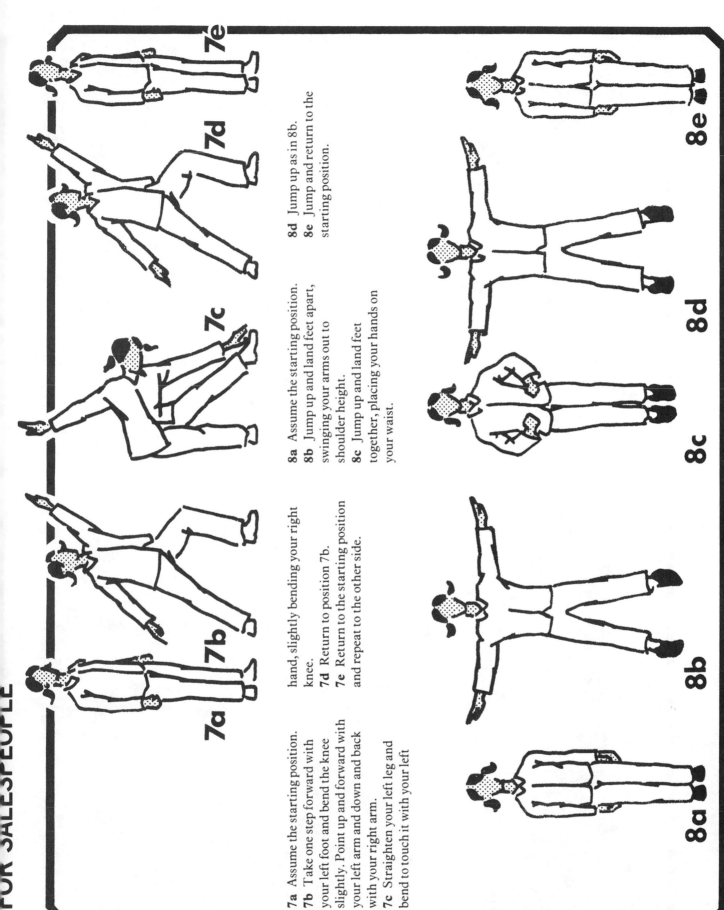

7a Assume the starting position.
7b Take one step forward with your left foot and bend the knee slightly. Point up and forward with your left arm and down and back with your right arm.
7c Straighten your left leg and bend to touch it with your left hand, slightly bending your right knee.
7d Return to position 7b.
7e Return to the starting position and repeat to the other side.

8a Assume the starting position.
8b Jump up and land feet apart, swinging your arms out to shoulder height.
8c Jump up and land feet together, placing your hands on your waist.
8d Jump up as in 8b.
8e Jump up and return to the starting position.

©DIAGRAM

Chinese program

FOR CHILDREN

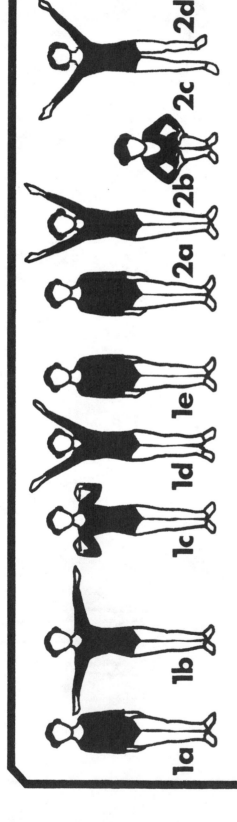

Always start by standing erect, feet together and arms by sides.
1a Assume the starting position.
1b Raise your arms sideways to shoulder level, palms down.
1c Bend your elbows and touch your shoulders.
1d Raise your arms up and out, palms in, while at the same time rising up onto your toes.
1e Return to the starting position and repeat.

2a Assume the starting position.
2b Raise both arms to the front and then above your head, palms inward.
2c Crouch down and place your hands on your knees.
2d Stand up straight, raising your arms to the sides and pointing your left foot back.
2e Return to the starting position. Then repeat, pointing your right foot back.

3a Assume the starting position.
3b Raise your arms sideways to shoulder level, palms down, while at the same time stepping forward onto your left foot and raising your right heel.
3c With your hands on your waist, raise your right leg as high in front as you can.
3d Return to position 3b.
3e Return to starting position. Repeat, raising your left leg.

4a Assume the starting position.
4b Place your hands on the back of your head, elbows in line with your body, and point your left foot to the side.
4c Bend to the left from the waist.
4d Stand upright and straighten your arms out to the side at shoulder level.
4e Return to the starting position and repeat to the right.

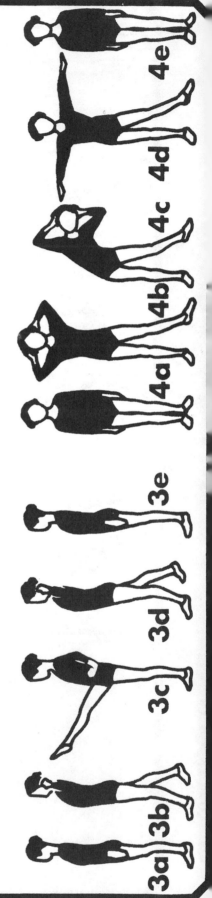

FOR CHILDREN

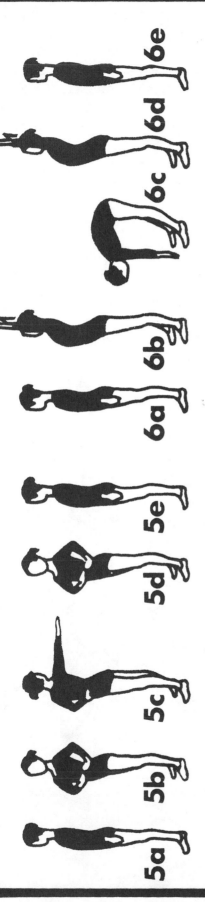

5a Assume the starting position.
5b Place your left hand on your waist and your right hand, palm up, across your body. Turn 45° to the left and place your left foot to the side.
5c Straighten your right arm to shoulder height and twist round to the right as far as possible.
5d Return to position 5b.
5e Return to starting position. Repeat to the other side.

6a Assume the starting position.
6b Take one step to the left and raise your arms forward and up so that your palms are forward and your back slightly arched.
6c Keeping your legs straight, bend forward and touch the ground by your left foot.
6d Return to position 6b.
6e Return to the starting position. Repeat, stepping and bending to the right.

7a Assume the starting position.
7b Take one step forward with your left leg while raising your arms above your head, palms in.
7c Swing your arms forward, down, and behind as far as possible, ending with your palms up; bend your body forward as shown.
7d Straighten up and slightly arch your back. Keeping your eyes fixed on your left hand and your back heel on the ground, swing your left arm up through 180° and your right arm round through 360°, ending with palms down.
7e Return to starting position. Repeat to the other side.

8a Assume the starting position.
8b Jump and land with your feet apart, hands on your waist.
8c Jump and land feet together.
8d Jump and land feet apart, clapping your hands overhead.
8e Return to start and repeat.

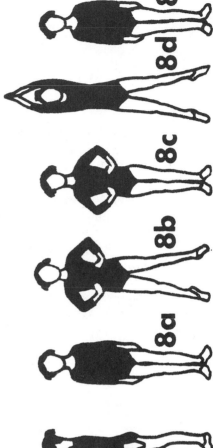

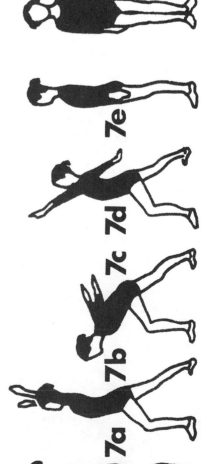

UK PROGRAM

This section is based on an exercise program published in the United Kingdom by the Health Education Council, following a series shown on BBC television. The Health Education Council, set up in 1968, works with Government backing in association with the National Health Service and area authorities. Its *Look After Yourself* campaign aims to show that "relatively simple adjustments to common contemporary life-styles, without being themselves burdensome, can produce real benefits to the quality of life now as well as longer life-expectancy."

UK exercise program
Two schedules — standard and advanced — are designed to meet the exercise requirements of persons of all degrees of fitness. Exercises are designed to increase mobility and strength, and to increase the efficiency of the heart and lungs. In the advanced schedule, strength and heart and lung exercises are combined in weight training.

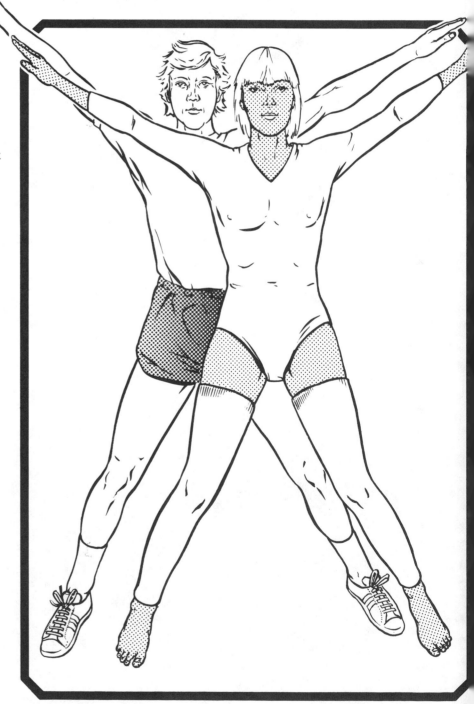

The standard schedule

Even people who have become quite unused to physical exercise can start this schedule, but check with your doctor first if you have any doubts about your health. Exercises in the standard schedule are carefully graded so that you can easily find your own level and then gradually improve your performance. Once you are familiar with the different parts of the schedule, you will be able to complete your personal program in a session lasting only 15 minutes; three sessions a week are sufficient to produce excellent results.

The standard schedule consists of three types of exercise: mobility exercises, strength exercises and exercises designed to increase the efficiency of the heart and lungs. Together these exercises will exercise your whole body, using muscles that remain unexercised in the course of most people's normal routine.

The mobility exercises have been selected to ensure that all the major joints and muscles are moved through their complete range of movement. These exercises should always be done first to warm up your body before the other exercises in the program. Attempt each exercise but do not overstrain yourself; aim to increase your flexibility by trying to push yourself just a little bit farther each session.

The strength exercises are designed to supply what the authors of this program describe as the "Plus Factor," that little extra bit of strength needed, for example, to run for a bus, lift a heavy log in the garden or take a long walk at the weekend. Exercising regularly against resistance, at a level slightly above normal requirements, will provide this extra strength and so help avoid torn muscles, ligaments or tendons, or even a slipped disk. Start with easy exercises in this section and substitute harder ones only as your strength improves.

Heart and lungs are exercised by stepping up the body's oxygen requirements, which is most easily done by exercising the large muscle groups of the legs, arms and trunk. After preliminary exercises, the schedule here incorporates jogging, cycling or swimming.

The advanced schedule

This is designed to meet the needs of fit people who can easily complete the exercises of the standard schedule. It retains the mobility exercises of the standard schedule but substitutes weight training in place of that schedule's exercises for strength and heart and lungs.

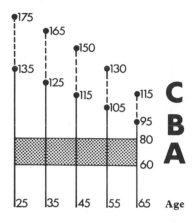

Your personal pulse rating

Monitoring your pulse is an essential feature of the part of this program designed to exercise the heart and lungs. The first step is to find out your own personal pulse rating. This represents the maximum number of beats per minute to which your pulse may be allowed to rise during the exercises. Personal ratings vary with age and fitness as summarized in the diagram above:

A shows the typical pulse range for persons at rest;

B shows pulse ratings by age for when you start the program;

C shows pulse ratings for when you are fitter—build up gradually, 5 or 10 beats per week.

Using your pulse rating

When you first start the heart and lung exercises, check your pulse every minute or so. (See p. 76 for how to do this.) If your pulse is at or below your personal pulse rating, continue exercising; if it is higher, stop and rest until your pulse comes down. Aim for 10 minutes continuous exercise without exceeding your personal rating.

©DIAGRAM

STANDARD SCHEDULE

Mobility exercises

These exercises are designed to increase your flexibility. They should be done in an even, relaxed way. Do not hurry or overstrain yourself. Breathing should be fitted to the rhythm of the movements. Repeat each exercise about 10—12 times. There is no need to increase the number of repetitions or to try to do the exercises more quickly. Progress is made by gently increasing and then maintaining your range of movement.

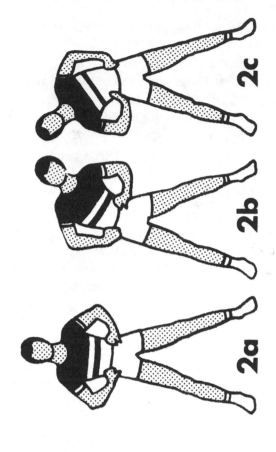

1a Stand with your feet apart and your arms hanging loosely by your sides.

1b Raise both arms in front of you.

1c Bring your arms up and past your ears. Then carry them back and around to complete a circle, finishing in the start position.

2a Stand with your feet wide apart and your hands on your hips, elbows bent.

2b Bend to the left from the waist, still facing forward and keeping your head in line with your body.

2c Straighten up, then bend to the right.

STANDARD SCHEDULE

Mobility exercises

3a Stand about 18in (50cm) behind a chair and rest your hands lightly on its back.

3b Raising your left knee, bring your forehead down to meet it. Do not hurry the movement.

3c Straighten up, lowering your leg.

3d Repeat with your right leg. Later you can try this exercise without using a chair.

4a Stand with your feet wide apart and stretch your arms out in front of you.

4b Bending your right arm across your chest, turn your head, arms and shoulders to the left as far as you can. Keep your body still.

4c Face the front again. Then repeat to the right.

5a Stand with your feet wide apart, resting both hands on the front of your left thigh.

5b Bend forward and slide your hands down your left leg as far as you can. Do not attempt to reach too far, especially if you suffer from back trouble.

5c Stand erect again and rest your hands on your right thigh.

5d Slide your hands down your right leg.

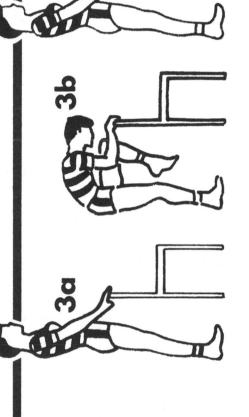

3a 3b 3c 3d

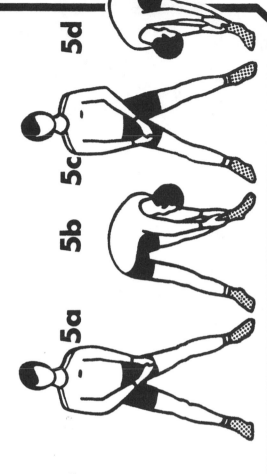

5a 5b 5c 5d

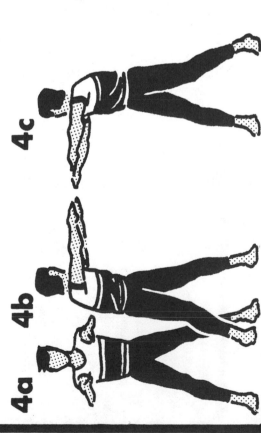

4a 4b 4c

©DIAGRAM

UK program

STANDARD SCHEDULE

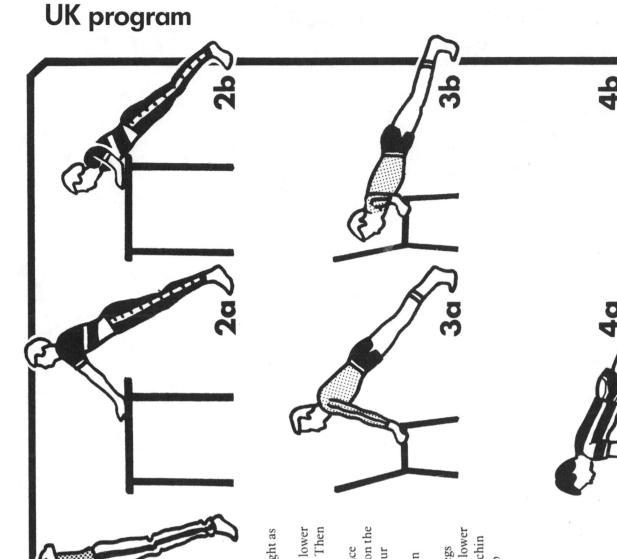

2b

2a

1b

1a

3b

3a

4b

4a

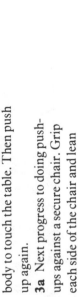

Strength exercises

There are three types of strength exercise in the UK standard schedule: push-ups, abdominal exercises and leg exercises. Exercises of each type are arranged progressively. Start with 10–12 repetitions of the easiest exercise of each type, increasing to 20 or 30. Only when you can do this easily should you substitute the next exercise.

Push-ups/press-ups

1a Stand with your arms out straight, your hands about 1ft (30cm) apart on a wall, at shoulder height.

1b Rise up on your toes. Keeping your body straight, bend your arms and lean forward until your chin and chest touch the wall. Straighten your arms to return to the starting position.

2a The next stage is to do push-ups leaning against a table. Make sure the table is secure. Stand about 3ft (90cm) away from the table and lean forward with your body and arms straight and your hands about 1ft (30cm) apart on the table.

2b Keeping your body straight, bend your arms and lower your body to touch the table. Then push up again.

3a Next progress to doing push-ups against a secure chair. Grip each side of the chair and lean forward with your arms straight as shown.

3b Bend your arms and lower your body to touch the chair. Then push up again.

4a This is a full push-up. Place your hands, fingers forward, on the floor immediately beneath your shoulders. With your arms straight, support your body on your hands and toes.

4b Keeping your body and legs straight, bend your arms and lower yourself until your chest and chin touch the floor. Then push up again.

STANDARD SCHEDULE

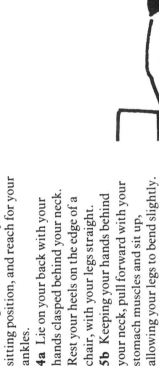
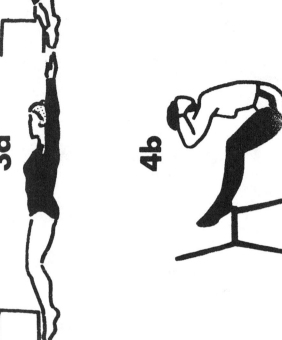
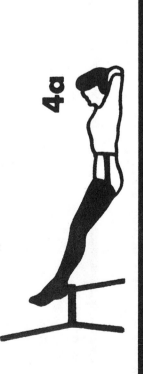
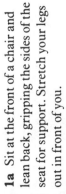

1a 2b 2a 1b

3b 3a

4b 4a

Strength exercises (abdomen)

As with the other strength exercises, start with the first exercise of the group and move on only when you are sure you are ready. Don't risk muscle strain by trying to proceed too quickly. Before you start, ensure that any items of furniture are firm and safe.

1a Sit at the front of a chair and lean back, gripping the sides of the seat for support. Stretch your legs out in front of you.

1b Bend your knees and lift your legs so that your thighs are brought up to your body.

2a Start as in 1a.

2b Keeping your legs straight, lift them as high as you can.

3a Lie on your back with your arms overhead and your feet tucked under a heavy chair.

3b Swing forward and up to a sitting position, and reach for your ankles.

4a Lie on your back with your hands clasped behind your neck. Rest your heels on the edge of a chair, with your legs straight.

5b Keeping your hands behind your neck, pull forward with your stomach muscles and sit up, allowing your legs to bend slightly.

©DIAGRAM

STANDARD SCHEDULE

Strength exercises (legs)

These exercises use a squatting movement to strengthen the leg muscles, which are inadequately exercised in the normal range of adult activity. Start with the first exercise and gradually work your way through the harder exercises as the strength of your legs improves.

1a Stand 18in (50cm) behind a chair and rest your hands lightly on its back. Sink down into a squat, keeping your back straight and, if possible, your feet flat on the floor. (At first you will probably find it easier to rise up onto your toes at this point.)
1b Straighten your legs and rise up onto your toes, using your arms to help you up if necessary.
2a As in 1a but with your hands on your hips.
2b Straighten your legs and rise up onto your toes.

3a Squat down with your hands on your hips.
3b Straighten your legs and rise quickly, pushing up so that your feet clear the ground by a few inches.

3c Squat down again.
3d As in 3b, but as your strength increases push up harder to make a higher jump.
4a Bend your knees and sink into a half-squat as shown.
4b Jump up, stretching your arms and legs out to make a star shape. As you land, let your knees bend slightly to absorb the shock.

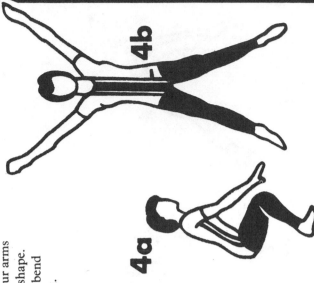

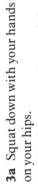

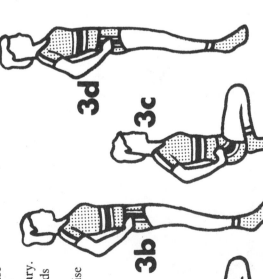

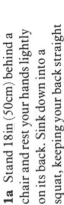

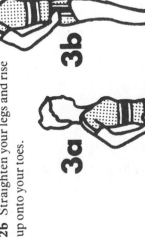

STANDARD SCHEDULE

Heart and lung exercises

These exercises are designed to improve your circulatory and respiratory systems. Like the strength exercises in this program, they are designed to be carried out progressively; only when you are satisfied with your performance at one exercise should you move on to the next one. Check your pulse frequently, and don't exceed your rating (see p. 283).

1 With your arms hanging loosely at your sides, gently run on the spot for about 30 seconds. As you improve, lift your knees up higher and gradually build up to 5–6 minutes.

2a With your hands on your hips, stand about 1ft (30cm) away from a low box or stool. Leading with your left foot, bring both feet up onto the box and then step down again. Repeat 15 times leading with the left foot, and then repeat 15 times leading with the right foot. Increase by one step per foot at each session until you can do 30 steps with each foot.

2b Gradually increase the height of the box to about 18in (46cm), or step up onto a low bench. When you can do this comfortably, build up the time spent on this exercise. Aim for 3–6 minutes continuous exercise without exceeding your pulse rating.

3a, b, c Once you can do exercise 2 comfortably, you are ready to include either jogging, cycling or swimming in your program. Pause for rest and pulse regulation as usual, aiming at 10 minutes continuous exercise.

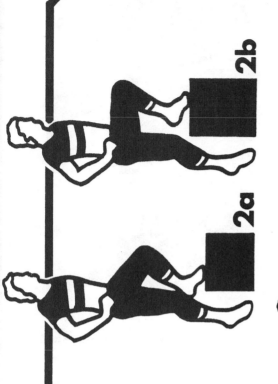

1

2a

2b

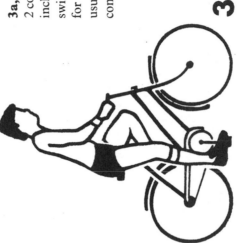

3a

3b

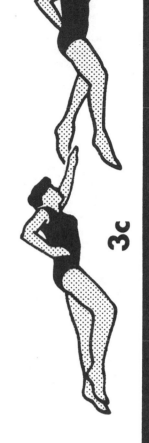

3c

©DIAGRAM

ADVANCED SCHEDULE

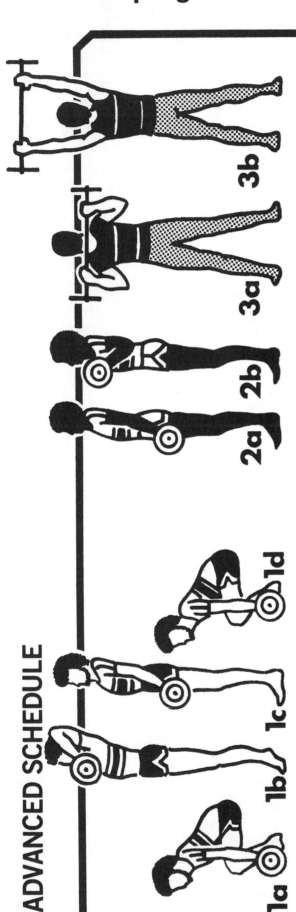

1a **1b** **1c** **1d**

2a **2b** **3a** **3b**

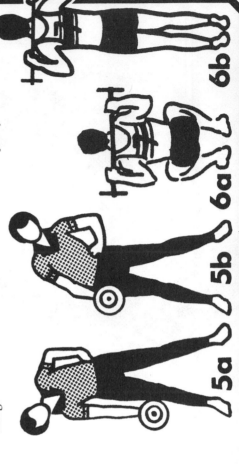

4a **4b**

5a **5b** **6a** **6b**

Weight training
The advanced schedule of the UK program combines mobility exercises (see p. 284) with weight training. This program should be started only by people who have completed the standard schedule. A barbell and dumb-bells are used (or substitute plastic bottles filled with water or sand). Start with weights of 3–5lb (1.4–3.5kg), increasing to a maximum of 30lb (13.6kg) for the very fit. Progress from 8–10 repetitions per exercise up to 20–30, checking your pulse rating frequently (see p. 283). Reduce rest periods between exercises as your stamina increases.

1a After doing the mobility exercises, stand with your feet about 10in (25cm) apart under a barbell. Lean forward with your back flat, and grip the bar with hands apart and knuckles forward.
1b Stand up, bringing the bar up to your chin in a straight line, close to your body.
1c Lower the bar to your thighs.
1d Bend your legs and return to the starting position.

2a Hold the bar in front of your thighs, palms forward.
2b Bend your elbows to bring the barbell up to your chest.
3a Star with the bar behind your neck, across your shoulders.
3b Extend your arms upward and hold the bar overhead.
4a Stand with your feet wide apart, holding the bar knuckles forward. Bend over, letting the bar hang.
4b Raise the bar to your chest.
5a Stand with your feet well apart, your left hand on your hip and your right hand holding a dumb-bell. Bend to the right.
5b Bend to the left. Repeat with the dumb-bell in your left hand.
6a Stand with the barbell behind your neck. Sink down until your thighs are almost level, keeping your back straight.
6b Rise up on your toes.

ADVANCED SCHEDULE

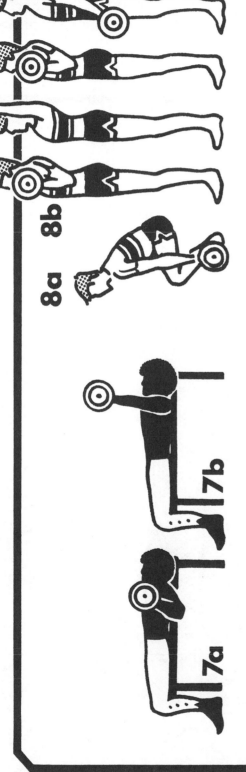

Weight training

7a Lie on your back on a firm bench or similar support, with your knees bent over the end. Let the barbell rest on your chest, holding it with your palms forward and your elbows bent.

7b Extend your arms upward to hold the bar above you. Then lower it again.

8a Crouch with the bar across your feet and grasp it with your knuckles facing forward.

8b Stand erect, pulling the bar straight up close to your body until it rests on the top of your chest.

8c Press up with your arms to hold the bar at arms' length overhead.

8d Bend your arms and lower the bar to your chest.

8e Bring the bar down across the front of your thighs.

8f Bend your legs and lower the bar back to the floor.

9a Lie flat on your back on the floor, with your arms stretched overhead.

9b Raise your legs, trunk and arms simultaneously to balance on your hips, bringing your arms forward as though attempting to grasp your ankles. (If you find this too difficult, work up to it by substituting the sit-up exercises from the standard schedule, see p. 287.)

10a Use only a very light weight for this quietening down exercise. Lie on your back on a firm bench, with your knees bent over the end. Hold the barbell across your thighs, with your palms downward.

10b Keeping your arms straight, raise the bar and swing it back over your head. Return to the starting position.

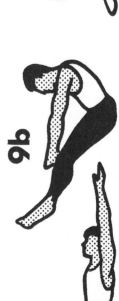

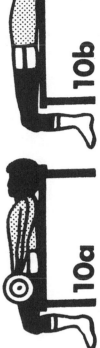

©DIAGRAM

US GENERAL PROGRAM

The program The following program is recommended for adults, both men and women, by the American Government. It was prepared by the President's Council on Physical Fitness, and its purpose is to improve the performer's overall physical fitness in the three areas of strength, stamina and flexibility. It is intended for people whose regular activities do not noticeably affect their heart or respiration rate, or for others whose regular sport affects only a limited set of muscles.

There are six groups of exercises, of increasing levels of

Before you begin
You should have a complete medical check-up at least once a year. If you are not used to exercise, have an examination before you start your program, and ask your doctor if he suggests any modifications.

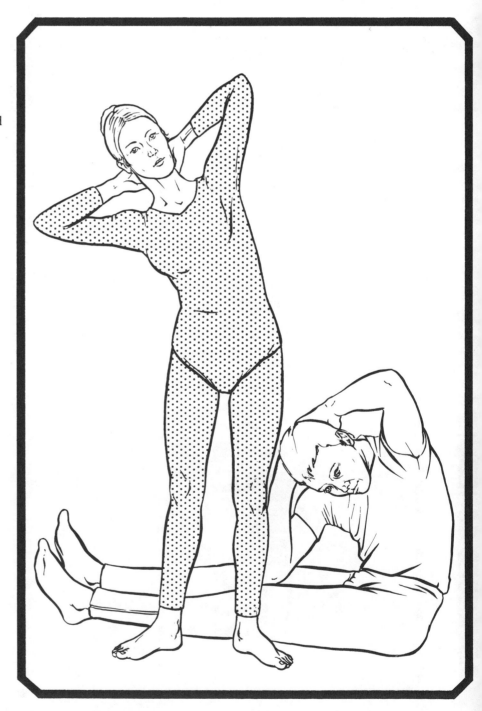

difficulty. The first group is an orientation program, intended for people unused to exercise, which is designed to tone up your muscles with mild exercises before you attempt the subsequent five levels. By gradually progressing from one level to another you will make sure that your fitness has a firm basis.

The exercises When you have passed to the first graded level, the six exercises from the orientation program should be performed before each workout. These prepare your circulation and tone your muscles for further exercise — they "warm up" your body. In each workout at a graded level these six warm-up exercises are followed by several "conditioning" exercises, planned to tone up and strengthen all the major muscle groups. Finally there is a circulatory activity, which stimulates and improves the respiratory and circulatory systems; the specific activity can be changed from day to day to provide variety.

Choosing your goal The first three levels should be attainable by most people through steady work and progress. The fourth level can be achieved by many with extra effort, and the fifth level is for very energetic and well-conditioned people. The level of fitness you can achieve depends on many factors (see pages 62–77); do not set your goals too high or you are likely to be disappointed. Allow your goals to develop as your ability improves. Remember that a positive attitude, which will be strengthened as you notice your progress, is half the battle. Whether you choose to maintain level 3, 4 or 5 your fitness will be considerably improved.

When and how often The exercises should be performed five times a week. They can be performed at any time of the day, but it may help you to make them part of your routine if you set aside the same time each day.

From level to level Start slowly and avoid strain. If you cannot complete an exercise, stop when it becomes difficult. When you have rested, resume the count until you have finished. Spend at least one week on the orientation program, and stay at each graded level for at least three weeks or until you pass the prove-out test.

The prove-out test This requires you to do the seven conditioning exercises without resting, and one satisfactory circulatory activity, on three consecutive days.

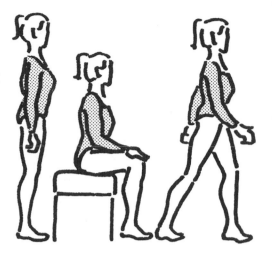

Posture
Good posture helps to ease tension, aids the functioning of internal organs, and helps the circulation (see also pp. 90–97). Good posture during exercise ensures that you will reap the maximum benefit from your exertion.

US general program

Measuring progress You will see your progress as the exercises become easier every day, and it can be measured between levels by the bench-stepping test. This measures the recovery rate of your cardio-vascular system — the surest measure of fitness. It should not be attempted until the orientation period has been completed. Keep a clear note of the recommended 15 workouts for each level, and of the results of step tests every two weeks.

Getting fit The program is designed to get you fit without strain or undue discomfort. When you start each new level, try to reduce the breathing spaces between the exercises until you can do the prove-out test. There is no need to rush; let your body improve at its own rate.

Staying fit When you have reached your desired level it may be maintained by three workouts a week, though it is much better to continue with workouts five times a week. After illness or a long interruption begin again at a lower level.

Daily opportunities Your training can be supplemented at every opportunity. Remember to walk or run whenever you can, instead of using the car. Walking provides exercise for the heart and legs and helps relieve tension. Use the stairs, not the elevator. Try a few exercises in spare moments and remember that isometric exercises can be performed very quickly anywhere at any time.

Step test
Use this test every 2 weeks to check your progress. For it you need a bench or chair about 16in (35cm) high.
a Place your right foot on the bench or chair.
b Bring your left foot alongside it and stand up straight.
c Lower your right foot to the floor.
d Lower your left foot to the floor. Repeat 30 times a minute for 2 minutes. Sit down for 2 minutes, then take your pulse for 30 seconds. Multiply the result by 2 to find the rate per minute; this will get lower as you get fitter.

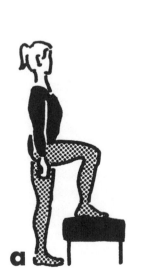
a

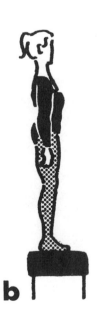
b

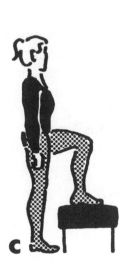
c

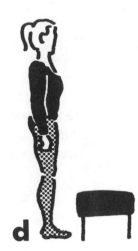
d

Water activities Swimming is one of the best all-round activities for people of all ages. The program recommends bobbing and swimming to supplement or replace the regular circulatory exercises. See the chart on this page for details of repetitions, times and distances for people at different levels of the program. For bobbing, take a deep breath, submerge to touch the bottom, and push up to the surface while exhaling. For swimming, use any stroke for the time given. For interval swimming, swim fast for the distance given, then swim slowly or walk back to the starting point before repeating as specified.

Weight training The program also recommends weight training as an excellent method of developing muscular strength and endurance, and suggests that where equipment is available it may be used as a supplement to the seven conditioning exercises. (In this book, see pages 234 and 290 for information on weight training.)

Sports Cycling, hiking, skating, tennis, running, cross-country skiing, rowing, canoeing, water skiing and skin diving are recommended in the program as examples of excellent conditioning and circulatory activities in which you can progress at your own rate. You can engage in them at any point in the program, if you start slowly. On days when you get a good workout in sports skip part or all of your exercise program — use your own judgment on this. Once the program has improved your fitness, you will be able to take part in sporting activities with renewed enthusiasm and vigor.

Water activities				
Level		Bobbing	Swimming	Interval swimming
1	M	10	5 min	
	F	10	5 min	
2	M	15	10 min	
	F	15	10 min	
3	M	25	15 min	
	F	20	15 min	
4	M	75		25yd × 20
	F	50		25yd × 10
5	M	100		50yd × 20
	F	125		25yd × 20

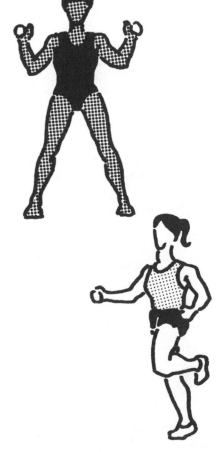

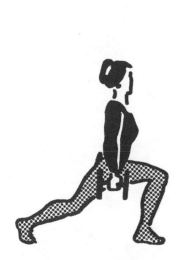

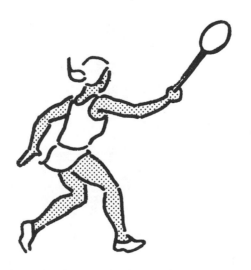

©DIAGRAM

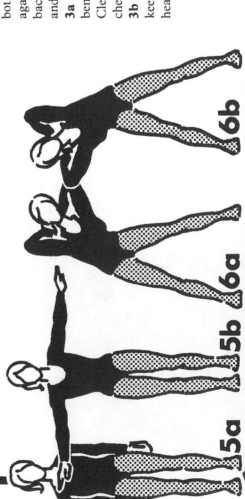

WOMEN'S ORIENTATION

1a **1b** **2a** **2b** **3a** **3b** **4a** **4b**

5a **5b** **6a** **6b**

Conditioning exercises
These simple exercises will prepare you for the progressive conditioning program. Exercises 1–6 are also used to warm up before each of the other levels. Stay at this level for at least a week, longer if you cannot do all the exercises easily and without fatigue.

1a Stand straight with your feet apart.
1b Bend forward and down, flexing your knees. Try to touch your toes, then rise again.
2a Stand upright, feet together and arms by your sides.
2b Raise your right knee as high as you can. Grasping your leg with both hands, pull your knee back against your body, keeping your back straight. Then lower your leg and repeat with the left.
3a Stand erect with your elbows bent and raised to shoulder level. Clench your fists in front of your chest.
3b Push your elbows back, keeping your back flat and your head up.

4a Stand with your hands on your hips.
4b Stretch your arms out in front of you and bend your knees half-way. Straighten up again.
5a Stand upright.
5b Extend your arms to the sides at shoulder height, palms up. Make small circles with your hands, 15 backward and 15 forward.
6a Stand with your hands clasped behind your neck, legs apart. Bend over to the left as far as you can.
6b Repeat to the right.

WOMEN'S ORIENTATION

Conditioning exercises

7a Lie facedown, with your hands tucked under your thighs.
7b Keeping your legs straight, lift them as high as you can. At the same time raise your head and shoulders.
8a Lie facedown with your legs together. Bending your knees, raise your feet from the floor. Place your hands beneath your shoulders, palms down.
8b Straighten your arms, pushing your upper body off the floor; keep your back rigid as shown.
9a Lie on your back, hands under the small of the back, palms down.
9b Use your stomach muscles to lift your head, shoulders and elbows. Hold the position.

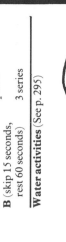

7a
7b
8a
8b
9a
9b

10a Stand on the edge of a book or stair. Raise your heels and balance on your toes with your arms outstretched to help you.
10b Lower your heels.

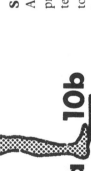

10a **10b**

Exercise	Uninterrupted repetitions
1	10
2	10 left, 10 right
3	20
4	10
5	15 each way
6	10 left, 10 right
7	10
8	6
9	5
10	15

Circulatory activity
(Choose one each workout)

A	$\frac{1}{2}$ mile
B (skip 15 seconds, rest 60 seconds)	3 series

Water activities (See p. 295)

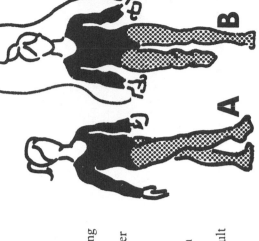

A **B**

Circulatory activities
A Walk with brisk strides, swinging your arms and breathing deeply.
B Skip or jump rope; move faster as your fitness improves.

Step test
After completing the orientation program, take the 2-minute step test (p. 294) and record your result to allow you to measure future improvement.

©DIAGRAM

US general program

WOMEN'S LEVEL 1

Warming up
Warm up by repeating exercises 1–6 of the orientation program.

Conditioning exercises

1a Stand with your arms by your sides and your feet together.
1b Keeping your legs straight, bend forward and down to touch your ankles. Bounce, then touch the tops of your feet. Bounce, then touch your toes.
2a Squat down, with your right leg bent and your left leg straight out behind you. Place your hands on the floor in front of you, fingers forward.
2b Bounce up and quickly change legs, extending your right leg and bringing your left foot up to your hands.

3a Sit with your legs apart and your hands on your knees.
3b Bend forward from the waist and stretch your arms out as far as possible.
4a Lie facedown with your legs together. Bend your knees and raise your feet. Place your hands under your shoulders, palms down.
4b Push your upper body off the floor, straightening your arms. Keep your back straight.

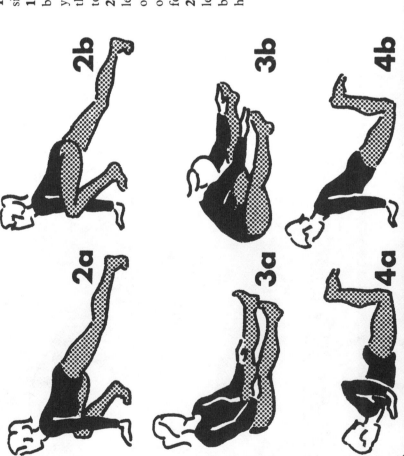

WOMEN'S LEVEL 1

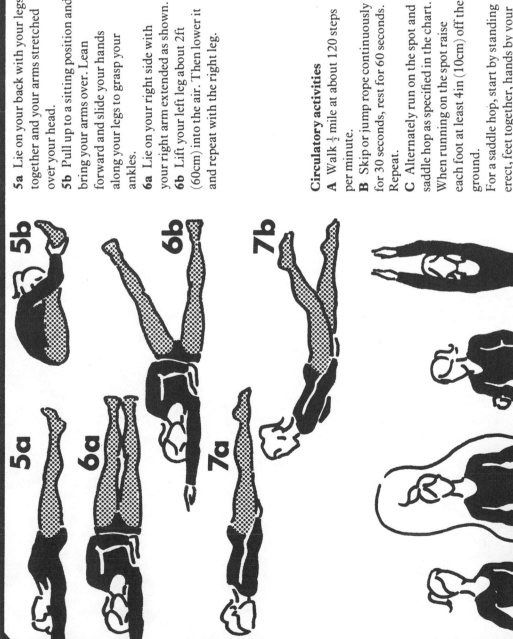

5a Lie on your back with your legs together and your arms stretched over your head.
5b Pull up to a sitting position and bring your arms over. Lean forward and slide your hands along your legs to grasp your ankles.

6a Lie on your right side with your right arm extended as shown.
6b Lift your left leg about 2ft (60cm) into the air. Then lower it and repeat with the right leg.

7a Lie facedown with your hands tucked under your thighs.
7b Arching your back, raise your chest and head. Lift your legs and kick rapidly up and down with alternate feet. Kick from the hips with your knees slightly bent.

Exercise	Uninterrupted repetitions
1	5
2	8
3	10
4	8
5	5
6	5 each leg
7	20

Circulatory activities
(Choose one each workout)

A (120 steps per minute)	$\frac{1}{2}$ mile
B (skip 30 seconds, rest 60 seconds)	2 series
C (run 50, straddle hop 10 — 2 cycles)	2 minutes

Water activities (See p. 295)

Step test
Check your progress every 2 weeks with the step test (p. 294).

Circulatory activities

A Walk $\frac{1}{2}$ mile at about 120 steps per minute.

B Skip or jump rope continuously for 30 seconds, rest for 60 seconds. Repeat.

C Alternately run on the spot and saddle hop as specified in the chart. When running on the spot raise each foot at least 4in (10cm) off the ground.

For a saddle hop, start by standing erect, feet together, hands by your sides. Count 1: swing your arms sideways and upward to touch hands above your head, arms straight, while at the same time moving your feet sideways and apart in a single jumping motion. Count 2: spring back to your starting position. Two counts in one hop.

© DIAGRAM

US general program

WOMEN'S LEVEL 2

Warming up
Don't forget to warm up by repeating exercises 1–6 of the orientation program.

Conditioning exercises

1a Stand straight with your arms by your sides.

1b Keeping your legs straight, bend over to touch your ankles. Then bounce to touch your feet, then your toes.

2a Squat with your right leg bent, left leg out behind you. Place your hands on the floor, fingers forward.

2b Bounce up and change legs to squat on your left leg, with your right leg out behind you.

3a Sit with your legs apart, hands on your knees.

3b Bend forward from the waist and extend your arms as far forward as possible.

4a Lie facedown with your legs together. Bend your knees and raise your feet. Place your hands under your shoulders, palms down.

4b Straighten your arms and push your upper body off the floor. Keep your back straight.

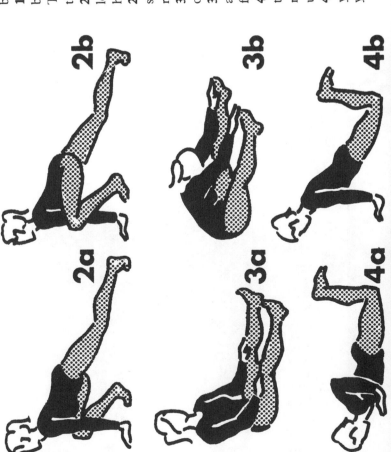

WOMEN'S LEVEL 2

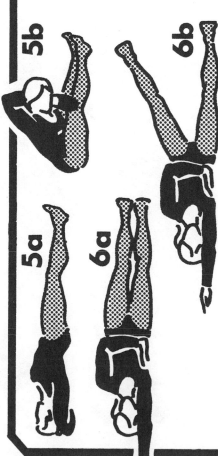

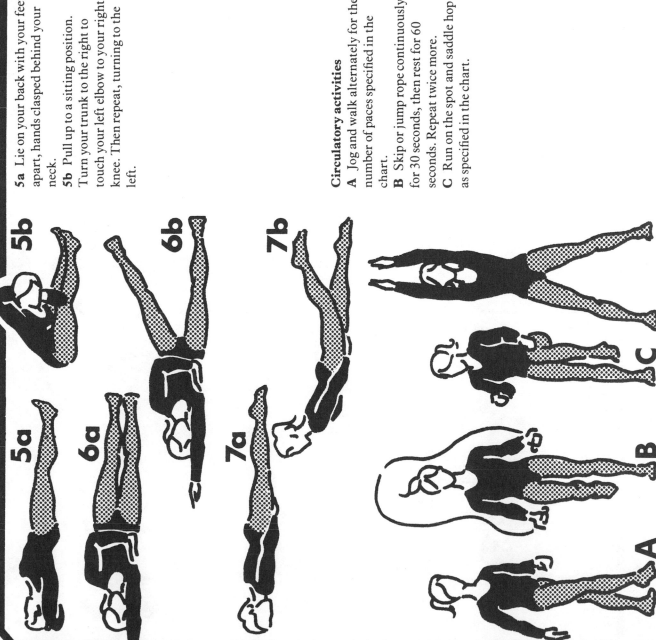

5a Lie on your back with your feet apart, hands clasped behind your neck.
5b Pull up to a sitting position. Turn your trunk to the right to touch your left elbow to your right knee. Then repeat, turning to the left.

6a Lie on your right side with your right arm extended as shown.
6b Lift your left leg about 2ft (60cm) into the air. Then lower it and repeat with the right leg.
7a Lie facedown with your hands tucked under your thighs.
7b Arching your back, raise your chest and head. Lift your legs and kick rapidly up and down. Kick from the hips with your knees slightly bent.

Circulatory activities

A Jog and walk alternately for the number of paces specified in the chart.
B Skip or jump rope continuously for 30 seconds, then rest for 60 seconds. Repeat twice more.
C Run on the spot and saddle hop as specified in the chart.

Exercise	Uninterrupted repetitions
1	10
2	12
3	15
4	12
5	10
6	10 each leg
7	30

Circulatory activities
(Choose one each workout)

A	(jog 50, walk 50	$\frac{1}{2}$ mile
B	(skip 30 seconds, rest 60 seconds)	3 series
C	(run 80, hop 15 — 2 cycles)	3 minutes

Water activities (See p. 295)

Step test
Check your progress every 2 weeks with the step test.

US general program

WOMEN'S LEVEL 3

Warming up
Warm up with exercises 1–6 of the orientation program.

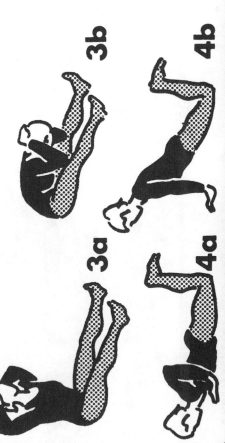

1a Stand straight with your arms by your sides.
1b Keeping your legs straight, bend over to touch your ankles. Then bounce to touch your feet, then your toes.
2a Squat with your right leg bent, left leg out behind you. Place your hands on the floor, fingers forward.
2b Bounce up and change legs to squat on your left leg, with your right extended behind you.
3a Sit with your legs apart, your hands clasped behind your head.
3b Bending forward from the waist, move your elbows as close to the floor as possible.
4a Lie facedown with your legs together. Bend your knees and raise your feet. Place your hands under your shoulders, palms down.
4b Straighten your arms and push your upper body off the floor. Keep your back straight.

WOMEN'S LEVEL 3

5a Lie on your back with your arms extended as shown and your legs straight.
5b Sit up and bend your knees. Put your arms round your knees, pulling them close to your chest.
6a Lie on your right side with your right arm extended as shown.
6b Lift your left leg about 2ft (60cm) into the air. Then lower it and repeat with the right leg.

7a Lie facedown with your hands tucked under your thighs.
7b Arching your back, raise your chest and head. Lift your legs and kick rapidly up and down. Kick from the hips with your knees slightly bent.

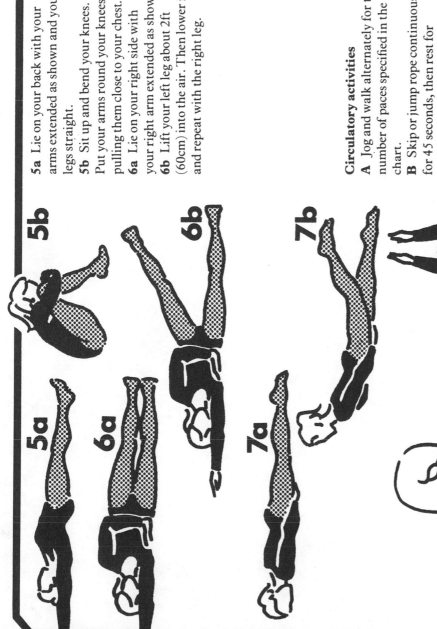

Circulatory activities

A Jog and walk alternately for the number of paces specified in the chart.
B Skip or jump rope continuously for 45 seconds, then rest for 30 seconds. Repeat 3 times.
C Run on the spot and saddle hop as specified in the chart.

Exercise	Uninterrupted repetitions
1	20
2	16
3	15
4	20
5	15
6	16 each leg
7	40

Circulatory activities
(Choose one each workout)

A (jog 50, walk 50)		$\frac{3}{4}$ mile
B (skip 45 seconds, rest 30 seconds)		3 series
C (run 110, hop 20— 2 cycles)		4 minutes

Water activities (See p. 295)

Step test
Monitor your progress every 2 weeks with the step test.

© DIAGRAM

US general program

Warming up
Remember to warm up with exercises 1–6 of the orientation program.

Conditioning exercises

1a Stand with your feet apart, your arms extended overhead, your thumbs interlocked.

1b Bend forward and down. Twist your body to touch the floor inside your right foot with both hands. Then touch outside your right toes and your right heel. Sweep upright in a wide arc. Repeat to the left.

2a Squat with your right leg bent and your left leg out behind you. Place your hands on the floor, fingers forward.

2b Bounce up and change legs to squat on your left leg, with your right leg extended behind you.

3a Sit with your legs apart, your fingers laced behind your neck.

3b Bend over from the waist, to touch your forehead to your left knee. Then repeat, bending to the right.

4a Lie facedown with your hands under your shoulders and your legs together.

4b Push up with your arms, with your body straight, resting on your hands and toes. Lower yourself so that your chest touches the floor.

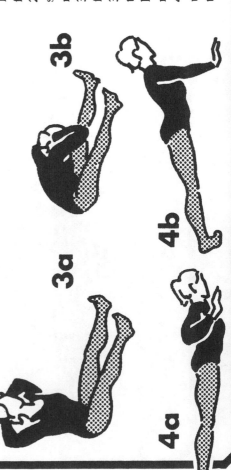

1a 1b 2a 2b 3a 3b 4a 4b

WOMEN'S LEVEL 4

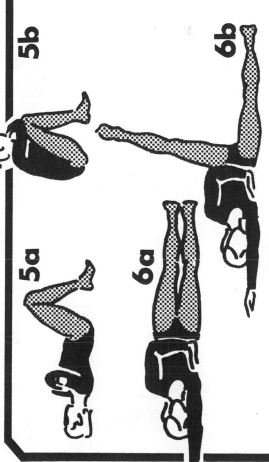

5a Lie on your back with your knees bent and your feet flat on the floor. Fold your arms across your chest and grasp opposite shoulders.
5b Keeping your arms crossed, pull up to a sitting position.
6a Lie on your right side, with your right arm extended as shown.
6b Whip your left leg rapidly up and down, reaching as high as you can. Repeat with your right leg.

7a Lie facedown with your legs together and your arms stretched out to the sides at shoulder level.
7b Arch your back, raising your arms, chest and head. At the same time lift your legs as high as possible, keeping them straight.

Circulatory activities
A Jog and walk as directed.
B Skip or jump rope continuously for 60 seconds, then rest for 30 seconds. Repeat 3 times.
C Run on the spot and saddle hop as specified in the chart.

Exercise	Uninterrupted repetitions
1	15 each side
2	20
3	20
4	8
5	20
6	10 each leg
7	15

Circulatory activities
(Choose one each workout)

A (jog 100, walk 50)	1 mile
B (skip 60 seconds, rest 30 seconds)	3 series
C (run 145, hop 25 — 2 cycles)	5 minutes

Water activities (See p. 295)

Step test
Remember to check your progress every 2 weeks with the step test.

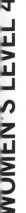
©DIAGRAM

US general program

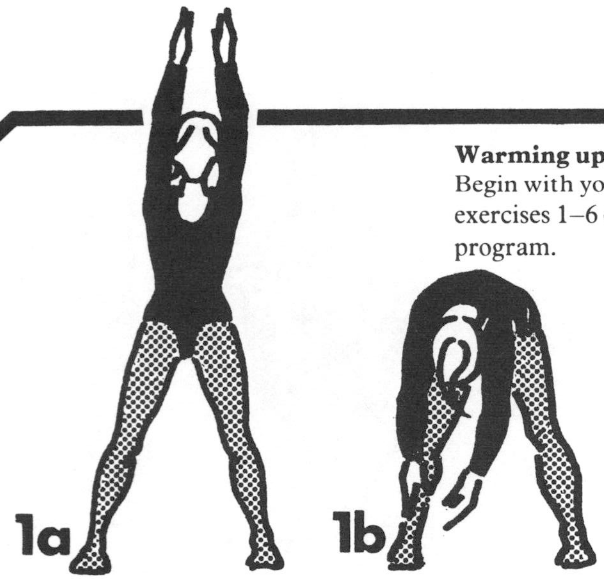

Warming up
Begin with your warm-up routine: exercises 1–6 of the orientation program.

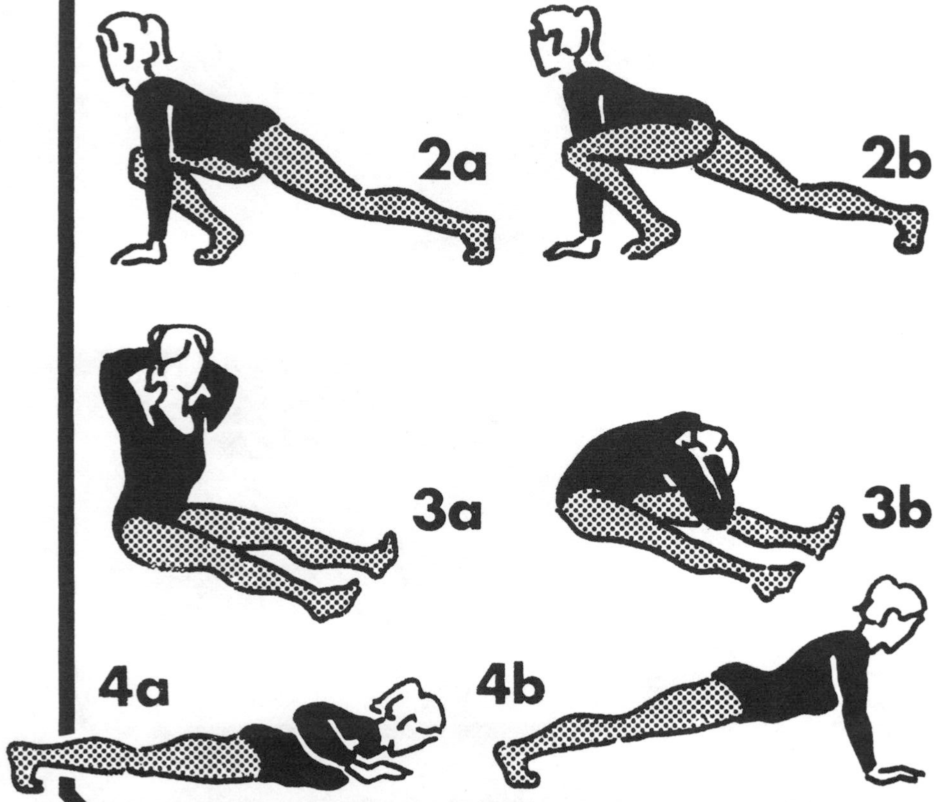

Conditioning exercises

1a Stand with your feet apart, your arms extended overhead with your thumbs interlocked.

1b Bend forward and down. Twist your body to touch the floor inside your right foot with both hands. Then touch outside your right toes and your right heel. Sweep upright in a wide arc. Repeat to the left.

2a Squat with your right leg bent and your left leg out behind you. Place your hands on the floor, fingers forward.

2b Bounce up and change legs to squat on your left leg, with your right extended behind you.

3a Sit with your legs apart, your fingers laced behind your neck.

3b Bend over from the waist, to touch your forehead to your left knee. Then repeat, bending to the right.

4a Lie facedown with your hands under your shoulders and your legs together.

4b Push up with your arms, with your body straight, resting on your hands and toes. Lower yourself so that your chest touches the floor.

1a

1b

2a

2b

3a

3b

4a

4b

WOMEN'S LEVEL 5

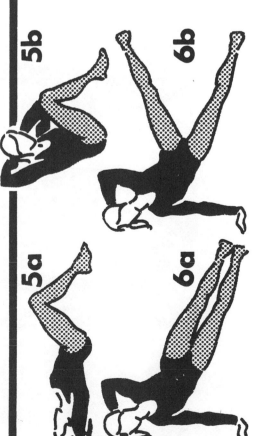

5a Lie on your back with your knees bent and your feet flat on the floor, with your fingers laced behind your neck.

5b Sit up and turn your trunk to the right, touching your right knee with your left elbow. Then repeat, touching your left knee with your right elbow.

6a Extend your right arm and lean to the right as shown. Hold your left hand behind your head.

6b Raise your left leg high.

7a Lie facedown with your fingers laced behind your neck.

7b Arch your back and raise your chest and legs. Extend your arms forward. Then clasp your hands behind your neck again and lower your body.

Exercise	Uninterrupted repetitions
1	25 each side
2	24
3	26
4	15
5	25
6	10 each side
7	25

Circulatory activities
(Choose one each workout)

A Jog-run	1 mile
B (skip 2 minutes, rest 45 seconds)	2 series
C (run 180, hop 30— 2 cycles)	6 minutes

Water activities (See p. 295)

Step test
Check your progress every 2 weeks with the step test.

Circulatory activities

A Jog and run alternately for the distance specified in the chart.

B Skip or jump rope continuously for 2 minutes, then rest for 45 seconds. Repeat twice.

C Run on the spot and saddle hop as specified in the chart.

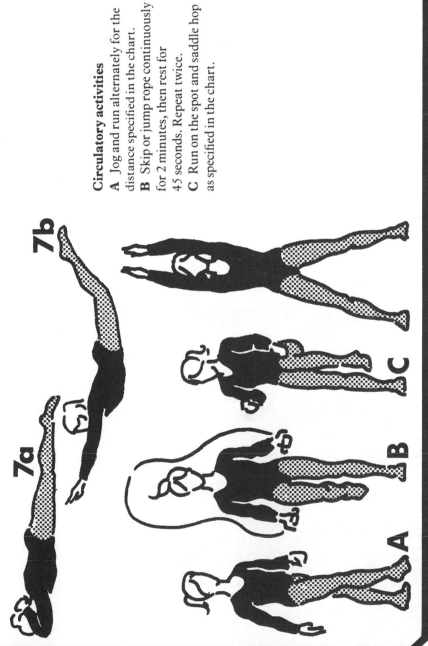

©DIAGRAM

US general program

MEN'S ORIENTATION

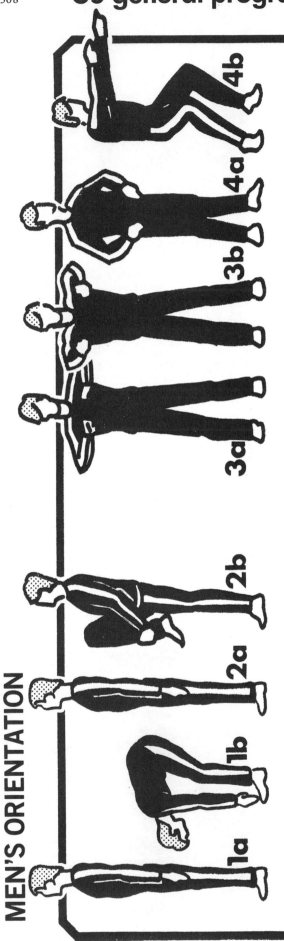

Conditioning exercises
These mild exercises are designed to prepare you for the full conditioning program. Spend at least a week on them. The first six exercises are also used to warm up before exercises at the other levels.

1a Stand with your feet slightly apart and your arms by your sides.
1b Bend forward and down from the waist, flexing your knees. Stretching gently, try to touch your toes, or the floor.
2a Stand with your feet together, arms by your sides.
2b Raise your right knee as high as you can. Keeping your back straight, pull your knee close to your body with both hands. Repeat with the left.
3a Stand with your elbows bent at shoulder height. Clench your fists in front of your chest.
3b Keep your back and neck straight and push your elbows back strongly.
4a Stand with your hands on your hips.
4b Bend your knees half-way and extend your arms forward, palms down.

5a Stand with your feet slightly apart and your arms by your sides.
5b Raise your arms to the sides, palms up, make 15 small backward circles with your hands, then 15 forward circles.
6a Stand with your feet slightly apart, your fingers laced behind your neck.
6b Keeping your hands behind your neck, bend your body to the left as far as possible. Then straighten up and bend to the right.

MEN'S ORIENTATION

7a Lie facedown with your hands tucked under your thighs.
7b Raise your head and shoulders from the floor. Keep your knees straight and lift your legs.

8a Lie facedown with your legs together and your hands beneath your shoulders, palms down. Bend your knees and lift your legs.
8b Straighten your arms, push your body up from the floor. Keep your back straight.

9a Lie on your back with your hands under the small of your back, palms down.
9b Pull up with your stomach muscles, lifting your head, shoulders and elbows from the floor.

10a Stand on your toes on the edge of a book or stair, with your heels raised.
10b Lower your heels.

Exercise	Uninterrupted repetitions
1	10
2	10 left, 10 right
3	20
4	10
5	15 each way
6	10 left, 10 right
7	10
8	6
9	5
10	15

Circulatory activities
(Choose one each workout)

A	½ mile
B (skip 15 seconds, rest 60 seconds)	3 series

Water activities (See p. 295)

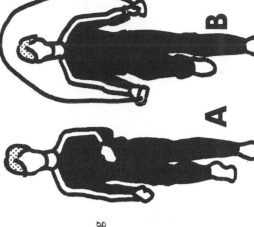

Circulatory activities
A Walk with brisk strides, swinging your arms and breathing deeply.
B Skip or jump rope; go faster as your skill and fitness improve.

Step test
After completing the orientation program, take the 2-minute step test (see p.294) and record your result to allow you to measure future improvement.

©DIAGRAM

US general program

MEN'S LEVEL 1

Warming up
Warm up with exercises 1–6 of the orientation program.

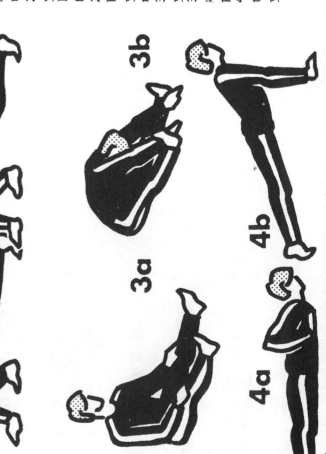

Conditioning exercises

1a Stand with your feet together and your arms by your sides.
1b Bend forward and down from the waist, with your knees straight. Touch your ankles, then bounce down to touch your feet, then your toes.

2a Squat on your right leg, with your left leg straight behind you. Place your hands on the floor, fingers forward.
2b Bounce up and change legs, bringing your left foot forward to your hands and extending your right leg behind you.

3a Sit with your legs apart and your hands on your knees.
3b Bend forward from the waist and stretch out your arms as far as possible.

4a Lie facedown, your legs together and your hands under your shoulders.
4b Straighten your arms and push up, with your body rigid, to rest on your hands and toes. Then lower yourself until your chest touches the floor.

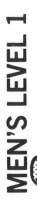

MEN'S LEVEL 1

5a Lie on your back with your legs together and your arms extended over your head.
5b Swing your arms forward and pull up to a sitting position. Slide your hands along your legs to grasp your ankles.
6a Lie on your right side, with your right arm stretched overhead.
6b Lift your left leg about 2ft (60cm) off the floor, then lower it.

7a Lie facedown, with your hands tucked under your thighs.
7b Arch your back, raising your head and chest. Lift your legs and kick rapidly with alternate feet. Kick from the hips and bend your knees slightly.

Exercise	Uninterrupted repetitions
1	10
2	12
3	12
4	4
5	5
6	12 each leg
7	30

Circulatory activities
(Choose one each workout)

A (120 steps per minute)		1 mile
B (skip 30 seconds, rest 30 seconds)		2 series
C (run 60, hop 10 — 2 cycles)		2 minutes

Water activities (See p. 295)

Step test
Check your progress every 2 weeks with the step test (p. 294).

Circulatory activities

A Walk for 1 mile at 120 steps per minute.
B Skip or jump rope continuously for 30 seconds, rest for 30 seconds. Repeat.
C Alternately run on the spot and saddle hop as specified in the chart. When running on the spot raise each foot at least 4in (10cm) off the ground. For a saddle hop, start by standing erect, feet together, hands by your sides. Count 1: swing your arms sideways and upward to touch hands above your head, arms straight, while at the same time moving your feet sideways and apart in a single jumping motion. Count 2: spring back to your starting position. Two counts in one hop.

©DIAGRAM

MEN'S LEVEL 2

Warming up
Warm up with the first six orientation exercises.

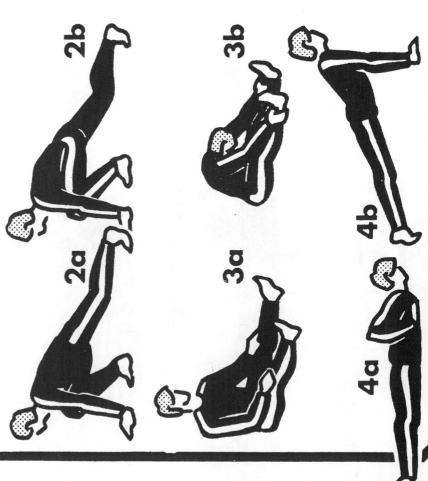

Conditioning exercises

1a Stand with your feet together and your arms by your sides.
1b Bend forward and down from the waist, with your knees straight. Touch your ankles, then bounce down to touch your feet, then your toes.
2a Squat on your right leg, with your left leg straight behind you. Place your hands on the floor, fingers forward.
2b Bounce up and change legs, bringing your left foot forward to your hands and extending your right leg behind you.
3a Sit with your legs apart and your hands on your knees.
3b Bend forward from the waist and stretch out your arms as far as possible.
4a Lie facedown, your legs together and your hands under your shoulders.
4b Straighten your arms and push up, with your body rigid, to rest on your hands and toes. Then lower yourself until your chest touches the floor.

MEN'S LEVEL 2

5a Lie on your back with your feet slightly apart and your fingers laced behind your neck.
5b Pull up to a sitting position and bend your body to the right until your left elbow touches your right knee. Then repeat to the other side.
6a Lie on your right side, with your right arm extended as shown.
6b Lift your left leg about 2ft (60cm) off the floor, then lower it.

7a Lie facedown, with your hands tucked under your thighs.
7b Arch your back, raising your head and chest. Lift your legs and kick rapidly with alternate feet. Kick from the hips and bend your knees slightly.

Exercise	Uninterrupted repetitions
1	20
2	16
3	18
4	10
5	20
6	16 each leg
7	40

Circulatory activities
(Choose one each workout)

A (jog 100, walk 100)	1 mile	
B (skip 60 seconds, rest 60 seconds)	3 series	
C (run 95, hop 15 — 2 cycles)	3 minutes	

Water activities (See p. 295)

Step test
Check your progress every 2 weeks with the step test.

Circulatory activities

A Jog and walk alternately for the number of paces indicated in the chart.
B Skip or jump rope continuously for 60 seconds, then rest for 60 seconds. Repeat twice more.
C Run on the spot and saddle hop as specified in the chart.

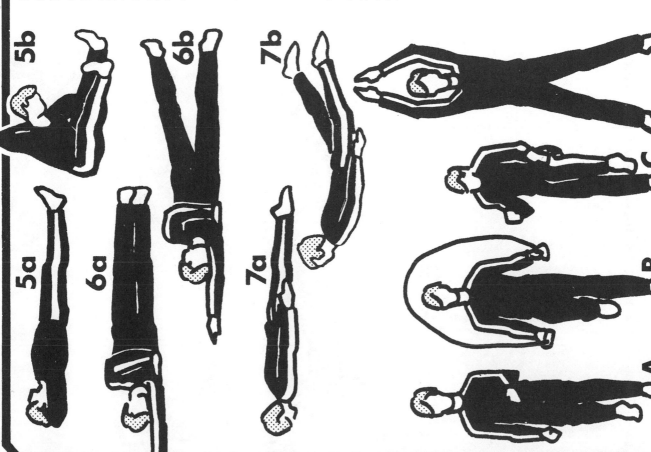

© DIAGRAM

MEN'S LEVEL 3

Warming up
Warm up with exercises 1–6 from the orientation program.

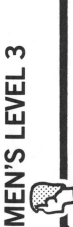

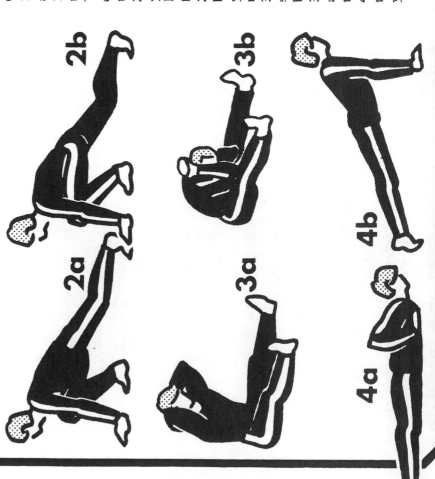

Conditioning exercises

1a Stand with your feet together and your arms by your sides.

1b Bend forward and down from the waist, with your knees straight. Touch your ankles, then bounce down to touch your feet, then your toes.

2a Squat on your right leg, with your left leg straight behind you. Place your hands on the floor, fingers forward.

2b Bounce up and change legs, bringing your left foot forward to your hands and extending your right leg behind you.

3a Sit with your legs apart, your shoulders back, and fingers laced behind your neck.

3b Bend forward from the waist and bring your elbows as close to the floor as possible.

4a Lie facedown, your legs together and your hands under your shoulders.

4b Straighten your arms and push up, with your body rigid, to rest on your hands and toes. Then lower yourself until your chest touches the floor.

MEN'S LEVEL 3

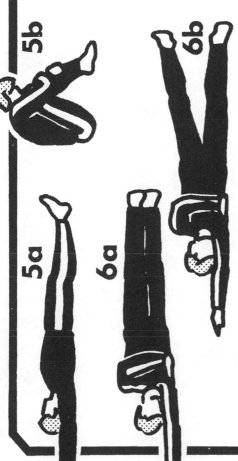

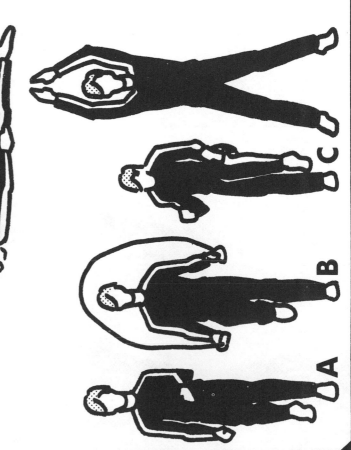

5a Lie on your back with your legs together and your arms extended over your head.
5b Swing your arms forward and pull up to a sitting position. Wrap your arms around your knees and pull them close to your body.
6a Lie on your right side, with your right arm extended as shown.
6b Lift your left leg about 2ft (60cm) off the floor, then lower it.
7a Lie facedown, with your hands tucked under your thighs.
7b Arch your back, raising your head and chest. Lift your legs and kick rapidly with alternate feet. Kick from the hips and bend your knees slightly.

Circulatory activities
A Jog and walk as specified.
B Skip or jump rope continuously for 60 seconds, then rest 60 seconds. Repeat 5 times.
C Run on the spot and saddle hop as specified.

Exercise	Uninterrupted repetitions
1	30
2	20
3	18
4	20
5	30
6	20 each leg
7	50

Circulatory activities
(Choose one each workout)

A	(jog 200, walk 100)	1½ miles
B	(skip 60 seconds, rest 60 seconds)	5 series
C	(run 135, hop 20) — 2 cycles	4 minutes

Water activities (See p. 295)

Step test
Check your progress every 2 weeks with the step test.

Warming up
Warm up with exercises 1–6 of the orientation program.

Conditioning exercises

1a Stand with your feet apart, your arms extended overhead and your thumbs interlocked.
1b Bend over and twist to touch the floor inside your right foot with both hands. Then touch the floor outside your right toes, then outside the heel. Swing up in a wide arc. Repeat to the left.
2a Squat on your right leg, with your left leg straight behind you. Place your hands on the floor, fingers forward.
2b Bounce up and change legs, bringing your left foot forward to your hands and extending your right leg behind you.
3a Sit with your legs apart and your fingers laced behind your neck.
3b Bend forward to the left and touch your left knee with your forehead. Repeat to the right.
4a Lie facedown, your legs together and your hands under your shoulders.
4b Straighten your arms and push up, with your body straight, to rest on your hands and toes. Then lower yourself until your chest touches the floor.

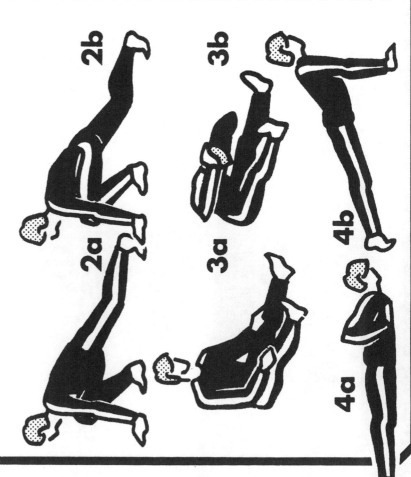

MEN'S LEVEL 4

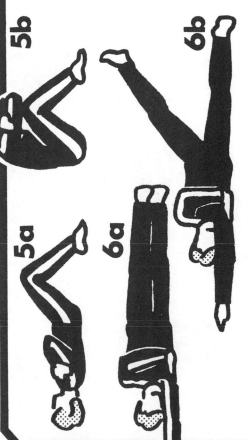

5a Lie on your back with your knees bent and your feet flat on the floor. Cross your arms over your chest to grasp opposite shoulders.
5b Keep your arms crossed and pull up to a sitting position.
6a Lie on your right side with your right arm extended as shown.
6b Whip your left leg up and down rapidly, reaching up as high as you can.
7a Lie facedown with your legs together and your arms straight out to the sides.
7b Arch your back to raise your arms, chest and head. Lift your legs as high as possible, keeping them straight.

Exercise	Uninterrupted repetitions
1	20 each side
2	28
3	24
4	30
5	30
6	20 each leg
7	20

Circulatory activities
(Choose one each workout)

A	1 mile
B (skip 90 seconds, rest 30 seconds)	3 series
C (run 180, hop 25 — 2 cycles)	5 minutes

Water activities (See p. 295)

Step test
Check your progress every 2 weeks with the step test.

Circulatory activities
A Jog continuously for 1 mile.
B Skip or jump rope continuously for 90 seconds, then rest for 30 seconds. Repeat 3 times.
C Run on the spot and saddle hop as specified in the chart.

©DIAGRAM

US general program

Warming up
Warm up with exercises 1–6 of the orientation program.

Conditioning exercises

1a Stand with your feet apart, your arms extended overhead and your thumbs interlocked.

1b Bend over and twist to touch the floor inside your right foot with both hands. Then touch the floor outside your right toes, then outside the heel. Swing up in a wide arc. Repeat to the left.

2a Squat on your right leg, with your left leg straight behind you. Place your hands on the floor, fingers forward.

2b Bounce up and change legs, bringing your left foot forward to your hands and extending your right leg behind you.

3a Sit with your legs apart and your fingers laced behind your neck.

3b Bend forward to the left and touch your left knee with your forehead. Repeat to the right.

4a Lie facedown, your legs together and your hands under your shoulders.

4b Straighten your arms and push up, with your body straight, to rest on your hands and toes. Then lower yourself until your chest touches the floor.

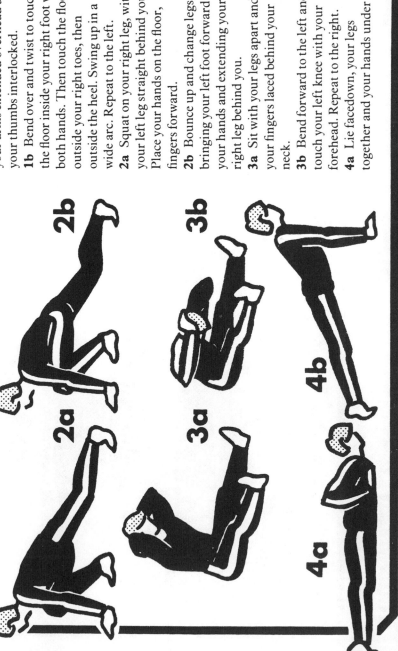

MEN'S LEVEL 5

5a Lie on your back with your knees bent and your feet flat on the floor, with your fingers laced behind your neck.

5b Sit up and turn to the right, until your left elbow touches your right knee. Then repeat, touching your left knee with your right elbow.

6a Extend your right arm and lean on it so that your weight rests on your arm and foot as shown.

Put your left hand behind your head.

6b Raise your left leg high. Repeat on the other side.

7a Lie facedown with your fingers laced behind your neck.

7b Arch your back to bring your legs and chest up. Extend your arms forward. Then link your fingers back behind your neck.

Circulatory activities

A Alternately jog and run for the distance specified; try to increase progressively the proportion of running.

B Skip or jump for 2 minutes, rest for 30 seconds. Repeat 3 times.

C Run on the spot and saddle hop as specified in the chart.

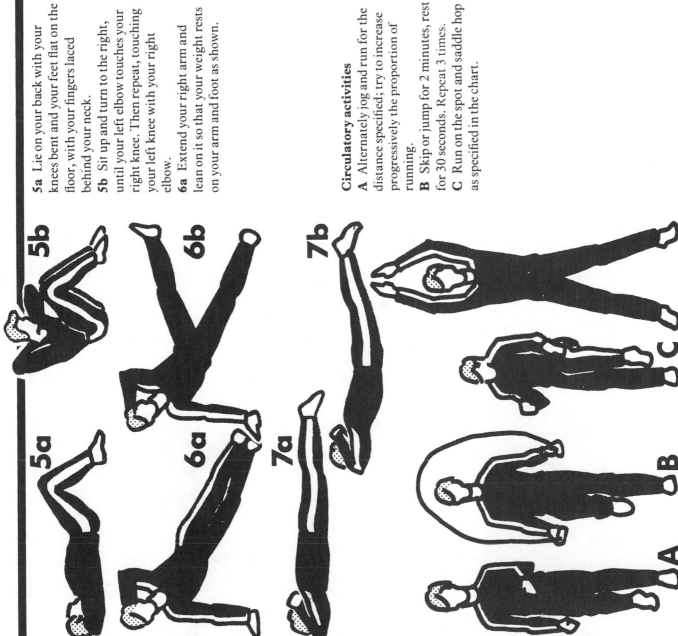

Exercise	Uninterrupted repetitions
1	30 each side
2	36
3	30
4	50
5	40
6	20 each side
7	30

Circulatory activities
(Choose one each workout)

A	3 miles
B (skip 2 minutes, rest 30 seconds)	3 series
C (run 216, hop 30 — 2 cycles)	6 minutes

Water activities (See p. 295)

Step test
Check your fitness every 2 weeks with the step test.

©DIAGRAM

US AEROBIC PROGRAM

This program is based on the information contained in the booklets *Physical Fitness and Health*, prepared by the President's Council on Physical Fitness and Sports, and *Fitness and Work Capacity*, recommended by the Council and prepared by the Forest Service of the US Department of Agriculture. *Fitness and Work Capacity* is oriented toward the achievement of fitness levels necessary for the efficient attainment of work goals without undue fatigue and with enough energy left over to enjoy leisure to the full. Because of this, it emphasizes "aerobic fitness," which it describes as "a well-developed oxygen delivery system." This delivery

Aerobic training session
The diagram shows the elements of an aerobic training session recommended by the President's Council. At every level of fitness the Council's program has three constituents: warming-up exercises, aerobic activity and cooling-down exercises. The particular session described in the diagram is that for a moderately fit man of 35. It consists of the following.

a A 5-minute warming-up period of exercises (see pp. 327–329), during which the heart rate is gradually built up from around 70 to around 140 beats per minute.

b 20 minutes jogging at a pace of 12 minutes per mile, during which time the heart rate is maintained at 145–157 beats per minute.

c A 5-minute cooling-down period of exercises, during which the heart rate decreases.

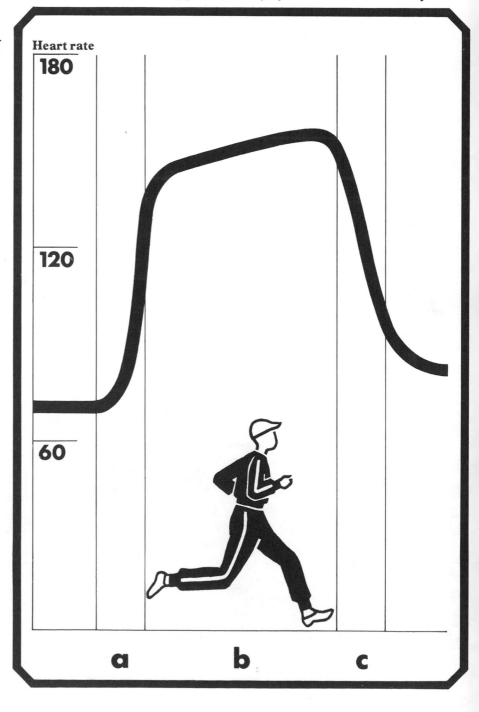

Heart rate

180

120

60

a   b   c

system comprises the cardio-vascular and respiratory systems — the heart, blood vessels and lungs. Aerobic fitness is therefore achieved by exercises that make the heart and lungs work harder to supply the working muscles with oxygen, via the blood. Increased aerobic fitness increases the efficiency of the cardio-vascular and respiratory systems, which in turn means that the heart has to work less. This reduces the risk of heart trouble and makes specific improvement in muscular and flexibility fitness easier.

Choose a program designed for your fitness-rating. Never attempt too high a level or you may risk heart strain and injury. The program is designed to improve your condition gradually, and can be adapted to your own needs. If one stage proves too difficult, stay on it longer before moving on. Fitness is equally beneficial to both sexes. For women, activities such as jogging can ease menstrual tension, both physical and mental, and the increased level of fitness can aid with childbirth and recovery. Combined with a proper diet running can help everyone to reduce and maintain a trim, firm figure.

Run wherever it is most convenient and enjoyable for you to do so. The most popular times are the early morning, lunch time, early evening, or last thing at night. Do not run for at least 2–3 hours after a meal, and once you have established a routine, stick to it at least three times a week in order to maintain your fitness level.

Jogging speeds
When jogging try to start off slowly, build up to a comfortable speed, and then slow down gradually as you near the end of your session.

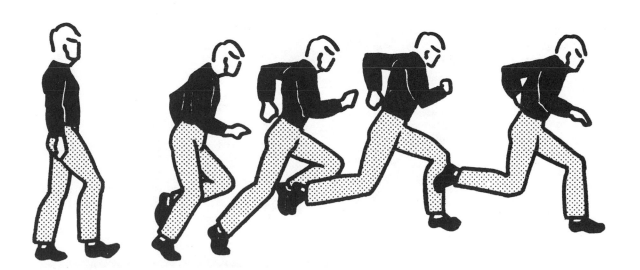

©DIAGRAM

US aerobic program

Summarized below are the starter aerobic exercise programs prepared by the President's Council on Physical Fitness and Sports. These programs are especially designed to help those who are unfit, and are first in a series that also includes intermediate and advanced programs. In the starter programs there is a gradual progression from walking to jogging; find the starting point to suit your fitness level and then proceed at your own rate. If at any time you cannot manage the stated pace, take that part of the program more slowly until your fitness improves.

Finding the right program
The following tests will help you to estimate your fitness and choose the most suitable program.
Walk test
Walk briskly on a level surface for up to 10 minutes.
If you cannot walk for at least 5 minutes without discomfort, begin exercising with program **A**.
If you can walk for more than 5 minutes but less than 10, begin exercising with week 3 of program **A**.
If you can walk for 10 minutes but have some difficulty, start with week 1 of program **B**.
If you have no trouble at all take the walk-jog test.
Walk-jog test
Alternately jog 50 steps and walk 50 steps for 10 minutes. Walk at the rate of 120 steps a minute and jog at the rate of 144 steps a minute.
If you cannot complete this test, start exercising with week 3 of program **B**.
If you can manage the 10 minutes but are tired and winded, start with week 4 of program **B** before starting program **C**.
If you complete the test with no difficulty start with program **C**.

	A Basic walking program
Week 1	Walk briskly 5 minutes (or less) Walk slowly 3 minutes Walk briskly 5 minutes (or less)
Week 2	Walk briskly 5 minutes* Walk slowly 3 minutes Walk briskly 5 minutes*
Week 3	Walk briskly 8 minutes Walk slowly 3 minutes Walk briskly 8 minutes
Week 4	Walk briskly 8 minutes* Walk slowly 3 minutes Walk briskly 8 minutes*
Week 5	
Week 6	
Week 7	
Week 8	

*Increase pace when you can walk for 5 minutes without getting tired.

Before beginning your program have a medical check-up.
Never overdo your exercise. Should you experience nausea,
trembling, breathlessness or pain, stop exercising at once; if
the symptoms persist, see a doctor. When you have
completed the first stage of the program move on to the
second stage and so on. The number of times that you
exercise a week will vary. Try to exercise every other day for
program **A**, four times a week for program **B**, and five times
a week for program **C**. After that, maintain your fitness
with three workouts a week.

B Walk-jog program	**C** Jogging program
Walk briskly 10 minutes (or less) Walk slowly 3 minutes Walk briskly 10 minutes (or less)	Jog 40 seconds (100yd) Walk 1 minute (100yd) Repeat 9 times
Walk briskly 15 minutes (or less) Walk slowly 3 minutes	Jog 1 minute (150yd) Walk 1 minute (100yd) Repeat 8 times
Jog 10 seconds (25yd) Walk 1 minute (100yd) Repeat 12 times	Jog 2 minutes (300yd) Walk 1 minute (100yd) Repeat 6 times
Jog 20 seconds (50yd) Walk 1 minute (100yd) Repeat 12 times	Jog 4 minutes (600yd) Walk 1 minute (100yd) Repeat 4 times
	Jog 6 minutes (900yd) Walk 1 minute (100yd) Repeat 3 times
	Jog 8 minutes (1200yd) Walk 2 minutes (200yd) Repeat 2 times
	Jog 10 minutes (1500yd) Walk 2 minutes (200yd) Repeat 2 times
	Jog 12 minutes (1 mile) Walk 2 minutes (200yd) Repeat 2 times

US aerobic program

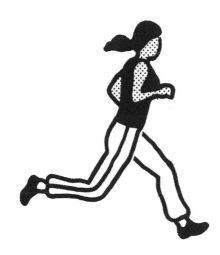

The human body is designed for running; primitive man relied on speed to catch food and to carry him out of danger. The best way to run is the natural way — that is, in a style that uses your body to the best advantage and doesn't impose undue strain on any part of it. There are as many styles of running as there are runners, and provided you follow certain guidelines there are no strict rules; the best style for you is the one in which you feel most comfortable and relaxed. This relaxation of body and mind is very important; remember that your aim is not speed, distance or competition, but health and enjoyment. Try to run as rhythmically and efficiently as you can to conserve your energy, because the more smooth and streamlined your action becomes, the easier running will be. Running will improve your posture and carriage, as well as benefiting your breathing and making your limbs strong and supple.

Breathing
Running increases your body's oxygen requirement, so you need to take in as much air as you can. Breathe through your mouth and inhale deeply. Practice breathing from the abdomen, so that your stomach expands as you breathe in and flattens as you exhale. Try to breathe rhythmically and regularly, not gasping for air. If you get out of breath, slow down; you should be able to talk as you run.

Posture
The first advice to beginners in running is to "run tall." Keep your body upright, your head up, your back straight, and your buttocks tucked in, but do not hold yourself stiffly. This is the most comfortable and efficient way to run. Let your arms swing loosely, balancing your leg movements, so that your right arm moves forward with your left leg. Swing your arms at your sides, not across your body; carry them low, with the fingers lightly clenched in a fist. The swing will help you to stride and breathe rhythmically, and increase your forward momentum.

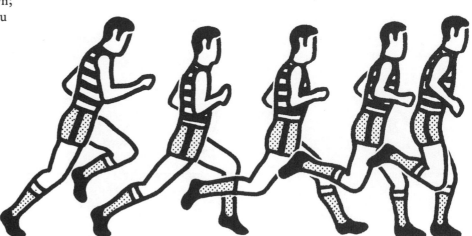

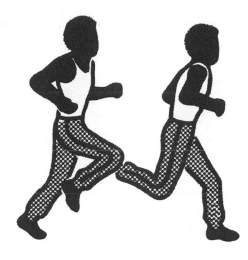

Stride

Length of stride varies with the individual, but keep it fairly short — do not overstride or force the length. Let your legs move freely and naturally from the hips. The faster you go, the more you will lengthen your stride and increase knee lift and back kick. An even, rhythmical movement is far more comfortable and efficient than straining for distance or using a choppy stride. Try to maintain an even pace, running so that you can hold a conversation comfortably — running with a friend can be fun, but don't risk injury through unnecessary competition.

Footstrike

Incorrect footstrike makes running more difficult and may result in injury. Many people try to run only on their toes or the ball of the foot. Correct footstrike is a rolling or rocking movement: landing on the heel (**a**), rocking onto the flat of the foot (**b**), and pushing off with the toes (**c**).

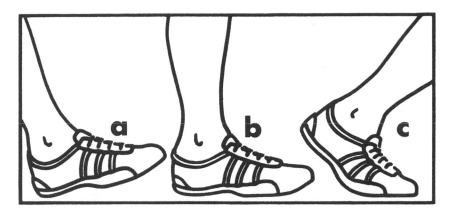

Injuries and ills from running

1 Back pain: often sciatica, a pinched nerve in the lower back.
2 Side stitch: a spasm caused by poor breathing during exercise.
3 Hip pain: can be caused by uneven leg length.
4 Runner's knee: pain perhaps caused by a structural imbalance.
5 Muscle soreness: common effect of exercise after long inactivity.
6 Shin splints: pain in the lower shin, often caused by running on hard surfaces.
7 Tendinitis: inflammation of the Achilles tendon above the heel.
8 Sprained ankle: can be caused by wearing low-topped shoes.
9 Blisters and calluses: caused by friction from poor footwear.
10 Bone bruises: painful bruises on the soles of the feet, a result of poor footwear or careless foot placement.

Treatment

If pain persists, or if you suspect a more serious injury, consult a doctor.

Most of the troubles mentioned can be prevented or alleviated with care and forethought. Back pain, muscle soreness and shin splints can all be avoided or eased by thoroughly warming up your body before running, using bending and stretching exercises. Begin your program gently, without trying to rush your progress. Well-fitting footwear that provides protection and support is essential, and can help you to avoid many injuries. Prevent heel bruising and shin splints by running on soft surfaces at first.

Discomfort caused by bodily defects or imbalance can often be eased by wearing strapping on a weak knee or ankle, by building up one shoe slightly, or even by surgery in severe cases. Ice packs and aspirin will offer temporary relief from pain and inflammation. As you become fitter and more supple, you will be considerably less susceptible to illness or injury.

US aerobic program

Before and after the run

An adequate warming-up and cooling-down routine is as vital to your aerobic fitness program as the exercise itself. It is tempting to neglect these periods and rush into the "real business" of running, but this can be dangerous. Spend a minimum of 5 minutes in preparing your body for the run, and in allowing it to adjust afterward. Also make sure that you wear warm clothing in cold or damp weather, so that you are not chilled after sweating.

Effects on heart and lungs

When you rush straight into a strenuous activity the muscles suddenly make heavy demands for more blood and oxygen. If you start "cold," particularly if you are in poor condition, the resulting shock and strain on your heart and lungs can be dangerous. If you stop your exercise abruptly, they continue to work hard, the heart pumping blood to the legs, away from the brain, which may lead to dizziness or fainting. In both cases the cardio-vascular system needs to be gently prepared for the change in work load. On the track, begin by walking briskly, then jog, and then run. Afterward, cool down slowly by slackening off gradually to a walk. Off the track, perform breathing and strengthening exercises before and after running.

Effects on muscles and joints

1 Your muscles and joints must be eased into action. When you get up, or after a day's work, you need to relax physically and mentally to disperse the tension and stiffness that have accumulated in your body. The exercises described on the following pages will warm up the three main muscle-groups used in running: the neck and shoulders, the back, and the legs. Stretching will loosen your muscles and ease tension in your joints. Do the exercises slowly and smoothly, breathing rhythmically. Never overdo things or strain to reach a position. Rest between movements, and vary the routine so that you use all parts of your body.

2 During running, various tensions build up in the body; back, shoulder and leg muscles tighten and need to be relaxed by gentle flexing and stretching. On the track, and as you run, shake your arms and legs to loosen them and help the circulation.

3 After running, cool down gradually by repeating exercises from your warming-up routine, or select other exercises from the program if you prefer. Such a cooling-down routine will refresh and revitalize your body, and help prevent injuries which often result from an inadequate workout that has left limbs and joints stiff. Aches and pains after running can also often be relieved by gentle exercise.

Between running

On the days when you don't run, you can substitute another form of aerobic exercise such as skipping or jumping rope, jogging on the spot, swimming or cycling. All these exercises will help maintain mobility. For overall fitness, aerobic exercises should be combined with exercises involving muscular strength and endurance.

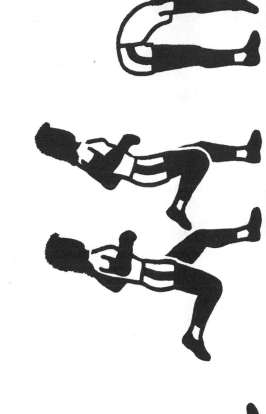

EXERCISES

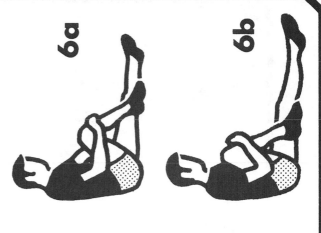

3

4

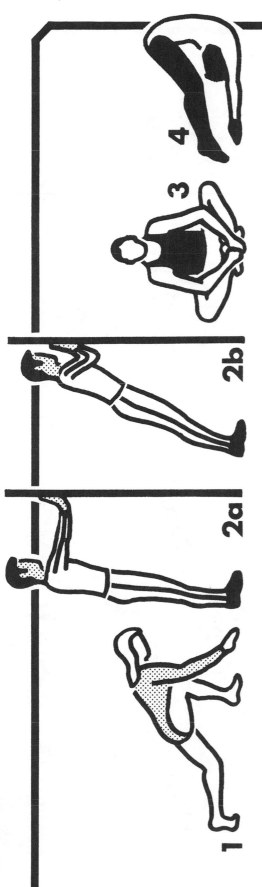

1

2a

2b

Warming-up and cooling-down exercises

These exercises will stretch and tone your muscles and help to prevent you from becoming sore and stiff after running. Always use the six exercises on this page as part of your routine, and add some from the following pages for variety.

1 Slowly slide into a stride position with your front foot almost flat and your rear foot resting on the toes. Balance with your hands on the floor. Hold for a count of 5, then repeat with the other leg forward.

2a Stand about 3ft (1m) from a wall, with your feet slightly apart and your hands on the wall.

2b Lean forward, bending your arms and keeping your heels flat on the floor so that your calves are stretched. Hold for 15–20 seconds; repeat several times.

3 Sit on the floor with your legs bent and your knees out to the sides. Hold your toes, and pull on them while pressing your legs downward with your elbows.

4 Lie on your back on the floor, with your arms stretched above your head. Bring your legs over your head and try and touch the floor with your toes. Hold for a count of 10; repeat several times.

5a Sit on the floor with your legs stretched in front of you, toes pointed. Stretch your arms forward.

5b Slide your hands down your legs and try to grasp your ankles; hold in a stretched position for several moments. Repeat 5 times.

6a Sit with your left leg stretched in front of you and your right leg bent up; grasp your right knee with both hands.

6b Pull your right knee toward your body 8–10 times. Repeat with the other leg.

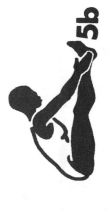

6a

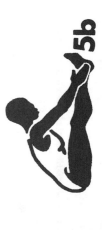

6b

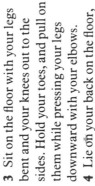

5a

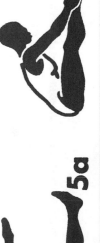

5b

US aerobic program

EXERCISES

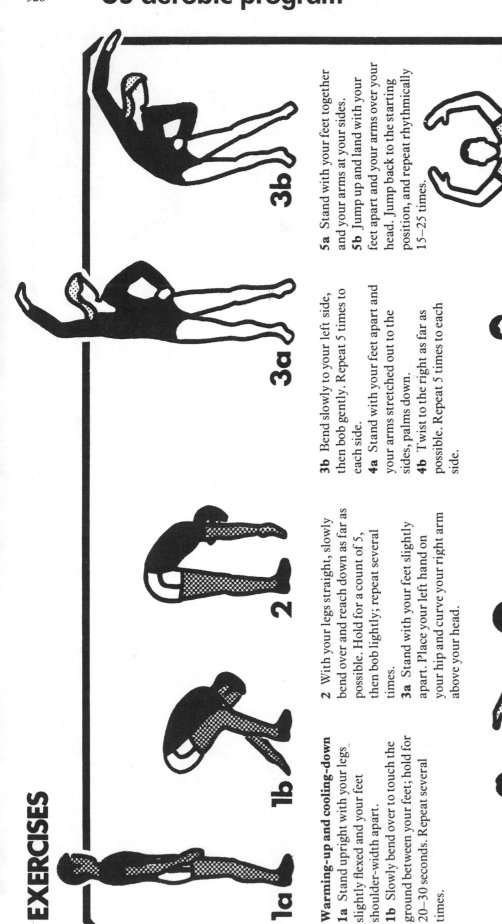

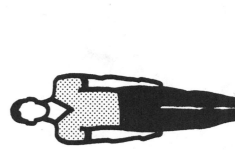

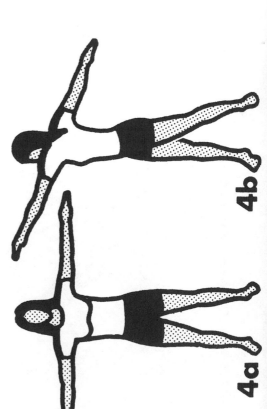

3b

3a

2

1b

1a

5b

5a

4b

4a

Warming-up and cooling-down
1a Stand upright with your legs slightly flexed and your feet shoulder-width apart.
1b Slowly bend over to touch the ground between your feet; hold for 20–30 seconds. Repeat several times.

2 With your legs straight, slowly bend over and reach down as far as possible. Hold for a count of 5, then bob lightly; repeat several times.
3a Stand with your feet slightly apart. Place your left hand on your hip and curve your right arm above your head.

3b Bend slowly to your left side, then bob gently. Repeat 5 times to each side.
4a Stand with your feet apart and your arms stretched out to the sides, palms down.
4b Twist to the right as far as possible. Repeat 5 times to each side.

5a Stand with your feet together and your arms at your sides.
5b Jump up and land with your feet apart and your arms over your head. Jump back to the starting position, and repeat rhythmically 15–25 times.

EXERCISES

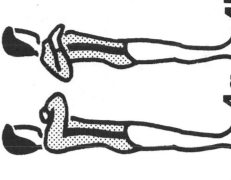

Warming-up and cooling-down
1a Stand with your feet apart, hands by your sides, and drop your chin down onto your chest.
1b, c, d Tilt your head to the left side, round to the back, to the right, and then to the front again in a complete circle. Repeat 3 times in each direction.

1a 1b 1c 1d

2a Run slowly on the spot, lifting your legs only a little way from the ground.
2b As your training progresses, lift your legs higher and increase your speed.
3a Stand upright.
3b Squat and place your hands on the floor, shoulder-width apart.
3c Thrust your legs backward, keeping your back straight, so that

you are in the push-up position. Return to the squat, and then stand upright again. Repeat 10–15 times.
4a Stand with your feet apart and your elbows bent, forearms across your chest.
4b Without arching your back, thrust your elbows backward, then return to the starting position. Repeat rhythmically 15 times.

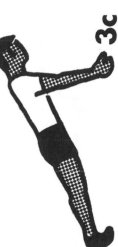
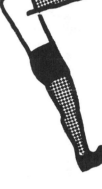
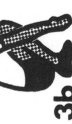
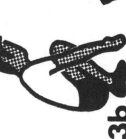
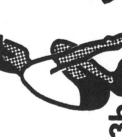
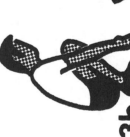
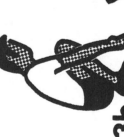
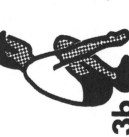
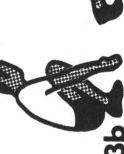
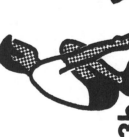
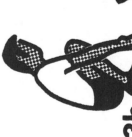

2a 2b 3a 3b 3c 4a 4b

©DIAGRAM

Further reading

Chapters 1–3

Campbell, W., Tucker, N. **An Introduction to Tests & Measurements in Physical Education** Bell

Clarke, H. Harrison **Application of Measurement to Health and Physical Education** Prentice Hall

Cooper, K. H. **Aerobics** Bantam Books

Diagram Group **Man's Body** Paddington Press

Diagram Group **Woman's Body** Paddington Press

DiGennaro, J. **Individualized Exercise and Optimal Physical Fitness** Lee & Febiger

Grandjean, E. **Fitting the Task to the Man (an Ergonomic Approach)** Taylor & Francis

Jones, K. L., Sharnberg, L. W., Byer, C.O. **Total Fitness** Canfield Press

Kuntzleman, C. T. **Rating the Exercises** William Morrow & Co

Mathews, D. K. **Measurement in Physical Education** W. B. Saunders Co

Shephard, R. J. **Endurance Fitness** University of Toronto Press

Shephard, R. J. **Physical Activity and Aging** Croom Helm

Singleton, W. T. **Introduction to Ergonomics** World Health Organization

Thomas, V. **Exercise Physiology** Crosby Lockwood Staples

Wessel, J. A. **Movement Fundamentals (Figure, Form, Fun)** Prentice Hall

Chapters 4, 5

Balaskas, A. **Bodylife** Sidgwick & Jackson

Bourne, G. **Pregnancy** Pan Books

Campbell, Greg **The Joy of Jumping** Richard Marek Publications

Downing, G. **The Massage Book** Penguin

Elrick, H., Crakes, J. **Living Longer and Better—Guide to Optimal Health** World Publications

Goleman, Daniel **The Varieties of the Medative Experience** E. P. Dutton

Higdon, H. **Fitness After Forty** World Publications

Jones, Frank, Pierce **"Body Awareness in Action" Study of the Alexander Technique** Churchill Livingstone

Lettvin, Maggie **Back Book: Healing the Hurt in your Lower Back** Souvenir Press

Montgomery, E. **At your Best for Birth and Later** John Wright & Sons

Nottridge, P., Lamplugh, D. **Slimnastics** Penguin

Ohashi, W. **Do-it-Yourself Shiatsu** Unwin Paperbacks

Roon, Karin **The New Way to Relax** Worlds Work

Tucker, W. E. **Home Treatment and Posture in Injury, Rheumatism and Osteoarthritis** Churchill Livingstone

Violin, M., Phelan, N. **Yoga Over Forty** Sphere

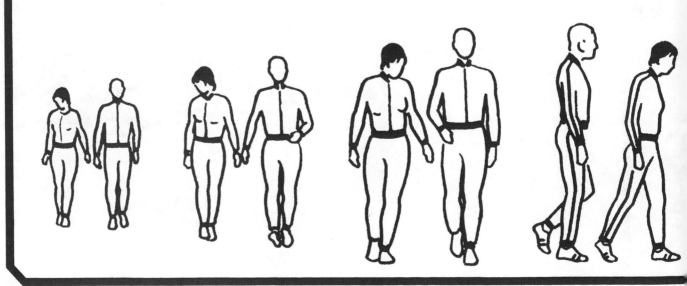

Chapter 6
Armbuster, D. A., Musker, F. F., Irwin, L. W. **Basic Skills in Sports for Men and Women** C. V. Mosby
Ballantin, R. **Richard's Bicycling Book** Pan Books
Blackburn, D., Jorgenson, M. **Zen and the Cross-Country Skier** Ward Ritchie Publications
Councilman, Dr J. E. **Competitive Swimming Manual for Coaches and Swimmers** Pelham Books
Diagram Group **Enjoying Combat Sports** Paddington Press
Diagram Group **Enjoying Racquet Sports** Paddington Press
Diagram Group **Enjoying Swimming** Paddington Press
Editors of Consumer Guide **The Running Book** Beekman House
Evans, H., Jackson, B., Ottaway, M. **The Sunday Times—We Learned to Ski** Collins
Pilss-Samek, H. **Exercise for Sports** Sterling Publishing Co
Sheeham, Dr G. **Running and Being the Total Experience** Simon and Schuster

Chapter 7
Dobbins, B., Sprague, K. **The Gold's Gym Weight Training Book** J. P. Tarcher Inc St Martin's Press
Frederic, Louis **Yoga Asanas** Thorsons Publishers
Heidenstam, O. **Modern Body-Building** Faber
Hittleman, Richard **Introduction to Yoga** Bantam Books
Hoare, Sophy **Yoga** Macdonald Guidelines
Kwong, Yin **T'ai Chi Ch'uan** Yin Kwong Herbalist
Man-ch'ing, Cheng, Smith, Robert W. **T'ai-Chi the "Supreme Ultimate" Experience for Health, Sport and Self-Defense** Charles E. Tuttle
Soo, Chee **The Chinese Art of K'ai Men** Gordon & Cremonesi
Wood, Ernest **Yoga** Pelican
Zane, C. **The Feminine Physique—Bodybuilding for the Woman** Christine Zane

Chapter 8
Adult Physical Fitness—A Program for Men and Women The President's Council on Physical Fitness and Sport
Fitness and Work Capacity Forest Service, US Department of Agriculture
Look After Yourself Health Education Council

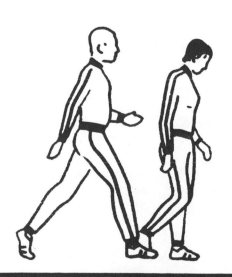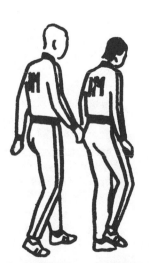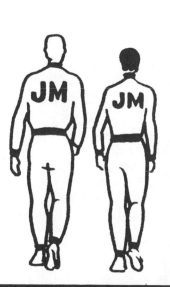

Index